PLATELET FUNCTION

CONTEMPORARY CARDIOLOGY

CHRISTOPHER P. CANNON, MD
SERIES EDITOR

Platelet Function: Assessment, Diagnosis, and Treatment, edited by *Martin Quinn*, MB BCh BAO, PhD, *and Desmond Fitzgerald*, MD, FRCPI, FESC, AAP, 2005

Cardiovascular Disease in the Elderly, edited by *Gary Gerstenblith*, MD, 2005

Diabetes and Cardiovascular Disease, Second Edition, edited by *Michael T. Johnstone*, MD, CM, FRCP(C), *and Aristidis Veves*, MD, DSc, 2005

Angiogenesis and Direct Myocardial Revascularization, edited by *Roger J. Laham*, MD, *and Donald S. Baim*, MD, 2005

Interventional Cardiology: Percutaneous Noncoronary Intervention, edited by *Howard C. Herrmann*, MD, 2005

Principles of Molecular Cardiology, edited by *Marschall S. Runge*, MD, *and Cam Patterson*, MD, 2005

Heart Disease Diagnosis and Therapy: A Practical Approach, Second Edition, by *M. Gabriel Khan*, MD, FRCP(C), FRCP(LONDON), FACP, FACC, 2005

Cardiovascular Genomics: Gene Mining for Pharmacogenomics and Gene Therapy, edited by *Mohan K. Raizada*, PhD, *Julian F. R. Paton*, PhD, *Michael J. Katovich*, PhD, *and Sergey Kasparov*, MD, PhD, 2005

Surgical Management of Congestive Heart Failure, edited by *James C. Fang*, MD *and Gregory S. Couper*, MD, 2005

Cardiopulmonary Resuscitation, edited by *Joseph P. Ornato*, MD, FAP, FACC *and Mary Ann Peberdy*, MD, FACC, 2005

CT of the Heart: Principles and Applications, edited by *U. Joseph Schoepf*, MD, 2005

Heart Disease and Erectile Dysfunction, edited by *Robert A. Kloner*, MD, PhD, 2004

Cardiac Transplantation: The Columbia University Medical Center/New York Presbyterian Hospital Manual, edited by *Niloo M. Edwards*, MD, *Jonathan M. Chen*, MD, *and Pamela A. Mazzeo*, 2004

Coronary Disease in Women: Evidence-Based Diagnosis and Treatment, edited by *Leslee J. Shaw*, PhD *and Rita F. Redberg*, MD, FACC, 2004

Complementary and Alternative Cardiovascular Medicine, edited by *Richard A. Stein*, MD *and Mehmet C. Oz*, MD, 2004

Nuclear Cardiology, The Basics: How to Set Up and Maintain a Laboratory, by *Frans J. Th. Wackers*, MD, PhD, *Wendy Bruni*, BS, CNMT, *and Barry L. Zaret*, MD, 2004

Minimally Invasive Cardiac Surgery, Second Edition, edited by *Daniel J. Goldstein*, MD *and Mehmet C. Oz*, MD, 2004

Cardiovascular Health Care Economics, edited by *William S. Weintraub*, MD, 2003

Platelet Glycoprotein IIb/IIIa Inhibitors in Cardiovascular Disease, Second Edition, edited by *A. Michael Lincoff*, MD, 2003

Heart Failure: A Clinician's Guide to Ambulatory Diagnosis and Treatment, edited by *Mariell L. Jessup*, MD *and Evan Loh*, MD, 2003

Management of Acute Coronary Syndromes, Second Edition, edited by *Christopher P. Cannon*, MD, 2003

PLATELET FUNCTION

Assessment, Diagnosis, and Treatment

Edited by

MARTIN QUINN

MB BCh BAO, PhD

Department of Cardiology
St. Vincent's University Hospital
Dublin, Ireland

DESMOND FITZGERALD

MD, FRCPI, FESC, AAP

Vice President of Research
University College Dublin
Dublin, Ireland

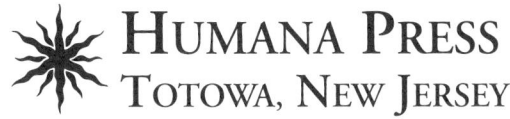 **HUMANA PRESS**
TOTOWA, NEW JERSEY

© 2005 Humana Press Inc.
999 Riverview Drive, Suite 208
Totowa, New Jersey 07512

www.humanapress.com

For additional copies, pricing for bulk purchases, and/or information about other Humana titles, contact Humana at the above address or at any of the following numbers: Tel.: 973-256-1699; Fax: 973-256-8341; E-mail: orders@humanapr.com; or visit our Website: www.humanapress.com

Cover design by Patricia F. Cleary.
Cover illustration: Platelet cytoskeleton at different stages of activation (Chapter 4, Fig. 10; *see* pp. 103–105).

This publication is printed on acid-free paper. ∞
ANSI Z39.48-1984 (American National Standards Institute) Permanence of Paper for Printed Library Materials.

Printed in the United States of America.   10 9 8 7 6 5 4 3 2 1

eISBN 1-59259-917-6

Library of Congress Cataloging-in-Publication Data

Platelet function : assessment, diagnosis, and treatment / edited by Martin
Quinn, Desmond Fitzgerald.
     p. ; cm. -- (Contemporary cardiology)
  Includes bibliographical references and index.
  ISBN 1-58829-244-4 (alk. paper)
  1. Blood platelet disorders--Diagnosis. 2. Blood platelets--Examination. [DNLM: 1. Blood Platelets--physiology. 2. Blood Platelet
Disorders--diagnosis. 3. Blood Platelet Disorders--physiopathology. 4. Blood Platelet Disorders--therapy.
WH 600 P716 2005] I. Quinn, Martin, PhD. II. Fitzgerald, Desmond, MD. III. Contemporary cardiology
(Totowa, N.J.: Unnumbered)
  RC647.B5P564 2005
  616.1'57--dc22   2004030476

PREFACE

Platelets are small anucleate blood-borne particles that play a central role in blood clot formation. In areas of endothelial damage or activation of the coagulation cascade, they change shape, release their granule contents, and activate. This process transforms the smooth discoid platelet into a sticky spiculated particle with the ability to bind to the plasma protein fibrinogen, forming a clot. Congenital or acquired defects of platelet function are rare and usually result in minor bleeding defects. Conversely, inadvertent or excessive platelet activation is common, for example, at the site of endothelial damage, and underlies many common cardiovascular disorders, such as myocardial infarction, unstable angina, and stroke. Antiplatelet agents play an important role in the management of these conditions, and a number of agents are now available to treat them.

Platelet function is difficult to assess, with many of the assays based on platelet aggregation. The relative paucity of approaches is a major limitation to the understanding of platelet biology, the assessment of thrombotic risk in patients, and the rational dosing of antiplatelet agents. *Platelet Function: Assessment, Diagnosis, and Treatment* focuses on platelet biology and reviews current methods of assessing platelet function.

The first section, on platelet physiology, provides the reader with an understanding of the platelet biology underlying functional analyses. The second section reviews means of assessing platelet function, including the commonly used platelet aggregation, thromboxane production, expression of platelet activation markers, procoagulant activity, and platelet function under-flow. Also discussed are the fast developing fields of proteomics and genomics and their application to platelet research. Chapters focus both on the technology and the outcome of research on platelets. The final section describes the clinical application of the various methods for the assessment of platelet function in vivo and provides an overview of antiplatelet therapy.

Platelet Function: Assessment, Diagnosis, and Treatment is aimed at an audience of scientists, clinical researchers, clinicians, and other health care workers with an interest in platelet biology.

Martin Quinn, MB BCh BAO, PhD
Desmond Fitzgerald, MD, FRCPI, FESC, AAP

CONTENTS

CONTRIBUTORS

ELAINE L. BEARER, MD, PhD • *Department of Pathology and Laboratory Medicine, Brown University Medical School, Providence, RI*

TATIANA BYZOVA, PhD • *Joseph J. Jacobs Center for Thrombosis and Vascular Biology, Department of Molecular Cardiology, Lerner Research Institute of the Cleveland Clinic Foundation, Cleveland, OH*

IAN DEL CONDE, MD • *Thrombosis Research Section, Department of Medicine, Baylor College of Medicine, Houston, TX*

DERMOT COX, PhD • *Department of Clinical Pharmacology, Royal College of Surgeons in Ireland, Dublin, Ireland*

JING-FEI DONG, MD, PhD • *Thrombosis Research Section, Department of Medicine, Baylor College of Medicine, Houston, TX*

DESMOND FITZGERALD, MD, FRCPI, FESC, AAP • *Vice President of Research, University College Dublin; formerly Department of Clinical Pharmacology, Royal College of Surgeons in Ireland, Dublin, Ireland*

MARK I. FURMAN, MD • *Center for Platelet Function Studies, Division of Cardiovascular Medicine, Department of Medicine, University of Massachusetts Medical School, Worcester, MA*

MEINRAD GAWAZ, MD • *Medizinische Universitätsklinik und Poliklinik, Klinikum auf dem Schnarrenberg, Universität Tübingen, Tübingen, Germany*

LISA K. JENNINGS, PhD • *Vascular Biology Center of Excellence, Departments of Medicine, Molecular Science, Surgery, and the Joint Program of Biomedical Engineering, The University of Tennessee Health Science Center, Memphis, TN*

MICHAEL KALAFATIS, PhD • *Joseph J. Jacobs Center for Thrombosis and Vascular Biology, Department of Molecular Cardiology, Lerner Research Institute of the Cleveland Clinic Foundation, Cleveland; Department of Chemistry, Cleveland State University, Cleveland, OH*

NEAL KLEIMAN, MD • *Director Cardiac Catheterization Laboratory, Methodist DeBakey Heart Center, Department of Medicine, Baylor College of Medicine, Houston, TX*

STEPHAN LINDEMANN, MD • *Department of Medicine, Johannes Gutenberg-University, Mainz, Germany,*

JOSÉ A. LÓPEZ, MD • *Thrombosis Research Section, Department of Medicine, Baylor College of Medicine, Houston, TX*

KATRIN MARCUS, PhD • *Medical Proteom-Center, Ruhr-University of Bochum, Bochum, Germany*

ANDREW MAREE, MD • *Department of Clinical Pharmacology, Royal College of Surgeons in Ireland, Dublin, Ireland*

THOMAS M. MCINTYRE, PhD • *Departments of Internal Medicine and Pathology and the Eccles Institute of Human Genetics, University of Utah, Salt Lake City, UT*

JAMES MCREDMOND, PhD • *The Conway Institute of Biomedical and Biomolecular Research, University College Dublin, Dublin, Ireland*

HELMUT E. MEYER, PhD • *Medical Proteom-Center, Ruhr-University of Bochum, Bochum, Germany*

ALAN D. MICHELSON, MD • *Center for Platelet Function Studies, Department of Pediatrics, University of Massachusetts Medical School, Worcester, MA*

DAVID J. MOLITERNO, MD • *Gill Heart Institute, Division of Cardiovascular Medicine, University of Kentucky Chandler Medical Center, Lexington, KY*

EMIL NEGRESCU, MD, PhD • *Joseph J. Jacobs Center for Thrombosis and Vascular Biology, Department of Molecular Cardiology, Lerner Research Institute of the Cleveland Clinic Foundation, Cleveland, OH*

CARLO PATRONO, MD • *Department of Pharmacology, University of Rome La Sapienza, Rome, Italy*

KARLHEINZ PETER, MD • *Department of Cardiology and Angiology, University of Freiburg, Freiburg, Germany*

EDWARD F. PLOW, PhD • *Joseph J. Jacobs Center for Thrombosis and Vascular Biology, Department of Molecular Cardiology, Lerner Research Institute of the Cleveland Clinic Foundation, Cleveland, OH*

STEPHEN M. PRESCOTT, MD • *Department of Internal Medicine and the Huntsman Cancer Institute, University of Utah, Salt Lake City, UT*

MARTIN QUINN, MB BCh BAO, PhD, MSc • *Department of Cardiology, St. Vincents University Hospital, Dublin, Ireland*

BIANCA ROCCA, MD • *Research Center on Physiopathology of Haemostasis, Department of Internal Medicine, Catholic University School of Medicine, Rome, Italy*

ZAVERIO M. RUGGERI, MD • *The Roon Research Center for Atherosclerosis and Thrombosis, Division of Experimental Hemostasis and Thrombosis, Department of Molecular and Experimental Medicine, The Scripps Research Institute, La Jolla, CA*

BRIAN SAVAGE, PhD • *The Roon Research Center for Atherosclerosis and Thrombosis, Division of Experimental Hemostasis and Thrombosis, Department of Molecular and Experimental Medicine, The Scripps Research Institute, La Jolla, CA*

JACQUELINE SAW, MD • *Laurel Cardiology, Vancouver General Hospital, Vancouver, British Columbia, Canada*

ANDREW S. WEYRICH, PhD • *Department of Internal Medicine and the Eccles Institute of Human Genetics, University of Utah, Salt Lake City, UT*

MELANIE M. WHITE, BS • *Vascular Biology Center of Excellence and the Department of Medicine, The University of Tennessee Health Science Center, Memphis, TN*

GUY A. ZIMMERMAN, MD • *Department of Internal Medicine and the Eccles Institute of Human Genetics, University of Utah, Salt Lake City, UT*

I PLATELET PHYSIOLOGY

1

Platelet Physiology

Martin Quinn, MB, BCh, BAO, PhD, MSc

INTRODUCTION

Platelets are anucleate circulating blood particles. They circulate around the body in an inactive state until they come into contact with areas of endothelial damage or activation of the coagulation cascade. Here they adhere to the endothelial defect, change shape, release their granule contents, and stick together to form aggregates. Physiologically these processes help to limit blood loss; however, inappropriate or excessive platelet activation results in an acute obstruction of blood flow, as occurs, for example, in an acute myocardial infarction. However, activated platelets also express and release molecules that stimulate a localized inflammatory response through the activation of leukocytes and endothelial cells, and it is now clear that platelet function is not merely limited to the prevention of blood loss. Indeed, platelets have been implicated in many pathological processes including host defense, inflammatory arthritis, adult respiratory distress syndrome, and tumor growth and metastasis. In this chapter I review our current understanding of platelet physiology in order to provide a global background for the more in-depth focused chapters later in this book.

From: *Contemporary Cardiology:*
Platelet Function: Assessment, Diagnosis, and Treatment
Edited by: M. Quinn and D. Fitzgerald © Humana Press Inc., Totowa, NJ

Table 1
Platelet Agonists

Adenosine diphosphate (ADP)
Thrombin
Thromboxane A_2
Epinephrine
Serotonin
Collagen
Shear stress
Prostaglandin E_2 (PGE_2; low concentration)
8-Iso-$PGF_{2\alpha}$

PLATELET ACTIVATION

Platelet activation describes the process that converts the smooth, nonadherent platelet into a sticky spiculated particle that releases and expresses biologically active substances and acquires the ability to bind the plasma protein fibrinogen. Activation occurs rapidly following exposure to chemical stimuli known as agonists. Activation can also occur as a result of the physical stimulus of high fluid shear stress, such as that found at the site of a critical arterial narrowing (1).

Platelet Agonists

Many agonists are generated, expressed, or released at the sites of endothelial injury or activation of the coagulation cascade (Table 1). Agonists differ in their ability to induce platelet activation; thrombin, collagen, and thromboxane A_2 (TXA_2) are all strong agonists and can produce aggregation independent of platelet granule secretion. Adenosine diphosphate (ADP) and serotonin are intermediate agonists and require granule secretion for full irreversible aggregation, whereas epinephrine is effective only at supraphysiological concentrations.

THROMBIN

Thrombin (factor II) is an enzyme, a serine protease to be exact, that has diverse physiological functions. In addition to stimulating platelet activation and the conversion of fibrinogen to fibrin, it is involved in the regulation of vessel tone, smooth muscle cell proliferation and migration, inflammation (2–5), angiogenesis (6), and embryonic development (7,8). It is generated from its inactive precursor prothrombin as a result of cleavage in the coagulation cascade. This reaction is greatly facilitated by the presence of activated platelets, which supply negatively charged phospholipids for the assembly of the prothrombinase complex.

The prothrombinase complex and thrombin biology are discussed in more detail in Chapter 12.

Thrombin signaling is mediated by a specialized family of G protein-linked receptors known as protease-activated receptors (PARs) (9). Thrombin stimulates these receptors by cleaving their amino-terminal extracellular domain. This unmasks a stimulatory sequence that autostimulates the receptor (10). Four separate PAR receptors have been described, PARs 1–4. Three of these are activated by thrombin, PAR-1, PAR-3, and PAR-4. PAR-2 is insensitive to thrombin but is activated by the enzyme trypsin. Two of the three PAR receptors activated by thrombin, PAR-1 (11) and PAR-4 (12), mediate thrombin's action on human platelets (13). The other one, PAR-3, is only expressed on mouse platelets. The PAR-1 and PAR-4 receptors differ in their affinities for thrombin and the time-course of their activation and deactivation. Lower concentrations of thrombin (~1 nM) stimulate PAR-1, and the response induced is more rapid and short lived than the response to PAR-4 stimulation, owing to internalization of the receptor (14). However, PAR-4 activation can also occur at low thrombin concentrations in the presence of PAR-3 owing to the phenomenon of *transactivation*, whereby thrombin binds to PAR-3, allowing it to cleave neighboring PAR-4 (15). Thrombin-induced aggregation is independent of Gi; however, its inhibition of adenylate cyclase is dependent on ADP secretion and Gi signaling through the P2Y$_{12}$ ADP receptor (16).

Thrombin also binds to the glycoprotein (GP)Ib-α subunit of the platelet von Willebrand factor (vWF) receptor, GPIb-IX-V, through its exocite II binding site, inducing platelet activation (17). This interaction results in allosteric inhibition of fibrinogen cleavage by thrombin (18) but enhances thrombin's activation of PAR-1 (19). The aggregation induced by the thrombin–GPIb interaction is dependent on platelet fibrin binding and is not inhibited by RGDS (17).

COLLAGEN

Endothelial damage exposes the extracellular matrix protein collagen, which is a potent platelet agonist. Platelets have three separate surface collagen receptors, GPIa-IIa (integrin α$_2$β$_1$), GPVI (a member of the immunoglobulin superfamily), and GPIb-IX-V (*see* Platelet Adhesion and GPIb-IX-V section below). The platelet immune receptor adaptor Fc receptor γ-chain (FcRγ) is required for collagen-induced signaling and non-covalently associates with GPVI (20). This association occurs in areas of the platelet membrane enriched with cholesterol, sphingolipids, and signaling molecules known as lipid rafts (21,22). A stepwise model of activation has been proposed with initial adhesion to collagen via

GPIa-IIa and subsequent interaction with GPVI/FcRγ for full platelet activation *(23)*. Signaling involves tyrosine phosphorylation of the immunoreceptor tyrosine-based activatory motif (ITAM) of the GPIV/ Fc complex by the Src family kinases Lyn and Fyn, leading to Syk binding and activation of phospholipase C *(24)*. Crosslinking of the transmembrane glycoprotein platelet endothelial cell adhesion molecule-1 (PECAM-1/CD31) inhibits ITAM signaling through the PECAM-1 immunoreceptor tyrosine-based inhibitory motif (ITIM) *(25)*. The small guanosine triphosphatase (GTPase) RAP-1, linked to GPIIb-IIIa activation, is also activated by GPVI/Fc signaling. This is to some extent dependent on ADP secretion and signaling through $P2Y_{12}$ *(26)*. Consistent with this finding, high concentrations of collagen can induce weak platelet aggregation independent of ADP release and TXA_2 production; however, maximal aggregation requires TXA_2 and secretion *(27)*.

THROMBOXANE A_2

TXA_2 is produced from arachidonic acid released from the membrane phospholipid by the action of phospholipase A_2. Arachidonic acid is metabolized to the intermediate product prostaglandin (PG)H_2 by the enzyme cyclooxygenase (COX), also referred to as PGH synthase. PGH_2 is further metabolized by a P450 enzyme, thromboxane synthase, to thromboxane A_2 or to a lesser extent in platelets, to PGE_2 *(28,29; see* Chapter 11 for a more in-depth discussion). TXA_2 is labile and has a very short half-life ($\approx$30 s). It is rapidly hydrolyzed to inactive TB_2. Two separate isoforms of the TXA_2 receptor have been identified, TXRα and TXRβ. The former is linked to Gq and the latter to Gi *(30,31)*. The TXA_2 precursor, PGH_2, also stimulates these receptors *(32)*. PGE_2 at low (nM) concentrations enhances platelet activation to subthreshold concentrations of certain agonists; conversely, at high (μM) concentrations, its actions are inhibitory.

ADENOSINE DIPHOSPHATE

ADP is released from the platelet dense granules upon activation and from red blood cells and damaged endothelial cells *(33,34)*. The platelet response to ADP is mediated by the $P2Y_1$ and $P2Y_{12}$ G protein-linked nucleotide receptors *(35,36)* (Fig. 1). ADP also stimulates the platelet $P2X_1$ ligand-gated ion channel, inducing transmembrane calcium flux. $P2X_1$ stimulation does not appear to play a major role in ADP-induced aggregation *(37,38)*; however, low concentrations of collagen (<1 μg/ mL) release ATP, which induces extracellular signal-regulated kinase (ERK)-2 activation via $P2X_1$ stimulation *(39)*. $P2Y_{12}$ stimulation is linked to inhibition of adenylate cyclase through Gi, and the Gq-coupled

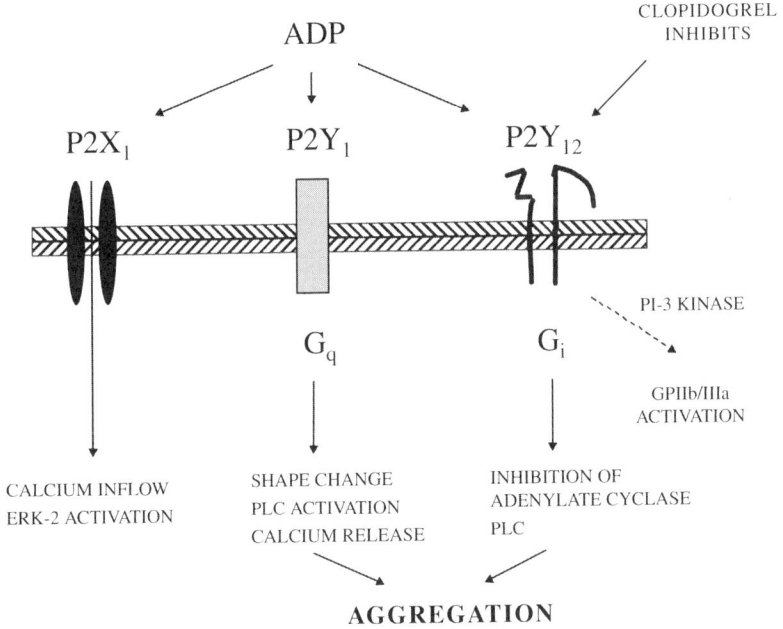

Fig. 1. Platelet ADP receptors. ERK-2, extracellular signal-regulated kinase 2; PLC, phospholipase C.

P2Y$_1$ is linked to activation of the β-isoform of phospholipase C, platelet shape change, and intracellular calcium mobilization *(35,40)*. Coordinated signaling through each receptor is required for full platelet activation and TXA$_2$ production *(36,41)*, although P2Y$_{12}$ can stimulate GPIIb-IIIa receptor activation independently at high concentrations of ADP through a phosphoinositide 3-kinase-dependent signaling pathway *(42)*. The ADP receptor antagonist clopidogrel irreversibly antagonizes the P2Y$_{12}$ receptor, probably through the formation of a disulphide bridge between Cys 17 and Cys 270 *(43)*.

SHEAR STRESS AND EPINEPHRINE

Epinephrine induces platelet activation through inhibition of adenylate cyclase via the Gi-linked α$_2$-adrenergic platelet receptor. It is a weak agonist and requires other agonists to induce full platelet aggregation. High shear stress, such as that found at the site of a severe coronary stenosis, can also lead to platelet activation. High shear induces vWF to bind to GPIb-IX-V, elevating intracellular calcium and activating a protein kinase G (PKG) signaling pathway that leads to mitogen-activated protein (MAP) kinase and GPIIb-IIIa activation *(44)*.

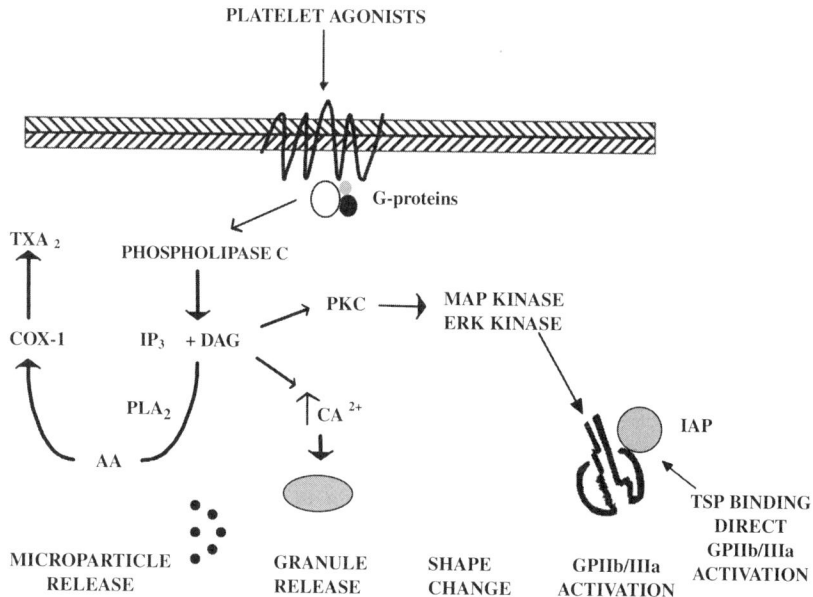

Fig. 2. Inside-out signaling. AA, arachidonic acid; COX-1, cyclooxygenase 1; DAG, diacylglycerol; ERK, extracellular signal-regulated kinase; IAP, integrin-associated protein; IP_3, inositol triphosphate; MAP, mitogen-activated protein; PKC, protein kinase C; PLA_2, phospholipase A_2; TSP, thrombospondin; TXA_2, thromboxane A_2.

Inside-Out Signal Transduction

Stimulation of platelet agonist receptors induces signals within the platelet, so-called inside-out signaling, which results in cytoskeletal rearrangement, shape change, protein synthesis, and granule secretion and ultimately alters the affinity of the platelet receptor for fibrinogen, GPIIb-IIIa (Fig. 2). The initial signal is transmitted through a number of different G proteins *(45)* including Gi, Gq, and G12/G13 *(46,47)*. Subsequent signals are mediated through activation of phospholipase Cβ, the hydrolysis of phosphatidylinositol into the second messengers inositol triphosphate (IP_3) and diacylglycerol (DAG), and the activation of nonreceptor protein tyrosine kinases (PTKs), leading to tyrosine and threonine phosphorylation of a number of platelet proteins. IP_3 stimulates calcium release and triggers phospholipase A_2 activation. Phospholipase A_2 releases arachidonic acid from the cell membrane, which is subsequently converted into TXA_2. DAG activates protein kinase C (PKC), leading to activation of isoforms of the MAP kinases and ERKs *(48)* and ultimately to GPIIb-IIIa activation *(49)*. Phosphatidylinositol 3-kinase (PI3K) also plays a role in integrin activation *(50,51)* through

Table 2
Platelet Secretions

Platelet-derived growth factor
P-selectin
RANTES
Platelet-activating factor
β-Thromboglobulin
Platelet factor 4
von Willebrand factor
α_2-Antiplasmin
Coagulation factor V
Fibrinogen
Fibronectin
Thrombospondin
ADP
Serotonin
CD40L
Matrix metalloproteinases 1 and 2
Vascular endothelial growth factor
Insulin-like growth factor
Epidermal and fibroblast growth factors
Transforming growth factor-β_1

the conversion of phosphatidylinositol (PtdIns) 4-phosphate and phosphatidyl 4-5-diphosphate to their 3-phosphorylated counterparts. These are membrane embedded and recruit phospholipase Cγ and Src to the membrane *(52)*.

Signaling-independent pathways of integrin activation have also been identified. Thrombospondin, specifically its carboxy-terminal cell binding domain (CBD), binds to integrin-associated protein (IAP/CD47). The thrombospondin/IAP complex interacts with GPIIb-IIIa, inducing its activation independent of intracellular signaling *(53)*. The thrombospondin/IAP interaction is also involved in platelet adhesion to tumor necrosis factor (TNF)-α-stimulated endothelial cells *(54)*, potentially helping to localize the activated platelet to areas of endothelial activation.

Platelet Secretion

Platelets release a number of biologically active substances upon activation (Table 2). These include the contents of their α and dense granules, lysozymes, and platelet-derived microparticles. In addition, activated platelets synthesize and secrete a number of biologically active products and express the inflammatory stimulant CD40L *(55)*. Platelet α-granules contain platelet-derived growth factor, P-selectin, vWF, α_2-

antiplasmin, β-thromboglobulin, platelet factor 4 coagulation factor V, and the adhesion molecules fibrinogen *(56)*, fibronectin, and thrombospondin; the dense granules contain ADP and serotonin. The released ADP provides a feedback loop for further platelet stimulation, and serotonin enables the binding of some of the proteins released from the α-granules to a subpopulation of platelets, through an as yet undefined receptor *(57)*. Platelet secretion requires the formation of soluble *N*-ethylmaleimide-sensitive factor attachment protein (SNAP) and receptor (SNARE) complexes among syntaxin 4, SNAP-25, and vesicle-associated membrane proteins (VAMP-3 and -8) *(58)*.

Activated platelets also release membrane microparticles. These contain GPIIb-IIIa, thrombospondin, and P-selectin, enhance local thrombin generation *(59)*, and induce COX-2 expression with the production of prostacyclin in monocytes and endothelial cells *(60)*.

PLATELET ADHESION AND GPIb-IX-V

In the high fluid stress environment of flowing arterial blood, the circulating platelet requires specialized receptors in order to adhere rapidly to damaged endothelium and its underlying subendothelial matrix. Initial adherence is mediated primarily by the platelet vWF receptor GPIb-IX-V *(61,62)*. Circulating vWF binds to collagen exposed in the subendothelium, allowing it to interact with GPIb-IX-V *(63)*, via the vWF A1-domain. This interaction is reversible; it allows the adherent platelets to roll and (probably through clustering of the receptor *[64]*), leads to platelet activation *(65)*. The activated platelets change shape and spread out over the endothelial defect, developing firm adherence through their GPIIb-IIIa, collagen, laminin ($\alpha_6\beta_1$), and fibronectin ($\alpha_5\beta_1$) receptors. In addition, the platelet adheres to endothelial cells through fibrinogen bound to activated GPIIb-IIIa, which bridges to the $\alpha_v\beta_3$ and intercellular adhesion molecule-1 (ICAM-1) *(66)* receptors expressed on activated endothelial cells and through the interaction of GPIb-IX-V with endothelial P-selectin.

Glycoprotein IIb-IIIa

GPIIb-IIIa is often referred to as the platelet receptor for fibrinogen; however, its binding is not restricted to fibrinogen, and other adhesive and nonadhesive ligands bind to it, including vWF, fibronectin, vitronectin, red cell ICAM-4 *(67)*, prothrombin, and thrombospondin. Fibrinogen is its principle ligand in vivo owing to its high plasma concentration. In the resting receptor the fibrinogen binding site is cryptic but is exposed on activation as a result of a conformational change in the receptor *(68)*. Fibrinogen is multivalent and crosslinks adjacent platelets to form an aggregate. The change in GPIIb-IIIa affinity with activation appears to be exerted by signals transmitted through the intracellular tails of the receptor *(69–71)*, probably as a result of a change in interaction of the integrin cytoplasmic tails with each other or with an activating or inhibitory intraplatelet factor *(72–76)*. The small GTPase RAP1b augments GPIIb-IIIa affinity, probably by modulating its interaction with the cytoskeleton *(77)*. Similarly, the small GTPase Rac3 interacts with the calcium- and integrin-binding protein (CIB) and promotes GPIIb-IIIa-mediated adhesion *(78)*.

GPIIb-IIIa is the most abundant platelet receptor, with 40–80,000 GPIIb-IIIa complexes per platelet *(79)*. It is an integrin receptor *(80)* composed of two subunits, α_{IIb} (CD41) and β_{III} (CD61). Each of these is the product of separate genes that lie on the long arm of chromosome 17 at q21-22 *(81,82)*. The subunits are combined noncovalently to form a globular amino-terminal head region from which the two carboxy-terminal tails extend, forming the transmembrane and intracellular portions of GPIIb-IIIa *(83)*. The α_{IIb} subunit is the larger of the two and consists of an extracellular heavy chain, $\alpha_{IIb}a$ (125 kDa), joined by a disulfide bond to the transmembrane and intracellular portion of the light chain, $\alpha_{IIb}b$ (25 kDa) *(84)*. The amino terminus of α_{IIb} contains seven approx 60 amino acid repeats, similar to the repeat pattern found in heterodimeric G proteins. In the recently crystallized $\alpha_v\beta_3$ receptor, these repeats form the blades of a β-propeller *(85,86)*. The β_3 chain (100 kDa) is composed of a single polypeptide chain with 28 disulphide bonds. These are important in maintaining the tertiary structure of GPIIb-IIIa. Disruption of these disulphide bonds results in receptor activation *(87,88)* and platelet aggregation *(89)*, indicating that these bonds may be involved in the conformational changes that occur upon platelet activation.

The exact ligand-binding domain on GPIIb-IIIa has not been defined; however regions on both α_{IIb} and β_3 have been implicated. The amino-terminus β-propeller of α_{IIb} appears to be important in ligand binding *(90–93)*. The ligand-binding domain resides on the upper surface of the propeller; calcium binding regions are found on the lower. The binding activity of GPIIIa has also been localized within its amino terminus *(94,95)*. This is within the proposed metal ion-coordinating site within GPIIIa, homologous to the inserted or I-domain seen in α (but not α_{IIb}) chains. Site-directed mutations in the oxygenated residues Ser 121 and Ser 123 surrounding this region impair ligand binding *(96)*, indicating the importance of this area in ligand binding.

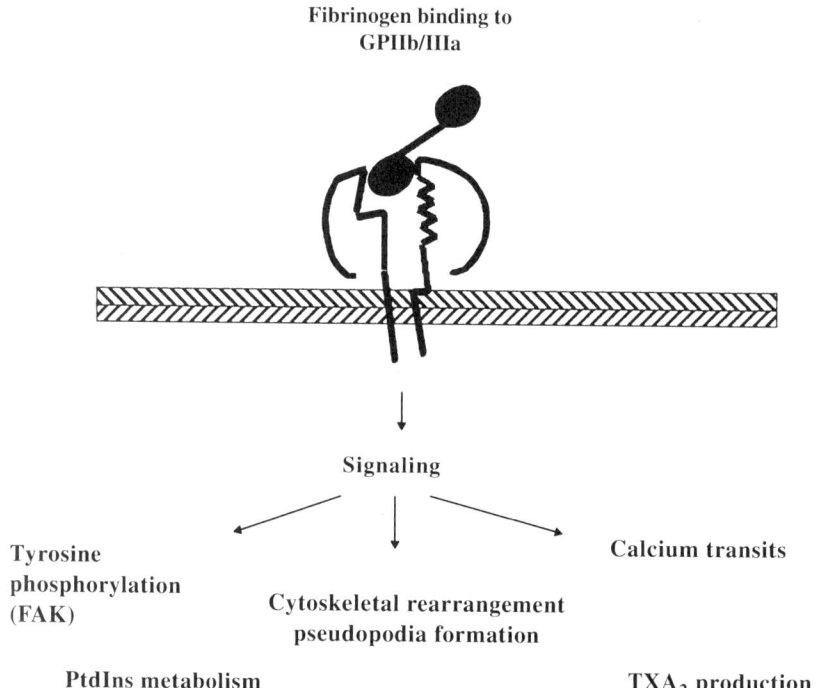

Fig. 3. Outside-in signaling. PtdIns, phosphatidylinositol; TXA$_2$, thromboxane A$_2$.

OUTSIDE-IN SIGNALING

GPIIb-IIIa is not merely a passive adhesion receptor for fibrinogen; it induces a number of intracellular signals upon ligand binding *(97)* leading to cytoskeletal rearrangement, pseudopodia formation, and spreading on solid-phase fibrinogen (Fig. 3). This outside-in signaling results in tyrosine phosphorylation of a number of platelet proteins and the formation of focal adhesion complexes of signaling proteins that amplify existing activation events, such as TXA$_2$ production and inositol phosphate metabolism *(98,99)*. These signals appear to be transmitted through a conformational change in the receptor subsequent to ligand binding, the so-called ligand-induced binding site (LIBS) *(100)*, leading to phosphorylation of the intracellular tail of the β-chain *(101)*. This growth factor receptor bound 2 probably allows its interaction with the signaling proteins growth factor receptor bound 2 (GRB2) and SHC, as well as the cytoskeletal protein myosin *(102,103)*. Other signaling molecules including the tyrosine kinase Src have been implicated in integrin signaling. Src associates with the intracellular tail of GPIIb-IIIa on adhesion to solid-phase fibrinogen. Inhibition of Src prevents phosphorylation of Syk and also prevents phosphorylation of the Syk substrates Vav1, Vav3, and SLP-76 and thus platelet spreading *(104)*. PtdIns $(3,4)P_2$ production has also been implicated in outside in signaling as it is dependent on fibrinogen binding to GPIIb-IIIa *(105)* and may play a role in actin assembly and pleckstrin phosphorylation *(106,107)*.

Fibrinogen

Fibrinogen is made up of three different pairs of identical subunits (α, β, and γ) and has six different sites that potentially interact with GPIIb-IIIa, two arginine-glycine-aspartate (RGD) domains at residues 95–97 and 572–574, respectively, in each of two α-chains and a dodecapeptide in the carboxy terminus (residues 400–411) of each γ-chain. The RGD and dodecapeptide peptides bind to separate sites on GPIIb-IIIa *(94,108,109)*. Although RGD inhibits fibrinogen binding, the dodecapeptide sequence appears to be the primary receptor binding domain in vivo *(110,111)*. In flowing conditions only the intact fibrinogen molecule supports adhesion, indicating that cooperative binding between the RGD and dodecapeptide sites or other, potentially unidentified, sites within the intact fibrinogen molecule are necessary for normal platelet function *(112)*.

PLATELETS AND INFLAMMATION

Activated platelets play an important role in inflammation and express or release a number of molecules that lead to leukocyte activation and secretion *(113)*. One of the most important immune mediators expressed by platelets is the CD40 ligand (L), a 33-kDa transmembrane protein related to TNF-α *(55)*. Platelets are the major intravascular source of CD40L which interacts with its receptor CD40, inducing endothelial expression of E-selectin, vascular cell adhesion molecule (VCAM)-1 and ICAM-1 and secretion of the chemokines interleukin-8 (IL-8) and monocyte chemoattractant protein (MCP-1). Platelet CD40L expression is rapidly downregulated through cleavage and release of its less active soluble form *(114)*. Released CD40L binds to GPIIb-IIIa and promotes platelet aggregation under shear. In animal models of atherosclerosis, CD40L inhibition *(115,116)* or knockout *(117)* dramatically limits the development and progression of atherosclerosis and reduces the stability of arterial thrombi *(118)*. The effect of platelet inhibitors on platelet CD40L release is variable. GPIIb-IIIa antagonists inhibit CD40L release at high levels of receptor occupancy but potentiate its release at lower levels of GPIIb-IIIa inhibition. Aspirin was shown to only partially inhibit CD40L release in collagen-stimulated platelets *(119)*.

Platelets also synthesize and release the inflammatory cytokine IL-1β from stored messenger RNA in a GPIIb-IIIa-dependent fashion. The IL-1β is released in membrane microvesicles and induces neutrophil endothelial binding *(120)*. In fact, surprisingly, the anucleate platelet can synthesize a vast array of proteins upon activation. The β-3 subunit of GPIIb-IIIa plays an important role in the control of platelet mRNA translation through the redistribution of eukaryotic initiation factor 4E, a mRNA cap-binding protein that controls global translation rates *(121)*.

CONCLUSIONS

Once considered merely a component of hemostasis, it is now clear that the tiny anucleate platelet influences many physiological and pathological processes. The underlying processes controlling these platelet functions are complex, and many are yet to be discovered. As our understanding of platelet physiology continues to progress, so to do the potential targets for platelet inhibition and it is likely that inhibition, of platelet function will continue to be one of the most important therapies in patients with atherosclerosis.

REFERENCES

1. Kroll MH, Hellums JD, McIntire LV, Schafer AI, Moake JL. Platelets and shear stress. Blood 1996;88:1525–1541.
2. Wenzel UO, Fouqueray B, Grandaliano G, et al. Thrombin regulates expression of monocyte chemoattractant protein-1 in vascular smooth muscle cells. Circ Res 1995;77:503–509.
3. DeMichele MA, Moon DG, Fenton JW, 2nd, Minnear FL. Thrombin's enzymatic activity increases permeability of endothelial cell monolayers. J Appl Physiol 1990;69:1599–1606.
4. Kranzhofer R, Clinton SK, Ishii K, Coughlin SR, Fenton JW, 2nd, Libby P. Thrombin potently stimulates cytokine production in human vascular smooth muscle cells but not in mononuclear phagocytes. Circ Res 1996;79:286–294.
5. McNamara CA, Sarembock IJ, Gimple LW, Fenton JW, 2nd, Coughlin SR, Owens GK. Thrombin stimulates proliferation of cultured rat aortic smooth muscle cells by a proteolytically activated receptor. J Clin Invest 1993;91:94–98.
6. Haralabopoulos GC, Grant DS, Kleinman HK, Maragoudakis ME. Thrombin promotes endothelial cell alignment in Matrigel in vitro and angiogenesis in vivo. Am J Physiol 1997;273:C239–C245.
7. Griffin CT, Srinivasan Y, Zheng YW, Huang W, Coughlin SR. A role for thrombin receptor signaling in endothelial cells during embryonic development. Science 2001;293:1666–1670.
8. Connolly AJ, Ishihara H, Kahn ML, Farese RV Jr, Coughlin SR. Role of the thrombin receptor in development and evidence for a second receptor. Nature 1996;381:516–519.

9. Molino M, Bainton DF, Hoxie JA, Coughlin SR, Brass LF. Thrombin receptors on human platelets. Initial localization and subsequent redistribution during platelet activation. J Biol Chem 1997;272:6011–6017.

10. Chen J, Ishii M, Wang L, Ishii K, Coughlin SR. Thrombin receptor activation. Confirmation of the intramolecular tethered liganding hypothesis and discovery of an alternative intermolecular liganding mode. J Biol Chem 1994;269:16041–16045.

11. Vu TK, Hung DT, Wheaton VI, Coughlin SR. Molecular cloning of a functional thrombin receptor reveals a novel proteolytic mechanism of receptor activation. Cell 1991;64:1057–1068.

12. Kahn ML, Zheng YW, Huang W, et al. A dual thrombin receptor system for platelet activation. Nature 1998;394:690–694.

13. Kahn ML, Nakanishi-Matsui M, Shapiro MJ, Ishihara H, Coughlin SR. Protease-activated receptors 1 and 4 mediate activation of human platelets by thrombin. J Clin Invest 1999;103:879–887.

14. Shapiro MJ, Weiss EJ, Faruqi TR, Coughlin SR. Protease-activated receptors 1 and 4 are shut off with distinct kinetics after activation by thrombin. J Biol Chem 2000;275:25216–25221.

15. Nakanishi-Matsui M, Zheng YW, Sulciner DJ, Weiss EJ, Ludeman MJ, Coughlin SR. PAR3 is a cofactor for PAR4 activation by thrombin. Nature 2000;404:609–613.

16. Kim S, Foster C, Lecchi A, et al. Protease-activated receptors 1 and 4 do not stimulate G(i) signaling pathways in the absence of secreted ADP and cause human platelet aggregation independently of G(i) signaling. Blood 2002;99:3629–3636.

17. Soslau G, Class R, Morgan DA, et al. Unique pathway of thrombin-induced platelet aggregation mediated by glycoprotein Ib. J Biol Chem 2001;276:21173–21183.

18. Li CQ, Vindigni A, Sadler JE, Wardell MR. Platelet glycoprotein Ib alpha binds to thrombin anion-binding exosite II inducing allosteric changes in the activity of thrombin. J Biol Chem 2001;276:6161–6168.

19. De Candia E, Hall SW, Rutella S, Landolfi R, Andrews RK, De Cristofaro R. Binding of thrombin to glycoprotein Ib accelerates the hydrolysis of Par-1 on intact platelets. J Biol Chem 2001;276:4692–4698.

20. Tsuji M, Ezumi Y, Arai M, Takayama H. A novel association of Fc receptor gamma-chain with glycoprotein VI and their co-expression as a collagen receptor in human platelets. J Biol Chem 1997;272:23528–23531.

21. Locke D, Chen H, Liu Y, Liu C, Kahn ML. Lipid rafts orchestrate signaling by the platelet receptor glycoprotein VI. J Biol Chem 2002;277:18801–18809.

22. Ezumi Y, Kodama K, Uchiyama T, Takayama H. Constitutive and functional association of the platelet collagen receptor glycoprotein VI-Fc receptor gamma-chain complex with membrane rafts. Blood 2002;99:3250–3255.

23. Kehrel B, Wierwille S, Clemetson KJ, et al. Glycoprotein VI is a major collagen receptor for platelet activation: it recognizes the platelet-activating quaternary structure of collagen, whereas CD36, glycoprotein IIb/IIIa, and von Willebrand factor do not. Blood 1998;91:491–499.

24. Poole A, Gibbins JM, Turner M, et al. The Fc receptor gamma-chain and the tyrosine kinase Syk are essential for activation of mouse platelets by collagen. EMBO J 1997;16:2333–2341.

25. Cicmil M, Thomas JM, Leduc M, Bon C, Gibbins JM. Platelet endothelial cell adhesion molecule-1 signaling inhibits the activation of human platelets. Blood 2002;99:137–144.

26. Larson MK, Chen H, Kahn ML, et al. Identification of P2Y12-dependent and -independent mechanisms of glycoprotein VI-mediated Rap1 activation in platelets. Blood 2003;101:1409–1415.

27. Cho MJ, Liu J, Pestina TI, et al. The roles of alpha IIb beta 3-mediated outside-in signal transduction, thromboxane A2, and adenosine diphosphate in collagen-induced platelet aggregation. Blood 2003;101:2646–26451.
28. Reilly M, Fitzgerald GA. Cellular activation by thromboxane A2 and other eicosanoids. Eur Heart J 1993;14:88–93.
29. FitzGerald GA. Mechanisms of platelet activation: thromboxane A2 as an amplifying signal for other agonists. Am J Cardiol 1991;68:11B–15B.
30. Hirata T, Ushikubi F, Kakizuka A, Okuma M, Narumiya S. Two thromboxane A2 receptor isoforms in human platelets. Opposite coupling to adenylyl cyclase with different sensitivity to Arg60 to Leu mutation. J Clin Invest 1996;97:949–956.
31. Narumiya S. Structures, properties and distributions of prostanoid receptors. Adv Prostaglandin Thromboxane Leukotriene Res 1995;23:17–22.
32. Halushka PV, Allan CJ, Davis-Bruno KL. Thromboxane A2 receptors. J Lipid Mediators Cell Signal 1995;12:361–378.
33. Meyers KM, Holmsen H, Seachord CL. Comparative study of platelet dense granule constituents. Am J Physiol 1982;243:R454–R461.
34. Gardner A, Jonsen J, Laland S, Hellem A, Owren P. Adenosine diphosphate in red blood cells as a factor in the adhesiveness of human blood platelets. Nature 1961;192:531–532.
35. Hollopeter G, Jantzen HM, Vincent D, et al. Identification of the platelet ADP receptor targeted by antithrombotic drugs. Nature 2001;409:202–207.
36. Jin J, Daniel JL, Kunapuli SP. Molecular basis for ADP-induced platelet activation. II. The P2Y1 receptor mediates ADP-induced intracellular calcium mobilization and shape change in platelets. J Biol Chem 1998;273:2030–2034.
37. Sun B, Li J, Okahara K, Kambayashi J. P2X1 purinoceptor in human platelets. Molecular cloning and functional characterization after heterologous expression. J Biol Chem 1998;273:11544–11547.
38. Savi P, Bornia J, Salel V, Delfaud M, Herbert JM. Characterization of P2x1 purinoreceptors on rat platelets: effect of clopidogrel. Br J Haematol 1997;98:880–886.
39. Oury C, Toth-Zsamboki E, Vermylen J, Hoylaerts MF. P2X(1)-mediated activation of extracellular signal-regulated kinase 2 contributes to platelet secretion and aggregation induced by collagen. Blood 2002;100:2499–2505.
40. Daniel J, Dangelmaier C, Jin J, Ashby B, Smith J, Kunapuli S. Molecular basis for ADP-induced platelet activation: evidence for three distinct ADP receptors on human platelets. J Biol Chem 1998;273:2024–2029.
41. Jin J, Quinton TM, Zhang J, Rittenhouse SE, Kunapuli SP. Adenosine diphosphate (ADP)-induced thromboxane A(2) generation in human platelets requires coordinated signaling through integrin alpha(IIb)beta(3) and ADP receptors. Blood 2002;99:193–198.
42. Kauffenstein G, Bergmeier W, Eckly A, et al. The P2Y(12) receptor induces platelet aggregation through weak activation of the alpha(IIb)beta(3) integrin—a phosphoinositide 3- kinase-dependent mechanism. FEBS Lett 2001;505:281–290.
43. Ding Z, Kim S, Dorsam RT, Jin J, Kunapuli SP. Inactivation of the human P2Y12 receptor by thiol reagents requires interaction with both extracellular cysteine residues, Cys17 and Cys270. Blood 2003;101:3908–3914.
44. Li Z, Xi X, Du X. A mitogen-activated protein kinase-dependent signaling pathway in the activation of platelet integrin alpha IIbbeta3. J Biol Chem 2001; 276:42226–42232.
45. Brass LF, Manning DR, Cichowski K, Abrams CS. Signaling through G proteins in platelets: to the integrins and beyond. Thromb Haemost 1997;78:581–589.
46. Dorsam RT, Kim S, Jin J, Kunapuli SP. Coordinated signaling through both G12/ 13 and G(i) pathways is sufficient to activate GPIIb/IIIa in human platelets. J Biol Chem 2002;277:47588–47595.

47. Nieswandt B, Schulte V, Zywietz A, Gratacap MP, Offermanns S. Costimulation of Gi- and G12/G13-mediated signaling pathways induces integrin alpha IIbbeta 3 activation in platelets. J Biol Chem 2002;277:39493–39498.

48. Nadal-Wollbold F, Pawlowski M, Levy-Toledano S, Berrou E, Rosa JP, Bryckaert M. Platelet ERK2 activation by thrombin is dependent on calcium and conventional protein kinases C but not Raf-1 or B-Raf. FEBS Lett 2002;531:475–482.

49. Blockmans D, Deckmyn H, Vermylen J. Platelet activation. Blood Rev 1995;9: 143–156.

50. Kovacsovics T, Bachelot C, Toker A, et al. Phosphoinositide 3-kinase inhibition spares actin assembly in activating platelets but reverses platelet aggregation. J Biol Chem 1995;270:11358–11366.

51. Hmama Z, Knutson K, Herrera-Velit P, Nandan D, Reiner N. Monocyte adherence induced by lipopolysaccharide involves CD14, LFA-1, and cytohesin-1. Regulation by Rho and phosphatidylinositol 3-kinase. J Biol Chem 1999;274:1050–1057.

52. Toker A, Cantley L. Signalling through the lipid products of phosphoinositide-3-OH kinase. Nature 1997;387:673–676.

53. Fujimoto TT, Katsutani S, Shimomura T, Fujimura K. Thrombospondin-bound integrin associated protein (CD47) physically and functionally modifies integrin alpha IIbbeta 3 by its extracellular domain. J Biol Chem 2003;7:7.

54. Lagadec P, Dejoux O, Ticchioni M, et al. Involvement of a CD47-dependent pathway in platelet adhesion on inflamed vascular endothelium under flow. Blood 2003;101:4836–4843.

55. Henn V, Slupsky JR, Grafe M, et al. CD40 ligand on activated platelets triggers an inflammatory reaction of endothelial cells. Nature 1998;391:591–594.

56. Keenan J, Solum N. Quantitative studies on the release of platelet fibrinogen by thrombin. Br J Haematol 1972;23:461–466.

57. Dale GL, Friese P, Batar P, et al. Stimulated platelets use serotonin to enhance their retention of procoagulant proteins on the cell surface. Nature 2002;415:175–179.

58. Polgar J, Chung SH, Reed GL. Vesicle-associated membrane protein 3 (VAMP-3) and VAMP-8 are present in human platelets and are required for granule secretion. Blood 2002;100:1081–1083.

59. Merten M, Pakala R, Thiagarajan P, Benedict C. Platelet microparticles promote platelet interaction with subendothelial matrix in a glycoprotein IIb/IIIa-dependent mechanism. Circulation 1999;99:2577–2582.

60. Barry O, Kazanietz M, Pratico D, FitzGerald G. Arachidonic acid in platelet microparticles up-regulates cyclooxygenase-2-dependent prostaglandin formation via a protein kinase C/mitogen-activated protein kinase-dependent pathway. J Biol Chem 1999;274:7545–7556.

61. Andrews RK, Shen Y, Gardiner EE, Dong JF, Lopez JA, Berndt MC. The glycoprotein Ib-IX-V complex in platelet adhesion and signaling. Thromb Haemost 1999;82:357–364.

62. Matsui H, Sugimoto M, Mizuno T, et al. Distinct and concerted functions of von Willebrand factor and fibrinogen in mural thrombus growth under high shear flow. Blood 2002;100:3604–3610.

63. Ruggeri ZM. von Willebrand factor. J Clin Invest 1997;99:559–564.

64. Kasirer-Friede A, Ware J, Leng L, Marchese P, Ruggeri ZM, Shattil SJ. Lateral clustering of platelet GP Ib-IX complexes leads to up-regulation of the adhesive function of integrin alpha IIbbeta 3. J Biol Chem 2002;277:11949–11956.

65. Zaffran Y, Meyer SC, Negrescu E, Reddy KB, Fox JE. Signaling across the platelet adhesion receptor glycoprotein Ib-IX induces alpha IIbbeta 3 activation both in platelets and a transfected Chinese hamster ovary cell system. J Biol Chem 2000;275:16779–16787.

66. Bombeli T, Schwartz BR, Harlan JM. Adhesion of activated platelets to endothelial cells: evidence for a GPIIbIIIa-dependent bridging mechanism and novel roles for endothelial intercellular adhesion molecule 1 (ICAM-1), alphavbeta3 integrin, and GPIbalpha. J Exp Med 1998;187:329–339.

67. Hermand P, Gane P, Huet M, et al. Red cell ICAM-4 is a novel ligand for platelet-activated alpha IIbbeta 3 integrin. J Biol Chem 2003;278:4892–4898.

68. Shattil SJ, Hoxie JA, Cunningham M, Brass LF. Changes in the platelet membrane glycoprotein IIb.IIIa complex during platelet activation. J Biol Chem 1985;260:11107–11114.

69. O'Toole T, Mandelman D, Forsyth J, Shattil SJ, Plow EF, Ginsberg MH. Modulation of the affinity of integrin alpha IIb beta 3 (GPIIb-IIIa) by the cytoplasmic domain of alpha IIb. Science 1991;254:845–847.

70. O'Toole T, Katagiri Y, Faull RJ, et al. Integrin cytoplasmic domains mediate inside-out signal transduction. J Cell Biol 1994;124:1047–1059.

71. Stephens G, O'Luanaigh N, Reilly D, et al. A sequence within the cytoplasmic tail of GpIIb independently activates platelet aggregation and thromboxane synthesis. J Biol Chem 1998;273:20317–20322.

72. Leisner TM, Wencel-Drake JD, Wang W, Lam SCT. Bidirectional transmembrane modulation of integrin alpha IIb beta 3 conformations. J Biol Chem 1999:12945–12949.

73. Chen Y, O'Toole T, Shipley T, et al. "Inside-out" signal transduction inhibited by isolated integrin cytoplasmic domains. J Biol Chem 1994;269:18307–18310.

74. Naik U, Patel P, Parise L. Identification of a novel calcium-binding protein that interacts with the integrin alphaIIb cytoplasmic domain. J Biol Chem 1997;272:4651–4654.

75. Naik UP, Naik MU. Association of CIB with GPIIb/IIIa during outside-in signaling is required for platelet spreading on fibrinogen. Blood 2003;24:24.

76. Tsuboi S. Calcium integrin-binding protein activates platelet integrin alpha IIbbeta 3. J Biol Chem 2002;277:1919–1923.

77. Bertoni A, Tadokoro S, Eto K, et al. Relationships between Rap1b, affinity modulation of integrin alpha IIbbeta 3, and the actin cytoskeleton. J Biol Chem 2002;277:25715–25721.

78. Haataja L, Kaartinen V, Groffen J, Heisterkamp N. The small GTPase Rac3 interacts with the integrin-binding protein CIB and promotes integrin alpha(IIb)beta(3)-mediated adhesion and spreading. J Biol Chem 2002;277:8321–8328.

79. Wagner CL, Mascelli MA, Neblock DS, Weisman HF, Coller BS, Jordan RE. Analysis of GPIIb/IIIa receptor number by quantification of 7E3 binding to human platelets. Blood 1996;88:907–914.

80. Hynes R. Integrins: a family of cell surface receptors. Cell 1987;48:549–554.

81. Bray PF, Rosa JP, Johnston GI, et al. Platelet glycoprotein IIb. Chromosomal localization and tissue expression. J Clin Invest 1987;80:1812–1817.

82. Rosa JP, Bray PF, Gayet O, et al. Cloning of glycoprotein IIIa cDNA from human erythroleukemia cells and localization of the gene to chromosome 17. Blood 1988;72:593–600.

83. Weisel J, Nagaswami C, Vilaire G, Bennett J. Examination of the platelet membrane glycoprotein IIb-IIIa complex and its interaction with fibrinogen and other ligands by electron microscopy. J Biol Chem 1992;267:16637–16643.

84. Calvete JJ. On the structure and function of platelet integrin alpha IIb beta 3, the fibrinogen receptor. Proc Soc Exp Biol Med 1995;208:346–360.

85. Springer T. An extracellular beta-propeller module predicted in lipoprotein and scavenger receptors, tyrosine kinases, epidermal growth factor precursor, and extracellular matrix components. J Mol Biol 1998;283:837–862.

86. Xiong JP, Stehle T, Diefenbach B, et al. Crystal structure of the extracellular segment of integrin alpha Vbeta3. Science 2001;294:339–345.

87. Kashiwagi H, Tomiyama Y, Tadokoro S, et al. A mutation in the extracellular cysteine-rich repeat region of the beta3 subunit activates integrins alphaIIbbeta3 and alphaVbeta3. Blood 1999;93:2559–2568.

88. Sun QH, Liu CY, Wang R, Paddock C, Newman PJ. Disruption of the long-range GPIIIa Cys(5)-Cys(435) disulfide bond results in the production of constitutively active GPIIb-IIIa (alpha(IIb)beta(3)) integrin complexes. Blood 2002; 100:2094–2101.

89. Peeschke E. Regulation of platelet aggregation by post-fibrinogen binding. Insights provided by dithiothreitol treated platelets. Thromb Haemost 1995:862–867.

90. Gulino D, Boudignon C, Zhang L, Concord E, Rabiet M, Marguerie G. Ca(2+)-binding properties of the platelet glycoprotein IIb ligand-interacting domain. J Biol Chem 1992;267:1001–1007.

91. Calvete J, Schafer W, Mann K, Henschen A, Gonzalez-Rodriguez J. Localization of the cross-linking sites of RGD and KQAGDV peptides to the isolated fibrinogen receptor, the human platelet integrin glycoprotein IIb/IIIa. Influence of peptide length. Eur J Biochem 1992;206:759–765.

92. D'Souza S, Ginsberg M, Burke T, Plow E. The ligand binding site of the platelet integrin receptor GPIIb-IIIa is proximal to the second calcium binding domain of its alpha subunit. J Biol Chem 1990;265:3440–3446.

93. D'Souza S, Ginsberg M, Matsueda G, Plow E. A discrete sequence in a platelet integrin is involved in ligand recognition. Nature 1991;350:66–68.

94. Cierniewski CS, Byzova T, Papierak M, et al. Peptide ligands can bind to distinct sites in integrin alphaIIbbeta3 and elicit different functional responses. J Biol Chem 1999;274:16923–16932.

95. Loftus J, O'Toole T, Plow E, Glass A, Frelinger A, Ginsberg M. A beta 3 integrin mutation abolishes ligand binding and alters divalent cation-dependent conformation. Science 1990;249:915–918.

96. Tozer E, Liddington R, Sutcliffe M, Smeeton A, Loftus J. Ligand binding to integrin alphaIIbbeta3 is dependent on a MIDAS-like domain in the beta3 subunit. Biol Chem 1996;271:21978–21984.

97. Yamada KM, Miyamoto S. Integrin transmembrane signaling and cytoskeletal control. Curr Opin Cell Biol 1995;7:681–689.

98. Fox JE, Lipfert L, Clark EA, Reynolds CC, Austin CD, Brugge JS. On the role of the platelet membrane skeleton in mediating signal transduction. Association of GP IIb-IIIa, pp60c-src, pp62c-yes, and the p21ras GTPase-activating protein with the membrane skeleton. J Biol Chem 1993;268:25973–25984.

99. Shattil S, Haimovich B, Cunningham M, et al J. Tyrosine phosphorylation of pp125FAK in platelets requires coordinated signaling through integrin and agonist recptors. J Biol Chem 1994;269:14738–14745.

100. Kouns WC, Kirchhofer D, Hadvary P, et al. Reversible conformational changes induced in glycoprotein IIb-IIIa by a potent and selective peptidomimetic inhibitor. Blood 1992;80:2539–2547.

101. Schaffner-Reckinger E, Gouon V, Melchior C, Plancon S, Kieffer N. Distinct involvement of beta3 integrin cytoplasmic domain tyrosine residues 747 and 759 in integrin-mediated cytoskeletal assembly and phosphotyrosine signaling. J Biol Chem 1998;273:12623–12632.

102. Jenkins A, Nannizzi-Alaimo L, Silver D, et al. Tyrosine phosphorylation of the beta3 cytoplasmic domain mediates integrin-cytoskeletal interactions. J Biol Chem 1998;273:13878–13885.

103. Law D, Nannizzi-Alaimo L, Phillips D. Outside-in integrin signal transduction. Alpha IIb beta 3-(GP IIb IIIa) tyrosine phosphorylation induced by platelet aggregation. J Biol Chem 1996;271:10811–10815.

104. Obergfell A, Eto K, Mocsai A, et al. Coordinate interactions of Csk, Src, and Syk kinases with [alpha]IIb[beta]3 initiate integrin signaling to the cytoskeleton. J Cell Biol 2002;157:265–275.
105. Sorisky A, King W, Rittenhouse S. Accumulation of PtdIns(3,4)P2 and PtdIns(3,4,5)P3 in thrombin-stimulated platelets. Different sensitivities to Ca2+ or functional integrin. Biochem J 1992;286:581–584.
106. Rittenhouse S. Phosphoinositide 3-kinase activation and platelet function. Blood 1996;89:4401–4414.
107. Toker A, Bachelot C, Chen C, et al. Phosphorylation of the platelet p47 phosphoprotein is mediated by the lipid products of phosphoinositide 3-kinase. J Biol Chem 1995;270:29525–29531.
108. D'Souza S, Ginsberg MH, Burke TA, Lam SC, Plow EF. Localization of an Arg-Gly-Asp recognition site within an integrin adhesion receptor. Science 1988;242:91–93.
109. D'Souza S, Ginsberg MH, Lam SC, Plow EF. Chemical cross-linking of arginyl-glycyl-aspartic acid peptides to an adhesion receptor on platelets. J Biol Chem 1988;263:3943–3951.
110. Farrell DH, Thiagarajan P, Chung DW, Davie EW. Role of fibrinogen alpha and gamma chain sites in platelet aggregation. Proc Natl Acad Sci USA 1992;89: 10729–10732.
111. Holmback K, Danton MJ, Suh TT, Daugherty CC, Degen JL. Impaired platelet aggregation and sustained bleeding in mice lacking the fibrinogen motif bound by integrin alpha IIb beta 3. EMBO J 1996;15:5760–5771.
112. Savage B, Bottini E, Ruggeri ZM. Interaction of integrin alpha IIb beta 3 with multiple fibrinogen domains during platelet adhesion. J Biol Chem 1995;270:28812–28817.
113. Gawaz M, Neumann FJ, Dickfeld T, et al. Activated platelets induce monocyte chemotactic protein-1 secretion and surface expression of intercellular adhesion molecule-1 on endothelial cells. Circulation 1998;98:1164–1171.
114. Henn V, Steinbach S, Buchner K, Presek P, Kroczek RA. The inflammatory action of CD40 ligand (CD154) expressed on activated human platelets is temporally limited by coexpressed CD40. Blood 2001;98:1047–1054.
115. Lutgens E, Cleutjens KB, Heeneman S, Koteliansky VE, Burkly LC, Daemen MJ. Both early and delayed anti-CD40L antibody treatment induces a stable plaque phenotype. Proc Natl Acad Sci USA 2000;97:7464–7469.
116. Mach F, Schonbeck U, Sukhova GK, Atkinson E, Libby P. Reduction of atherosclerosis in mice by inhibition of CD40 signalling. Nature 1998;394:200–203.
117. Lutgens E, Gorelik L, Daemen MJ, et al. Requirement for CD154 in the progression of atherosclerosis. Nat Med 1999;5:1313–1316.
118. Andre P, Prasad KS, Denis CV, et al. CD40L stabilizes arterial thrombi by a beta3 integrin—dependent mechanism. Nat Med 2002;8:247–252.
119. Nannizzi-Alaimo L, Alves VL, Phillips DR. Inhibitory effects of glycoprotein IIb/IIIa antagonists and aspirin on the release of soluble CD40 ligand during platelet stimulation. Circulation 2003;107:1123–1128.
120. Lindemann S, Tolley ND, Dixon DA, et al. Activated platelets mediate inflammatory signaling by regulated interleukin 1beta synthesis. J Cell Biol 2001;154:485–490.
121. Lindemann S, Tolley ND, Eyre JR, Kraiss LW, Mahoney TM, Weyrich AS. Integrins regulate the intracellular distribution of eukaryotic initiation factor 4E in platelets. A checkpoint for translational control. J Biol Chem 2001;276:33947–33951.

2 Platelet Integrins and Signaling

Karlheinz Peter, MD

INTRODUCTION

The term *integrin* describes an adhesion molecule family and origi-nates from the integrative function of these molecules between extracel-lular ligands and the intracellular cytoskeleton *(1,2)*. Integrins mediate cell–cell, cell–extracellular matrix, and cell–pathogen interactions. Integrins have two major functions: First, they mechanically couple the cytoskeleton to the extracellular matrix or to surface receptors of other cells. Second, they transmit signals from the inside of the cell to the outside of the cell and vice versa *(3)*. At least 24 different integrins are known in vertebrates (Fig. 1). Resting platelets express integrins $\alpha_2\beta_1$, $\alpha_5\beta_1$, $\alpha_6\beta_1$, $\alpha_v\beta_3$, and $\alpha_{IIb}\beta_3$ *(4)*. In addition to these, $\alpha_L\beta_2$ and $\alpha_M\beta_2$ expression on activated platelets has been reported *(5)*.

INTEGRIN STRUCTURE

All integrins consist of two subunits (α and β) that are noncovalently linked to each other (Fig. 2). Both subunits are type I membrane glyco-

From: *Contemporary Cardiology:*
Platelet Function: Assessment, Diagnosis, and Treatment
Edited by: M. Quinn and D. Fitzgerald © Humana Press Inc., Totowa, NJ

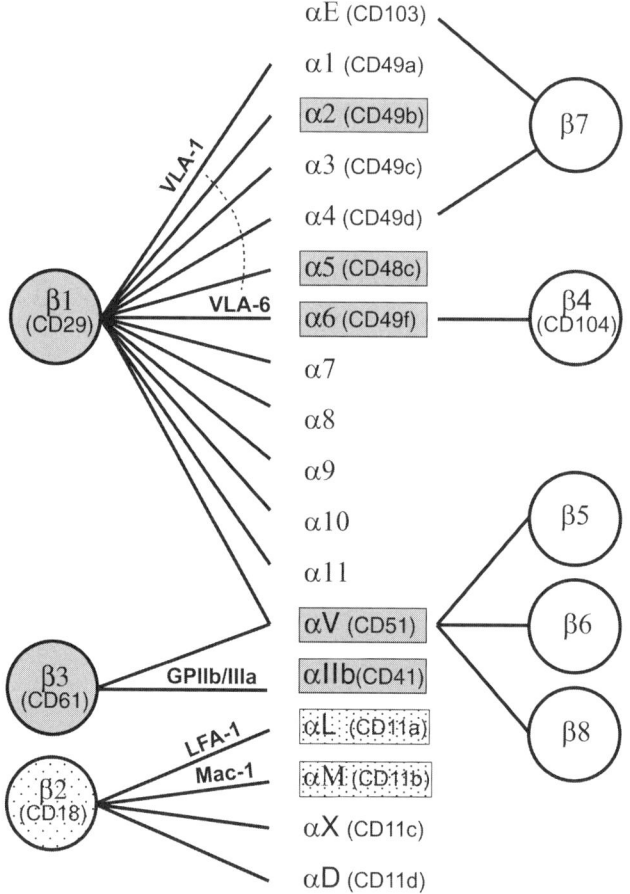

Fig. 1. Integrin α/β heterodimers. Integrin nomenclature and CD numbers are given. Integrins expressed on resting platelets are in dark gray. Integrins reported to be expressed only on activated platelets are in light gray. LFA-1, leukocyte function-associated antigen-1; VLA, very late activation antigen.

proteins. Eighteen different α-subunits and 8 different β-subunits have so far been identified (Fig. 1) *(1,2)*. With the exception of α_4, all integrin subunits have a short cytoplasmic tail, a transmembraneous region, and a large extracellular domain. Both subunits of integrins are rich in cysteine residues; and their pairing in disulfide bonds has been shown to be important in the structure of integrins and may also play a role in the conformational changes during their activation *(6,7)*. In addition, integrins may possess an endogenous thiol isomerase activity that itself may be part of the integrin activation process *(8)*. Their characteristics

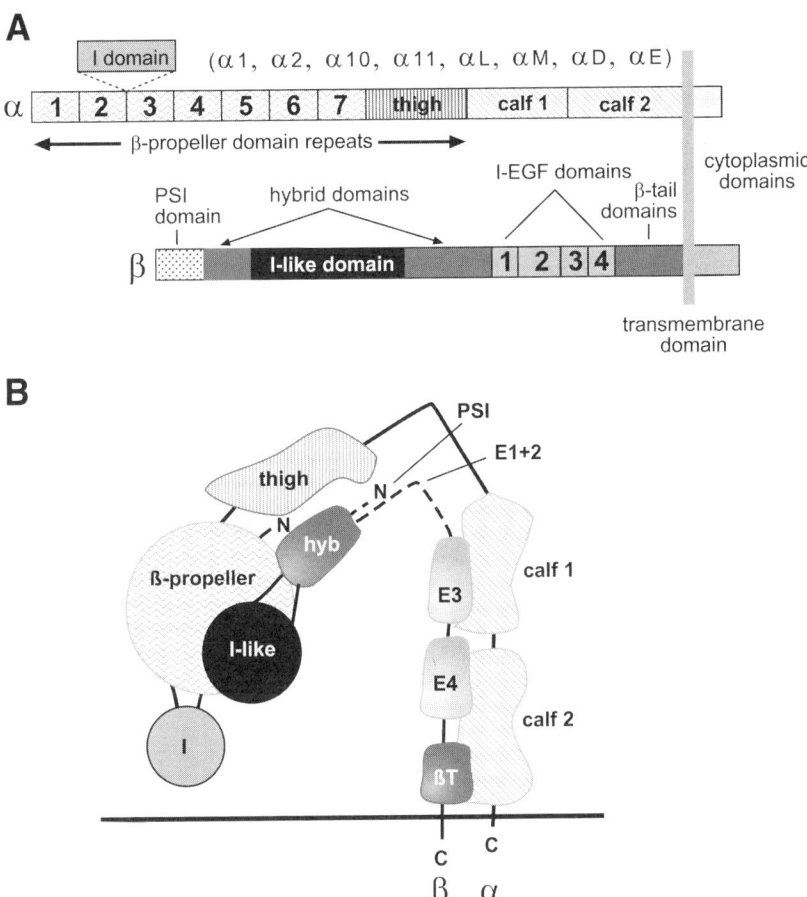

Fig. 2. Integrin structure. Proposed domain organization within the primary structure **(A)** and within the 3D structure **(B)** of integrins according to Takagi and Springer *(9,45)*. For a detailed description *see* text. hyd, hybrid; I-EGF, integrin epidermal growth factor; PSI, plexin, semaphorin, and integrin domain.

in respect to cell type expression, ligand specificity, cytoplasmic inter-action partners, and signaling pathways are often overlapping and are the subject of extensive scientific work in many laboratories. For several of these integrins, different conformational states have been demonstrated *(2,9)*. Upon cell stimulation, integrins can change their conformation rapidly from a low- to a high-affinity state in respect to their ligand binding properties. This is of particular importance for integrins on leu-kocytes and platelets, since these cells have to be recruited from the blood stream by the rapid activation of their integrins.

Figure 2 shows proposed models for integrin structures. The extracellular part of both integrin subunits seems to form a "globular head" and two long "legs" or "stalks." In the middle of the stalks a "knee" or "genu" region has been postulated at which the extracellular integrin domains seem to be bend. The globular head contains the ligand binding regions *(10,11)*.

Structure of the α-Subunits

The N termini of the α-subunits contain seven segments of around 60 amino acids each, which have weak homologies to one another, and these segments are proposed to form a β-propeller with seven four-stranded β-sheets arranged like the blades of a propeller around a pseudosymmetry axis *(11,12)*. Mapping of epitopes, which are far apart in the primary sequence but close in the predicted structure, and X-ray crystallography have confirmed the β-propeller model *(13,14)*. The C-terminal 4-strands of the seven repeats are similar to the so-called EF-hand structure, which is composed of a divalent cation-binding motif *(15,16)*. The problem of the β-propeller model and the finding that EF-hand motifs are based on α-helical structures was recently elucidated by the finding that a Ca^{2+}-binding β-hairpin loop resembles integrin sequence motifs better than the EF hand *(16,17)*. Furthermore, the recently published crystal structure of $α_V$ *(13)* indeed revealed a β-propeller structure, as predicted by Springer *(11,12)*. Mutagenesis studies suggest that ligand-binding residues cluster in one portion of the top and side of the β-propeller and that the Ca^{2+}-binding domains are in loops on the lower, bottom face of the propeller *(18)*.

Half of the integrin α-subunits ($α_1$, $α_2$, $α_{10}$, $α_{11}$, $α_L$, $α_M$, $α_X$, $α_D$, $α_E$) contain a domain of around 200 amino acids that is inserted between β-sheets 2 and 3 of the β-propeller structure. This domain is called the I- or A-domain because of its homology to the von Willebrand factor A1-, A2-, and A3-domains and it is the major integrin binding site in the integrins containing an I-domain *(19–21)*. The 3D structure of the dinucleotide-binding or Rossmann fold, with α-helices surrounding a central β-sheet, is adopted by the I-domain *(22)*. A metal ion-dependent adhesion site (MIDAS) within the I-domain binds negatively charged residues in ligands. The I-domain of $α_L$, expressed solely on the cell surface, is able to mediate cell adhesion, providing strong evidence for the central role of the I-domain in ligand binding *(23)*.

Corresponding to the stalk or leg region is a large portion of around 500 residues that is predicted to consist of three two-layer β-sandwich domains, designated the thigh, calf-1, and calf-2 domains *(13,24)*.

The transmembrane domains of the α-subunit as well as the β-subunit are predicted to form α-helical coiled coils; the hand of the coiled coil seems to be uncertain *(25)*. 3D models suggest a close juxtaposition of the transmembrane domains of both subunits *(25–27)*.

Cytoplasmic domains of the α-subunits are generally between 20 and 40 amino acids in length. There are several sequence similarities between the different α-subunits including completely conserved motifs. The GFFKR region, which is directly adjacent to the transmembrane domain, is highly conserved, and its direct role in platelet activation has been demonstrated *(28–31)*. A number of signaling, adaptor, and cytoskeletal proteins have been demonstrated to interact with integrin cytoplasmic domains, some of which are able to regulate the integrin activation state. Recent nuclear magnetic resonance (NMR) studies suggest that the N-terminal part of the α_{IIb}-subunit is an extension of the helical structure of the transmembrane region up to the middle of the cytoplasmic domain (P998), followed by a turn that allows the acidic C-terminal portion to fold back and interact with the positively charged N-terminal region *(32)*. Interestingly, the cytoplasmic domains of both integrin subunits seem to interact directly with each other, and the disturbance of this interaction seems to be one of the central mechanisms of inside-out signaling in integrins *(28,29,33–35)*.

Structure of the β-Subunits

The N-terminal residues 1–50 of all β-subunits share sequence homology with other membrane proteins, and therefore the region has been termed the PSI domain for plexins, semaphorins, and integrins (Fig. 2) *(36)*. The PSI domain is predicted to form two α-helices. It is a cystein-rich region with seven cysteins in integrins, with the first forming a long-range disulfide bond to the cystein-rich C-terminal region of the β-subunit extracellular domains *(37)*. The region of approximately residues 100–340 is termed the *I-like domain*, since this evolutionarily conserved region contains a putative metal-binding sequence similar to the MIDAS domain in the α-subunit I-domain, its secondary structure is similar, and its sequence is homologous to the I-domain. In the α_V crystal structure a large interface between the β-propeller and the I-like domain could be seen *(13)*. In integrins lacking the I-domain, the I-like domain seems to regulate ligand binding directly, whereas in integrins containing the I-domain, the I-like domain seems to be indirectly involved in ligand binding. On either side of the I-like domain, there is a so-called hybrid domain, which forms β-sandwich domains. Without constituting the N terminus in the primary structure, this insertion between the hybrid domains positions the I-like domain in a loop at the end of the extracellular domain in the integrin tertiary structure. From around residue 435–600, four cystein-rich repeats were termed integrin-epidermal growth factor domains (I-EGF) because of their homology to EGF domains. The C-terminal part of the extracellular domain of integrin subunits, termed the β-tail domain, is cystein-rich and contains an α-helix and a β-sheet.

Cytoplasmic domains of the β-subunits generally contain 45–60 amino acids. Recent NMR studies suggest that the N-terminal part of the β_3-subunit forms a helical structure as an extension of the transmembrane region up to the middle of the cytoplasmic domain (K735) *(32)*. As in the α-subunits, in the cytoplasmic domains of β-subunits there are sequence similarities and completely conserved motifs between the various integrins. One of these motifs, the NPXY/F motif, is found twice in most β-subunit cytoplasmic domains. Indeed, very recently several phosphotyrosine-binding (PTB) domain-containing proteins have been shown to bind to β-subunit cytoplasmic domains, revealing a common regulatory mechanism for integrin activation *(38)*. In addition, several other intracellular molecules have been shown to interact with the β-subunit cytoplasmic domains, including calcium- and integrin-binding protein (CIB), β_3-endonexin, cytohesin-1 and talin *(39)*.

Conformational Changes of Integrins in Inside-Out and Outside-In Signaling

Control of the activation state of integrins is vital for cells and needs to be tightly regulated in a coordinated and fast manner (Figs. 2 and 3). This is especially true for cells that circulate in blood such as leukocytes and platelets. GPIIb-IIIa on circulating platelets needs to be maintained in a conformation that does not allow binding of natural ligands, e.g., fibrinogen. However, upon vessel injury, platelets are activated, and they have to change the activation status of GPIIb-IIIa within the shortest possible time to allow fibrinogen binding, platelet aggregation, and thus vessel sealing. Similarly, integrins expressed on the surface of leukocytes are maintained in a low-affinity state for their ligands until they are activated by the immune response. Inappropriate ligand binding of leukocyte integrins would cause chronic inflammation *(40)*.

In integrin activation induced by cell activation, an activating stimulus is transferred from the inside of the cell to the outside and is therefore termed inside-out signaling (Fig. 3). Cell activation results in the binding of signaling molecules to the cytoplasmic domains of integrins. Thus the association between the transmembrane and cytoplasmic domains of the α- and β-subunits is disturbed and both are separated, which finally results in integrin activation *(32,35,41)*. The cytoskeletal protein talin

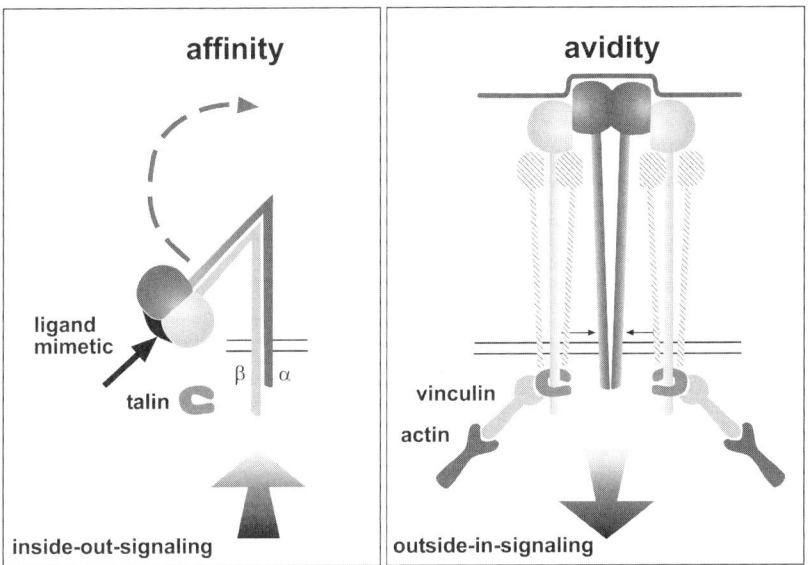

Fig. 3. Affinity and avidity regulation in inside-out and outside-in signaling in integrins. **(Left)** Inside-out signaling. The transmembrane and cytoplasmic domains of an α- and β-subunit are associated with each other. The binding of a signaling, adaptor, or cytoskeletal molecule results in separation of the cytoplasmic and transmembrane domains and causes a conformational change from the bend to the extended structure of the extracellular integrin "legs." Thus the ligand-binding sites within the integrin head pieces are fully exposed and bind native ligands. Integrin clustering with cytoskeletal anchorage is induced by homodimerization of the α-subunit and a homotrimerization of the β-subunit. High-affinity binding and avidity modulation (cytoskeletal crosslinking) in combination result in a high adhesive strength. **(Right)** Outside-in signaling. Ligand-mimetic peptides can bind to integrins in the bended form. Thus the integrin extracellular domain undergoes a conformational change into the extended form, which enables the head piece to bind native ligands and which can be accompanied by a separation of the transmembrane and cytoplasmic domains and cytoskeletal rearrangements.

may be considered a prototype for regulatory function in integrin activation via its binding to the cytoplasmic integrin domains *(2)*. The head domain of talin is able to bind to the cytoplasmic domain of the β_3-subunit. For exposure of the head domain, talin can be cleaved either by calpain or by phosphatidyl inositols, linking platelet activation directly to the activation of GPIIb-IIIa *(38,42,43)*. The binding of the head of talin results in the conformational change of GPIIb-IIIa from a low-affinity to a high-affinity receptor *(43)*. Furthermore, via the adaptor molecule vinculin, talin mediates the cytoskeletal anchorage of GPIIb-

IIIa to the actin cytoskeleton. This cytoskeletal anchorage is the basis for integrin clustering, whereby integrin avidity is greatly increased. In very elegant recent work, it could be demonstrated that separation of the integrin α- and β-subunits results in homodimerization of α-subunits and homotrimerization of β-subunits and that this process runs parallel with the upregulation of ligand affinity and the initiation of receptor clustering *(41)*. This important work thus links affinity and avidity regulation of integrins.

One of the most fascinating areas in integrin research is the question of how the conformational change of the cytoplasmic domains of integrins is transferred to the ligand binding site in the headpiece of the integrins. Over a decade ago it was already realized that platelet activation or ligand binding causes the exposure of so-called ligand-induced binding sites (LIBS; epitopes) at the C-terminal end of the extracellular domains of GPIIb-IIIa, especially on the β-subunit *(44)*. Thus, it was recognized early that there are long-range conformational changes within integrin molecules. However, only very recently, based on studies with NMR, crystallography, and electron microscopy, was a generally accepted model for this conformational change in integrins developed. In this model, the low-affinity integrin is bent at the so-called genu region (α-subunit: between the tight and the calf-1 domains; β-subunit: between I-EGF1 and I-EGF2), bringing the headpiece in direct contact with the tailpiece. In this bent conformation, the headpiece is accessible for small-ligand mimetics but not for the multivalent macromolecules. Inside-out signaling then results in the transition of the bent form into an extended form, in which the stalk regions of integrins parallel each other.

This extended form has been seen earlier in electron micrographs *(44)*. Initially, it was postulated that the headpieces of the α- and β-subunits are then separated to allow ligand binding. However, very recent data suggest that the headpieces stay together but the shift from the bent to the extended conformation causes a change in the angle between the hybrid domains of the α-subunit and the I-like domain of the β-subunit *(45,46)*. The I-domain is the major integrin binding site in those integrins that contain this domain. Crystallographic studies suggest two conformations of the isolated I-domain, an open and a closed conformation. Indeed, the finding of two conformational states in two I-domains (α_2 and α_M) that are most distantly related regarding their sequence homologies within the group of integrins implies a general principle of regulation of ligand binding to I-domains *(9)*. Elegant expression studies of the I-domain on the cell membrane alone proved the central role of this domain, since it is sufficient to mediate ligand binding *(23)*. An initial model of I-domain activation from the closed to the open state proposes a movement of the C-terminal α-helix within the I-domain, resulting in the exposure of a high-affinity MIDAS *(9)*.

GPIIb-IIIa is best studied example of the integrins that do not contain an I-domain. Both subunits seem to demonstrate ligand binding sites located in the β-propeller in the α-subunit and the I-like domain in the β-subunit. Epitope mapping suggests that putative ligand binding sites on the top surface of the I-like domain interact with the β-propeller near β-sheets 2 and 3, thus creating a tertiary ligand binding pocket *(47)*. Indeed, in the crystal structure of $α_V β_3$ together with an RGD peptide, the model of a tertiary ligand binding pocket consisting of both subunits was confirmed. The Asp of RGD coordinated to the MIDAS bound metal in the I-like domain of $β_3$, and the Arg coordinated to the β-propeller within the $α_V$-subunit *(48)*.

THE ROLE OF AFFINITY AND AVIDITY REGULATION IN INTEGRIN FUNCTION

Avidity modulation describes changes in lateral mobility and integrin clustering that strengthen the binding of cells to multivalent ligands and matrices (Fig. 3). The sole expression of integrin binding domains (the I-domain of leukocyte function-associated antigen-1 [LFA-1]) and the monovalent binding of ligands are sufficient to mediate cell adhesion *(23)*. However, the intracellular crosslinking and cytoskeletal anchorage of integrins provide a means to regulate cell adhesion further. The integrin/cytoskeleton association can modulate cell adhesion by coupling of the adhesive forces of the individual integrin/ligand pairs. To break adhesion, all the cytoskeleton-coupled integrin receptors have to be separated from their ligands simultaneously. This would require more physical force than disengagement of individual integrin/ligand bonds. Indeed, for LFA-1, a central role of avidity modulation in the regulation of cell adhesion independent on the affinity regulation could be demonstrated *(28,49)*. Furthermore, in a recent report it was elegantly demonstrated that integrin clustering and conformational changes to high-affinity ligand binding, e.g., avidity and affinity changes, are simultaneously induced by homodimerization and homotrimerization of GPIIb-IIIa subunits *(41)*. For the interaction of integrins with fibronectin, it was proposed that integrins may be regulated in two distinct manners. Affinity changes may be used for the binding of soluble fibronectin and avidity changes for the binding of immobilized, multimeric fibronectin *(50)*. In conclusion, integrin-mediated cell adhesion can be mediated by both affinity change and avidity modulation. Most probably, both together are regulated simultaneously and only the combination of both provides the basis for strong cell adhesion.

SPECIFIC PLATELET INTEGRINS
$\alpha_2\beta_1$ *(GPIa-IIa, VLA-2, CD49b/CD29)*

$\alpha_2\beta_1$ is the major collagen receptor on platelets that mediates stable adhesion on collagen, and 2000–4000 $\alpha_2\beta_1$ molecules are found per platelet. Expression of $\alpha_2\beta_1$ seems to be dependent on α_2-alleles, and, interestingly, atherothrombotic risk is influenced by α_2 polymorphisms, arguing for an important role of $\alpha_2\beta_1$ *(51)* in thrombosis. As in other integrins, it is postulated that $\alpha_2\beta_1$ is expressed in a low-affinity default state for collagen binding. Upon platelet activation, outside-in signaling at the receptor is supposed to result in a conformational change of the I-domain of α_2, which was clearly shown to constitute the collagen binding site *(52,53)*. Indeed, in recent X-ray crystallographic studies, the α_2 I-domain revealed an open and closed conformation depending on the presence of ligands *(54,55)*. Similar to other integrins (LFA-1, Mac-1, and GPIIb-IIIa), the highly conserved GFFKR region within the α-subunit cytoplasmic domain seems to play a crucial role in the activation of integrin $\alpha_2\beta_1$ *(28,29,31,56)*.

$\alpha_2\beta_1$ has long been considered *the* major collagen receptor of platelets. However, the most recent model of platelet adhesion to collagen proposes that the initial contact with collagen under high shear stress is made by GPVI *(57–59)*. The fast off-rate of the interaction between GPVI and collagen allows tethering of platelets but no firm adhesion. However, collagen binding to GPVI causes platelet activation, which by inside-out signaling results in a conformational change of $\alpha_2\beta_1$ from a low- to a high-affinity receptor and which by receptor clustering (avidity modulation) finally allows stable platelet adhesion on collagen *(59)*. Indeed, in mice with β_1-deficient platelets, clot stability on collagen was decreased, resulting in frequent emboli originating from those unstable thrombi *(60)*. Recent data also describe outside-in signaling in $\alpha_2\beta_1$ similar to that of GPIIb-IIIa *(61)*. $\alpha_2\beta_1$-mediated spreading of platelets on collagen results in tyrosine phosphorylation of proteins such as Src, Syk, SLP-76, and focal adhesion kinase *(61)*. Interestingly as in the interaction between fibrinogen and GPIIb-IIIa, outside-in signaling does not occur with the binding of monovalent collagen or collagen peptide but does occur on immobilized, multivalent collagen, arguing for the central role of integrin clustering *(61)*.

$\alpha_v\beta_3$ *(CD51/CD61)*

Integrin $\alpha_v\beta_3$ is expressed at a low copy number of only a few hundred molecules per platelet. Its role, especially relative to the GPIIb-IIIa receptor, which is expressed 50–500-fold as often compared with $\alpha_v\beta_3$, has not yet been defined. Osteopontin, a glycoprotein expressed in atherosclerotic plaques and in injured arteries but not in normal arteries, is a ligand for $\alpha_v\beta_3$. Activated platelets, but not nonactivated platelets, adhere to immobilized osteopontin, mediated solely by the $\alpha_v\beta_3$ receptor *(62)*. These findings argue that the default state of $\alpha_v\beta_3$ expressed on platelets is also a low-affinity state comparable to the low-affinity state of GPIIb-IIIa on unstimulated platelets. Interestingly, in other cell types the default state of $\alpha_v\beta_3$ seems be a high-affinity state, indicating a cell type-specific regulation of the $\alpha_v\beta_3$ affinity states, as was described for other integrins *(33,63)*. Indeed, it seems to be reasonable that a cell circulating in the blood has a low-affinity default state of its integrins and a cell embedded in tissue has a high-affinity default state of its integrins.

$\alpha_5\beta_1$ *(VLA-5, CD49c/CD29) and* $\alpha_6\beta_1$ *(VLA-6, CD49f/CD29)*

$\alpha_5\beta_1$ and $\alpha_6\beta_1$ mediate platelet adhesion to fibronectin and laminin, respectively. Both are thought to have supplementary roles in platelet adhesion at injured vessel areas *(4,64)*. However, no information on the relative roles of $\alpha_5\beta_1$ and $\alpha_6\beta_1$, compared with other platelet adhesion receptors, is available.

$\alpha_L\beta_2$ *(LFA-1, CD11a/CD18) and* $\alpha_M\beta_2$ *(Mac-1, CD11b/CD18)*

Activated but not resting platelets have been reported to express β_2-integrins (LFA-1 and Mac-1). The role of these β_2-integrins in platelet adhesion or aggregation is not known. However, they seem to modulate caspase activation and consequently the life span of mouse platelets *(5,65)*.

GPIIb-IIIa $(\alpha_2\beta_1,$ *CD41/CD61)*

The term GPIIb-IIIa originates from platelet protein gel electrophoresis describing band numbers IIb and IIIa *(66)*. GPIIb consists of two chains (a heavy chain of 105 kDa and a light chain of 25 kDa) linked by a disulfide bond *(67,68)*. GPIIIa is a single-chain protein of 95 kDa *(67,68)*. Cloning of the genes was achieved in the late 1980s, and GPIIb and GPIIIa are both located in close physical proximity on chromosome 17 *(69,70)*. GPIIb-IIIa is the most abundant platelet membrane receptor, with 50,000–80,000 molecules per platelet, thus constituting up to 2% of the amount of total platelet protein and 15% of total surface protein *(71,72)*. The genetic defect of Glanzmann's disease helped to identify the role of this glycoprotein for fibrinogen binding and for platelet aggregation *(73,74)*. Direct binding experiments with fibrinogen *(75,76)*, blocking experiments with monoclonal antibodies *(77)*, and reconstitution of GPIIb-IIIa binding function either after purification of the protein

(78) or by expression of the transfected cDNA on model cell lines *(79)* provided definite proof of the binding of fibrinogen and the consequent role of GPIIb-IIIa in platelet aggregation. In addition to fibrinogen, several other ligands that bind to GPIIb-IIIa (von Willebrand factor, fibronectin, vitronectin, thrombospondin, CD40 ligand) have been identified *(80,81)*. The two glycoproteins GPIIb and GPIIIa were later shown to be identical to the antibody epitopes CD41 and CD61. At the end of the 1980s, it was recognized that GPIIb-IIIa is a member of the adhesion molecule family of integrins, and their integrative function between extracellular ligands and the intracellular cytoskeleton was described *(82)*. According to the original term, GPIIb-IIIa, $\alpha_{IIb}\beta_3$ was chosen as the term within the integrin nomenclature *(82)*.

INSIDE-OUT SIGNALING OF GPIIb-IIIa

The signaling pathways from platelet membrane receptors to the cytoplasmic domains of GPIIb-IIIa are far from being completely understood, but it is well accepted that activation of GPIIb-IIIa is the common final pathway of platelet activation. Small G protein GTPases such as Rac and Rho may regulate GPIIb-IIIa activation *(83)*. Tyrosine kinases such as Src and Syk, phospholipases, and protein kinase C (PKC) may be involved in this signaling. For two proteins that bind directly to the β_3-cytoplasmic domain, a direct effect on affinity regulation could be demonstrated. The binding of the N-terminal head of talin to the β_3-cytoplasmic domain causes a direct upregulation of fibrinogen binding to GPIIb-IIIa *(43)*. Also, the binding of β_3-endonexin to the β_3-cytoplasmic domain causes an increase in GPIIb-IIIa affinity for fibrinogen *(84)*.

OUTSIDE-IN SIGNALING OF GPIIb-IIIa

Ligand binding to GPIIb-IIIa results in outside-in signaling in platelets. Platelets can adhere to immobilized fibrinogen without being activated and thus without the precondition of a high-affinity GPIIb-IIIa receptor. In contrast to soluble fibrinogen, which only binds to the activated, high-affinity GPIIb-IIIa, immobilized fibrinogen exposes so-called receptor-induced binding site (RIBS) epitopes that allow binding to the nonactivated, low-affinity GPIIb-IIIa receptor *(85)*. Ligand binding causes conformational changes of the cytoplasmic domains and integrin clustering *(30,86–88)*. However, only the combination of both results in full outside-in signaling *(89)*. At least three different signaling pathways have been identified:

1. Activation of the tyrosine kinase Syk is triggered by integrin clustering within seconds after cell attachment *(90)*. One of the targets of Syk is the multifunctional adaptor molecule SLP-76, which directly relays signals from GPIIb-IIIa to the actin cytoskeleton *(91)*.

2. Activation of pp125^{FAK} requires integrin clustering and platelet activation. pp125^{FAK} seems to play a regulatory role in dynamic changes of focal contacts and actin stress fibers (92).
3. Platelet aggregation causes tyrosine phosphorylation of two NXXY motifs within the β_3-cytoplasmic domain (93). Indeed, the importance of this pathway for outside-in signaling was demonstrated in a knockout mouse model in which both tyrosines of the β_3-cytoplasmic domain were substituted by phenylalanines (94). A diminished stability of platelet aggregates and a reduced clot retraction was reflected in a pronounced tendency to rebleed (94). Furthermore, the protein Shc has been identified as a direct downstream signaling partner of GPIIb-IIIa in phosphorylation-dependent signaling (95).

The GPIIb-IIIa Ligand Fibrinogen

Fibrinogen is a 340,000-Dalton dimeric macromolecule consisting of three pairs of disulfide-bonded polypeptide chains, designated Aα-, Bβ-, and γ-chain. Fibrinogen is transformed to fibrin monomers by the cleavage of fibrinopeptides A and B. The symmetric bivalent structure of fibrinogen provides the basis for its bridging function between two GPIIb-IIIa receptors and thus for platelet aggregation. Three sites on fibrinogen that are potentially involved in binding to GPIIb-IIIa have been identified: two RGD sequences within the α-chain and a sequence of 12 amino acids (HHLGGAKQAGDV) close to the carboxy terminal end of the γ-chain (96). The γ-chain sequence seems to be the primary interaction site. Fibrinogen molecules without this sequence did not mediate binding to GPIIb-IIIa and platelet aggregation (97,98), whereas recombinant fibrinogen molecules designed to contain RGE sequences instead of the native RGD sequences still support fibrinogen binding and platelet aggregation (97). In addition, blocking experiments with peptide-specific antibodies provided further evidence for the primary role of the γ-chain sequence but not the RGD sequences (99). Nevertheless, peptides based on both sequences block fibrinogen binding to GPIIb-IIIa. Interestingly, naturally occurring GPIIb-IIIa inhibitors, e.g., in snake venoms and pharmaceutically designed drugs, are imitating the RGD sequence, as discussed in the next section.

Glanzmann's Thrombasthenia: GPIIb-IIIa Blockade by Nature

In 1918, Glanzmann first described patients with a hereditary form of hemorrhagic thrombasthenia. Abnormalities in GPIIb-IIIa have been defined beginning in the 1970s as the basis of the autosomal recessive inheritance of Glanzmann's thrombasthenia (73). Meanwhile, several mutations have been identified on GPIIb or GPIIIa resulting either in total loss or considerable reduction in platelet surface expression of GPIIb-IIIa or in the expression of nonfunctional GPIIb-IIIa (74,100,101).

The clinical features of these patients are quite interesting, since their situation resembles a chronic blockade of GPIIb-IIIa. The vast majority of these patients suffer from easy bruising, purpura, epistaxis, and gingival bleeding. In women, menorrhagia is a major problem. Gastrointestinal hemorrhage is seen in only a few patients. Intracranial bleeding is described in three patients. Two of these had a trauma, and the circumstances for the third patient are not reported *(100)*. Many of these patients needed blood transfusions during life. Indeed, some patients, especially at younger age, died of hemorrhagic problems mostly combined with trauma *(100)*. Interestingly, no myocardial infarctions or strokes have been reported *(100)*. Nevertheless, since most of these patients are at younger age, conclusions have to be drawn with caution.

Overall, the clinical sequelae of the loss of the platelets' ability to aggregate via GPIIb-IIIa are astonishingly mild. Indeed, the clinical features of Glanzmann's disease resemble the clinical consequences of pharmaceutical blockade of GPIIb-IIIa. Spontaneous bleeding is of minor concern, whereas bleeding with trauma constitutes a major problem that very often can only be managed with blood transfusions. Spontaneous cerebral bleeding in Glanzmann's thrombasthenia as well as in pharmaceutical blockade of GPIIb-IIIa fortunately is not a concern. Certainly, this advantageous safety profile is one of the major reasons for the broad use of GPIIb-IIIa blockers.

IMPORTANCE OF STRUCTURAL KNOWLEDGE FOR ANTI-INTEGRIN DRUG DEVELOPMENT

Integrins are attractive targets for therapeutic agents. Anti-GPIIb-IIIa agents have already been used successfully in hundred of thousands of patients during coronary angioplasty. Three different agents are used, all of which can be considered ligand mimetics. Abciximab, a humanized Fab fragment, binds at or near the binding pocket of fibrinogen, and the original antibody 7E3 was described as presenting some degree of specificity for the activated GPIIb-IIIa receptor *(102)*. Eptifibatide, a cyclic KGD peptide mimetic, was designed based on the snake venom disintegrin barbourin, which inhibits GPIIb-IIIa by its ligand-mimetic binding *(103)*. Tirofiban is a chemical modeled after the RGD binding sequence within fibrinogen and therefore by its design is a pure ligand mimetic. The consequence of the strategy to block GPIIb-IIIa with ligand mimetics is the induction of a conformational change of GPIIb-IIIa by these agents, similar to the conformational change induced by RGD peptides *(104)*. Indeed, as a measure of this conformational change, all three clinically used GPIIb-IIIa blockers induce binding of anti-LIBS antibodies *(104,105)*. Binding of these GPIIb-IIIa blockers is expected to change the GPIIb-IIIa structure from the bent to the extended form.

This conformational change may result in two unwanted and thus paradoxical effects of the ligand-mimetic GPIIb-IIIa blockers. First, after dissociation of the blockers, the GPIIb-IIIa receptor may stay in the extended form and may be able to bind fibrinogen *(104)*. For $\alpha_v\beta_3$, induction of ligand binding could be induced by RGD peptides, and the authors proposed a mechanism of conformational memory of the integrin after dissociation of the ligand-mimetic blockers *(106)*. Second, outside-in signal transduction may be induced by the binding of GPIIb-IIIa blockers, which may then result in platelet activation. Indeed, platelet activation has been observed in trials with oral GPIIb-IIIa blockers *(107–110)*.

In conclusion, structural knowledge of the conformational changes within the integrin GPIIb-IIIa gives rise to the question of whether ligand mimetics are optimal candidates as therapeutic GPIIb-IIIa blockers. Indeed, the importance of this question is emphasized since it became clear that the benefits of the intravenous use of GPIIb-IIIa blockers are less than expected and the trials with oral GPIIb-IIIa blockers showed an increase in mortality, resulting in a halt of further development of these agents *(110–112)*. Thus, future strategies for the therapeutic blockade of GPIIb-IIIa should consider the now available structural knowledge of integrin receptors and might thereby avoid the development of agents that cause conformational changes of GPIIb-IIIa.

Interestingly, newly developed anti-integrin agents directed against LFA-1 and Mac-1 already follow a different strategy. Several anti-α_L-subunit agents have been developed that bind between the C-terminal α-helix and the β-sheet of the I-domain, a site that is distant from the ligand binding site at the MIDAS *(9,23,113–115)*. Thus these agents favor the closed state of the I-domain but do not directly compete with ligand binding. Another class of compounds that inhibit ligand binding to Mac-1 and LFA-1 to the same extent has been demonstrated to bind to the MIDAS domain of the β_2-subunit I-like domain, thereby only indirectly inhibiting ligand binding to the I-domain *(9,116,117)*. A recent report describing an antibody (4F8) that binds to a ligand-attenuated binding site (LABS) on GPIIb-IIIa and thus prevents platelet aggregation may indeed define a potential binding site for anti-GPIIb-IIIa agents that may be able to lock the receptor in a low-affinity state for fibrinogen *(118)*. A similar epitope has also been described for $\alpha_5\beta_1$ *(119)*. Overall, these anti-integrin agents are not prone to induce conformational changes and potential outside-in signaling, as has been shown for ligand-mimetics drugs.

REFERENCES

1. Hynes RO. Integrins: versatility, modulation, and signaling in cell adhesion. Cell 1992;69:11–25.
2. Hynes RO. Integrins: bidirectional, allosteric signaling machines. Cell 2002; 110:673–687.
3. Springer TA. Adhesion receptors of the immune system. Nature 1990;346:425–434.
4. Faull RJ, Du X, Ginsberg MH. Receptors on platelets. Methods Enzymol 1994;245:183–194.
5. Philippeaux MM, Vesin C, Tacchini-Cottier F, Piguet PF. Activated human platelets express beta2 integrin. Eur J Haematol 1996;56:130–137.
6. Davis G, Camarillo C. Regulation of integrin-mediated myeloid cell adhesion to fibronectin: influence of disulfide reducing agents, divalent cations and phorbol ester. J Immunol 1993;151:7138–7150.
7. Edwards B, Curry M, Southon E, Chong A, Graf LJ. Evidence for a dithiol-activated signaling pathway in natural killer cell avidity regulation of leukocyte function antigen-1: structural requirements and relationship to phorbol ester- and CD16-triggered pathways. Blood 1995;86:2288–2301.
8. O'Neill S, Robinson A, Deering A, Ryan M, Fitzgerald DJ, Moran N. The platelet integrin alpha IIbbeta 3 has an endogenous thiol isomerase activity. J Biol Chem 2000;275:36984–36990.
9. Takagi J, Springer TA. Integrin activation and structural rearrangement. Immunol Rev 2002;186:141–163.
10. Arnaout MA. Integrin structure: new twists and turns in dynamic cell adhesion. Immunol Rev 2002;186:125–140.
11. Springer TA. Predicted and experimental structures of integrins and beta-propellers. Curr Opin Struct Biol 2002;12:802–813.
12. Springer TA. Folding of the N-terminal, ligand-binding region of integrin alpha-subunits into a beta-propeller domain. Proc Natl Acad Sci USA 1997;94:65–72.
13. Xiong JP, Stehle T, Diefenbach B, et al. Crystal structure of the extracellular segment of integrin alpha Vbeta3. Science 2001;294:339–345.
14. Oxvig C, Springer TA. Experimental support for a beta-propeller domain in integrin alpha-subunits and a calcium binding site on its lower surface. Proc Natl Acad Sci USA 1998;95:4870–4875.
15. Gulino D, Boudignon C, Zhang LY, Concord E, Rabiet MJ, Marguerie G. Ca(2+)-binding properties of the platelet glycoprotein IIb ligand-interacting domain. J Biol Chem 1992;267:1001–1007.
16. Tuckwell DS, Brass A, Humphries MJ. Homology modelling of integrin EF-hands. Evidence for widespread use of a conserved cation-binding site. Biochem J 1992;285:325–331.
17. Springer TA, Jing H, Takagi J. A novel Ca^{2+} binding beta hairpin loop better resembles integrin sequence motifs than the EF hand. Cell 2000;102:275–277.
18. Kamata T, Tieu KK, Irie A, Springer TA, Takada Y. Amino acid residues in the alpha IIb subunit that are critical for ligand binding to integrin alpha IIbbeta 3 are clustered in the beta-propeller model. J Biol Chem 2001;276:44275–44283.
19. Michishita M, Videm V, Arnaout MA. A novel divalent cation-binding site in the A domain of the beta 2 integrin CR3 (CD11b/CD18) is essential for ligand binding. Cell 1993;72:857–867.
20. Diamond MS, Garcia-Aguilar J, Bickford JK, Corbi AL, Springer TA. The I domain is a major recognition site on the leukocyte integrin Mac-1 (CD11b/CD18) for four distinct adhesion ligands. J Cell Biol 1993;120:1031–1043.
21. Peter K, Schwarz M, Conradt C, et al. Heparin inhibits ligand binding to the leukocyte integrin Mac-1 (CD11b/CD18). Circulation 1999;100:1533–1539.

22. Lee JO, Rieu P, Arnaout MA, Liddington R. Crystal structure of the A domain from the alpha subunit of integrin CR3 (CD11b/CD18). Cell 1995;80:631–638.

23. Lu C, Shimaoka M, Zang Q, Takagi J, Springer TA. Locking in alternate conformations of the integrin alphaLbeta2 I domain with disulfide bonds reveals functional relationships among integrin domains. Proc Natl Acad Sci USA 2001;98:2393–2398.

24. Lu C, Oxvig C, Springer TA. The structure of the beta-propeller domain and C-terminal region of the integrin alphaM subunit. Dependence on beta subunit association and prediction of domains. J Biol Chem 1998;273:15138–15147.

25. Adair BD, Yeager M. Three-dimensional model of the human platelet integrin alpha IIbbeta 3 based on electron cryomicroscopy and x-ray crystallography. Proc Natl Acad Sci USA 2002;99:14059–14064.

26. Li R, Babu CR, Lear JD, Wand AJ, Bennett JS, DeGrado WF. Oligomerization of the integrin alphaIIbbeta3: roles of the transmembrane and cytoplasmic domains. Proc Natl Acad Sci USA 2001;98:12462–12467.

27. Schneider D, Engelman DM. GALLEX, a measurement of heterologous association of transmembrane helices in a biological membrane. J Biol Chem 2003; 278:3105–3111.

28. Peter K, O'Toole TE. Modulation of cell adhesion by changes in alpha L beta 2 (LFA-1, CD11a/CD18) cytoplasmic domain/cytoskeleton interaction. J Exp Med 1995;181:315–326.

29. Peter K, Bode C. A deletion in the alpha subunit locks platelet integrin alpha IIb beta 3 into a high affinity state. Blood Coagul Fibrinolysis 1996;7:233–236.

30. Stephens G, O'Luanaigh N, Reilly D, et al. A sequence within the cytoplasmic tail of GPIIb independently activates platelet aggregation and thromboxane synthesis. J Biol Chem 1998;273:20317–20322.

31. Schuler P, Assefa D, Ylanne J, et al. Adhesion of monocytes to medical steel as used for vascular stents is mediated by the integrin receptor Mac-1 (CD11b/CD18; aMb2) and can be inhibited by semiconductor coating. Cell Comm Adhes 2003;10:17–26.

32. Vinogradova O, Velyvis A, Velyviene A, et al. A structural mechanism of integrin alpha(IIb)beta(3) "inside-out" activation as regulated by its cytoplasmic face. Cell 2002;110:587–597.

33. O'Toole TE, Katagiri Y, Faull RJ, et al. Integrin cytoplasmic domains mediate inside-out signal transduction. J Cell Biol 1994;124:1047–1059.

34. Hughes PE, Diaz-Gonzalez F, Leong L, et al. Breaking the integrin hinge. A defined structural constraint regulates integrin signaling. J Biol Chem 1996;271:6571–6574.

35. Travis MA, Humphries JD, Humphries MJ. An unraveling tale of how integrins are activated from within. Trends Pharmacol Sci 2003;24:192–197.

36. Bork P, Doerks T, Springer TA, Snel B. Domains in plexins: links to integrins and transcription factors. Trends Biochem Sci 1999;24:261–263.

37. Calvete JJ, Arias J, Alvarez MV, Lopez MM, Henschen A, Gonzalez-Rodriguez J. Further studies on the topography of the N-terminal region of human platelet glycoprotein IIIa. Localization of monoclonal antibody epitopes and the putative fibrinogen-binding sites. Biochem J 1991;274:457–463.

38. Calderwood DA, Fujioka Y, de Pereda JM, et al. Integrin beta cytoplasmic domain interactions with phosphotyrosine-binding domains: a structural prototype for diversity in integrin signaling. Proc Natl Acad Sci USA 2003;100:2272–2277.

39. Liu S, Calderwood DA, Ginsberg MH. Integrin cytoplasmic domain-binding proteins. J Cell Sci 2000;113:3563–3571.

40. Hogg N, Henderson R, Leitinger B, McDowall A, Porter J, Stanley P. Mechanisms contributing to the activity of integrins on leukocytes. Immunol Rev 2002;186:164–171.

41. Li R, Mitra N, Gratkowski H, et al. Activation of integrin alphaIIbbeta3 by modulation of transmembrane helix associations. Science 2003;300:795–798.

42. Martel V, Racaud-Sultan C, Dupe S, et al. Conformation, localization, and integrin binding of talin depend on its interaction with phosphoinositides. J Biol Chem 2001;276:21217–21227.

43. Calderwood DA, Zent R, Grant R, Rees DJ, Hynes RO, Ginsberg MH. The Talin head domain binds to integrin beta subunit cytoplasmic tails and regulates integrin activation. J Biol Chem 1999;274:28071–28074.

44. Du X, Gu M, Weisel JW, et al. Long range propagation of conformational changes in integrin alpha IIb beta 3. J Biol Chem 1993;268:23087–23092.

45. Takagi J, Petre BM, Walz T, Springer TA. Global conformational rearrangements in integrin extracellular domains in outside-in and inside-out signaling. Cell 2002;110:599–511.

46. Luo BH, Springer TA, Takagi J. High affinity ligand binding by integrins does not involve head separation. J Biol Chem 2003;278:17185–17189.

47. Puzon-McLaughlin W, Kamata T, Takada Y. Multiple discontinuous ligand-mimetic antibody binding sites define a ligand binding pocket in integrin alpha(IIb)beta(3). J Biol Chem 2000;275:7795–7802.

48. Xiong JP, Stehle T, Zhang R, et al. Crystal structure of the extracellular segment of integrin alpha Vbeta3 in complex with an Arg-Gly-Asp ligand. Science 2002;296:151–155.

49. van Kooyk Y, van Vliet SJ, Figdor CG. The actin cytoskeleton regulates LFA-1 ligand binding through avidity rather than affinity changes. J Biol Chem 1999;274:26869–26877.

50. Faull RJ, Kovach NL, Harlan JM, Ginsberg MH. Stimulation of integrin-mediated adhesion of T lymphocytes and monocytes: two mechanisms with divergent biological consequences. J Exp Med 1994;179:1307–1316.

51. Kunicki TJ. The influence of platelet collagen receptor polymorphisms in hemostasis and thrombotic disease. Arterioscler Thromb Vasc Biol 2002;22:14–20.

52. Kamata T, Puzon W, Takada Y. Identification of putative ligand binding sites within I domain of integrin alpha 2 beta 1 (VLA-2, CD49b/CD29) [published erratum appears in J Biol Chem 1996;271:19008]. J Biol Chem 1994;269:9659–9663.

53. Jung SM, Moroi M. Platelets interact with soluble and insoluble collagens through characteristically different reactions. J Biol Chem 1998;273:14827–14837.

54. Emsley J, King SL, Bergelson JM, Liddington RC. Crystal structure of the I domain from integrin alpha 2beta 1. J Biol Chem 1997;272:28512–28517.

55. Emsley J, Knight CG, Farndale RW, Barnes MJ, Liddington RC. Structural basis of collagen recognition by integrin alpha2beta1. Cell 2000;101:47–56.

56. Wang Z, Leisner TM, Parise LV. Platelet {alpha}2{beta}1 integrin activation: contribution of ligand internalization and the {alpha}2 cytoplasmic domain. Blood 2003;2002–2009, 2753.

57. Nieswandt B, Brakebusch C, Bergmeier W, et al. Glycoprotein VI but not {{alpha}}2{beta}1 integrin is essential for platelet interaction with collagen. EMBO J 2001;20:2120–2130.

58. Massberg S, Gawaz M, Gruner S, et al. A crucial role of glycoprotein VI for platelet recruitment to the injured arterial wall in vivo. J Exp Med 2003;197:41–49.

59. Nieswandt B, Watson SP. Platelet-collagen interaction: is GPVI the central receptor? Blood 2003;102:449–461.

60. Kuijpers MJE, Schulte V, Bergmeier W, et al. Complementary roles of glycoprotein VI and {alpha}2{beta}1 integrin in collagen-induced thrombus formation in flowing whole blood ex vivo FASEB J 2003;17:685–687.

61. Inoue O, Suzuki-Inoue K, Dean WL, Frampton J, Watson SP. Integrin alpha2beta1 mediates outside-in regulation of platelet spreading on collagen through activation of Src kinases and PLCgamma2. J Cell Biol 2003;160:769–780.

62. Bennett JS, Chan C, Vilaire G, Mousa SA, DeGrado WF. Agonist-activated alpha vbeta 3 on platelets and lymphocytes binds to the matrix protein osteopontin. J Biol Chem 1997;272:8137–8140.

63. Helluin O, Chan C, Vilaire G, Mousa S, DeGrado WF, Bennett JS. The activation state of alpha vbeta 3 regulates platelet and lymphocyte adhesion to intact and thrombin-cleaved osteopontin. J Biol Chem 2000;275:18337–18343.

64. Hindriks G, Ijsseldijk MJ, Sonnenberg A, Sixma JJ, de Groot PG. Platelet adhesion to laminin: role of Ca^{2+} and Mg^{2+} ions, shear rate, and platelet membrane glycoproteins. Blood 1992;79:928–935.

65. Piguet PF, Vesin C, Rochat A. Beta2 integrin modulates platelet caspase activation and life span in mice. Eur J Cell Biol 2001;80:171–177.

66. Phillips DR, Jennings LK, Edwards HH. Identification of membrane proteins mediating the interaction of human platelets. J Cell Biol 1980;86:77–86.

67. Phillips DR, Charo IF, Parise LV, Fitzgerald LA. The platelet membrane glycoprotein IIb-IIIa complex. Blood 1988;71:831–843.

68. Calvete JJ. Platelet Integrin GPIIb/IIIa: Structure-function correlations. An update and lessons from other integrins. Proc Soc Exp Biol Med 1999;222:29–38.

69. Bray PF, Rosa JP, Johnston GI, et al. Platelet glycoprotein IIb. Chromosomal localization and tissue expression. J Clin Invest 1987;80:1812–1817.

70. Rosa JP, Bray PF, Gayet O, et al. Cloning of glycoprotein IIIa cDNA from human erythroleukemia cells and localization of the gene to chromosome 17. Blood 1988;72:593–600.

71. Jennings L, Phillips D. Purification of glycoproteins IIb and III from human platelet plasma membranes and characterization of a calcium-dependent glycoprotein IIb-III complex. J Biol Chem 1982;257:10458–10466.

72. Wagner CL, Mascelli MA, Neblock DS, Weisman HF, Coller BS, Jordan RE. Analysis of GPIIb/IIIa receptor number by quantification of 7E3 binding to human platelets. Blood 1996;88:907–914.

73. Nurden AT, Caen JP. Specific roles for platelet surface glycoproteins in platelet function. Nature 1975;255:720–722.

74. Nurden AT, Nurden P. Inherited defects of platelet function. Rev Clin Exp Hematol 2001;5:314–334; quiz following 431.

75. Mustard JF, Packham MA, Kinlough-Rathbone RL, Perry DW, Regoeczi E. Fibrinogen and ADP-induced platelet aggregation. Blood 1978;52:453–466.

76. Marguerie GA, Plow EF, Edgington TS. Human platelets possess an inducible and saturable receptor specific for fibrinogen. J Biol Chem 1979;254:5357–5363.

77. Bennett JS, Hoxie JA, Leitman SF, Vilaire G, Cines DB. Inhibition of fibrinogen binding to stimulated human platelets by a monoclonal antibody. Proc Natl Acad Sci USA 1983;80:2417–2421.

78. Parise L, Phillips D. Reconstitution of the purified platelet fibrinogen receptor. Fibrinogen binding properties of the glycoprotein IIb-IIIa complex. J Biol Chem 1985;260:10698–10707.

79. O'Toole TE, Loftus JC, Du XP, et al. Affinity modulation of the alpha IIb beta 3 integrin (platelet GPIIb-IIIa) is an intrinsic property of the receptor. Cell Regul 1990;1:883–893.

80. Kamata T, Takada Y. Platelet integrin alphaIIbbeta3-ligand interactions: what can we learn from the structure? Int J Hematol 2001;74:382–389.

81. Andre P, Prasad KS, Denis CV, et al. CD40L stabilizes arterial thrombi by a beta3 integrin-dependent mechanism. Nat Med 2002;8:247–252.

82. Hynes RO. Integrins: a family of cell surface receptors. Cell 1987;48:549–554.

83. Hughes PE, Renshaw MW, Pfaff M, et al. Suppression of integrin activation: a novel function of a Ras/Raf-initiated MAP kinase pathway. Cell 1997;88:521–530.

84. Kashiwagi H, Schwartz MA, Eigenthaler M, Davis KA, Ginsberg MH, Shattil SJ.
    Affinity modulation of platelet integrin alpha IIbbeta 3 by beta 3-endonexin, a
    selective binding partner of the beta 3 integrin cytoplasmic tail. J Cell Biol
    1997;137:1433–1443.
85. Ugarova T, Budzynski A, Shattil S, Ruggeri Z, Ginsberg M, Plow E. Conforma-
    tional changes in fibrinogen elicited by its interaction with platelet membrane gly-
    coprotein GPIIb-IIIa. J Biol Chem 1993;268:21080–21087.
86. Hantgan RR, Lyles DS, Mallett TC, Rocco M, Nagaswami C, Weisel JW. Ligand
    binding promotes the entropy-driven oligomerization of integrin alpha IIbbeta 3. J
    Biol Chem 2003;278:3417–3426.
87. Hantgan RR, Paumi C, Rocco M, Weisel JW. Effects of ligand-mimetic peptides
    Arg-Gly-Asp-X (X = Phe, Trp, Ser) on alphaIIbbeta3 integrin conformation and
    oligomerization. Biochemistry 1999;38:14461–14474.
88. Leisner TM, Wencel-Drake JD, Wang W, Lam SC. Bidirectional transmembrane
    modulation of integrin alphaIIbbeta3 conformations. J Biol Chem 1999;
    274:12945–12949.
89. Miyamoto S, Akiyama SK, Yamada KM. Synergistic roles for receptor occupancy
    and aggregation in integrin transmembrane function. Science 1995;267:883–885.
90. Clark EA, Brugge JS. Integrins and signal transduction pathways: the road taken.
    Science 1995;268:233–239.
91. Obergfell A, Judd BA, del Pozo MA, Schwartz MA, Koretzky GA, Shattil SJ. The
    molecular adapter SLP-76 relays signals from platelet integrin alpha IIbbeta 3 to the
    actin cytoskeleton. J Biol Chem 2001;276:5916–5923.
92. Shattil S, Haimovich B, Cunningham M, et al. Tyrosine phosphorylation of
    pp125FAK in platelets requires coordinated signaling through integrin and agonist
    receptors. J Biol Chem 1994;269:14738–14745.
93. Law DA, Nannizzi-Alaimo L, Phillips DR. Outside-in integrin signal transduction.
    Alpha IIb beta 3-(GP IIb IIIa) tyrosine phosphorylation induced by platelet aggre-
    gation. J Biol Chem 1996;271:10811–10815.
94. Law DA, DeGuzman FR, Heiser P, Ministri-Madrid K, Killeen N, Phillips DR.
    Integrin cytoplasmic tyrosine motif is required for outside-in alphaIIbbeta3 signal-
    ling and platelet function. Nature 1999;401:808–811.
95. Cowan KJ, Law DA, Phillips DR. Identification of shc as the primary protein bind-
    ing to the tyrosine-phosphorylated beta 3 subunit of alpha IIbbeta 3 during outside-
    in integrin platelet signaling. J Biol Chem 2000;275:36423–36429.
96. Andrieux A, Hudry-Clergeon G, Ryckewaert J, et al. Amino acid sequences in
    fibrinogen mediating its interaction with its platelet receptor, GPIIbIIIa. J Biol
    Chem 1989;264:9258–9265.
97. Farrell D, Thiagarajan P, Chung D, Davie E. Role of fibrinogen {alpha}
    and {gamma} chain sites in platelet aggregation. Proc Natl Acad Sci USA
    1992;89:10729–10732.
98. Farrell D, Thiagarajan P. Binding of recombinant fibrinogen mutants to platelets. J
    Biol Chem 1994;269:226–231.
99. Liu Q, Matsueda G, Brown E, Frojmovic M. The AGDV residues on the gamma
    chain carboxyl terminus of platelet-bound fibrinogen are needed for platelet aggre-
    gation. Biochim Biophys Acta 1997;1343:316–326.
100. George JN, Caen JP, Nurden AT. Glanzmann's thrombasthenia: the spectrum of
    clinical disease. Blood 1990;75:1383–1395.
101. French DL, Seligsohn U. Platelet glycoprotein IIb/IIIa receptors and Glanzmann's
    thrombasthenia. Arterioscler Thromb Vasc Biol 2000;20:607–610.

102. Coller BS. A new murine monoclonal antibody reports an activation-dependent change in the conformation and/or microenvironment of the platelet glycoprotein IIb/IIIa complex. J Clin Invest 1985;76:101–108.

103. Scarborough RM, Naughton MA, Teng W, et al. Design of potent and specific integrin antagonists. Peptide antagonists with high specificity for glycoprotein IIb-IIIa. J Biol Chem 1993;268:1066–1073.

104. Peter K, Schwarz M, Ylanne J, et al. Induction of fibrinogen binding and platelet aggregation as a potential intrinsic property of various glycoprotein IIb/IIIa (alphaIIbbeta3) inhibitors. Blood 1998;92:3240–3249.

105. Dickfeld T, Ruf A, Pogatsa-Murray G, et al. Differential antiplatelet effects of various glycoprotein IIb-IIIa antagonists. Thromb Res 2001;101:53–64.

106. Legler DF, Wiedle G, Ross FP, Imhof BA. Superactivation of integrin alphavbeta3 by low antagonist concentrations. J Cell Sci 2001;114:1545–1553.

107. Cox D, Smith R, Quinn M, Theroux P, Crean P, Fitzgerald DJ. Evidence of platelet activation during treatment with a GPIIb/IIIa antagonist in patients presenting with acute coronary syndromes. J Am Coll Cardiol 2000;36:1514–1519.

108. Schneider DJ, Taatjes DJ, Sobel BE. Paradoxical inhibition of fibrinogen binding and potentiation of alpha-granule release by specific types of inhibitors of glyco-protein IIb-IIIa. Cardiovasc Res 2000;45:437–446.

109. Holmes MB, Sobel BE, Cannon CP, Schneider DJ. Increased platelet reactivity in patients given orbofiban after an acute coronary syndrome: an OPUS-TIMI 16 substudy. Orbofiban in Patients with Unstable Coronary Syndromes. Thrombolysis in Myocardial Infarction. Am J Cardiol 2000;85:491–493, A10.

110. Quinn MJ, Plow EF, Topol EJ. Platelet glycoprotein IIb/IIIa inhibitors: recognition of a two-edged sword? Circulation 2002;106:379–385.

111. Chew DP, Bhatt DL, Sapp S, Topol EJ. Increased mortality with oral platelet glycoprotein IIb/IIIa antagonists: a meta-analysis of phase III multicenter random-ized trials. Circulation 2001;103:201–206.

112. Bhatt DL, Topol EJ. Scientific and therapeutic advances in antiplatelet therapy. Nat Rev Drug Discov 2003;2:15–28.

113. Liu G, Huth JR, Olejniczak ET, et al. Novel p-arylthio cinnamides as antagonists of leukocyte function-associated antigen-1/intracellular adhesion molecule-1 in-teraction. 2. Mechanism of inhibition and structure-based improvement of pharma-ceutical properties. J Med Chem 2001;44:1202–1210.

114. Weitz-Schmidt G, Welzenbach K, Brinkmann V, et al. Statins selectively inhibit leukocyte function antigen-1 by binding to a novel regulatory integrin site. Nat Med 2001;7:687–692.

115. Woska JR Jr, Shih D, Taqueti VR, Hogg N, Kelly TA, Kishimoto TK. A small-molecule antagonist of LFA-1 blocks a conformational change important for LFA-1 function. J Leukoc Biol 2001;70:329–334.

116. Welzenbach K, Hommel U, Weitz-Schmidt G. Small molecule inhibitors induce conformational changes in the I domain and the I-like domain of lymphocyte func-tion-associated antigen-1. Molecular insights into integrin inhibition. J Biol Chem 2002;277:10590–10598.

117. Gadek TR, Burdick DJ, McDowell RS, et al. Generation of an LFA-1 antagonist by the transfer of the ICAM-1 immunoregulatory epitope to a small molecule. Science 2002;295:1086–1089.

118. Quinn MJ, Fullard J, Kerrigan S, Harriott P, Cox D, Fitzgerald DJ. Characterization of a ligand-attenuated binding site on glycoprotein IIb/IIIa. Thromb Haemost 2002;88:811–816.

119. Mould AP, Akiyama SK, Humphries MJ. The inhibitory anti-beta1 integrin monoclonal antibody 13 recognizes an epitope that is attenuated by ligand occupancy. Evidence for allosteric inhibition of integrin function. J Biol Chem 1996;271:20365–20374.

3 Platelet Adhesion

Brian Savage, PhD,
and Zaverio M. Ruggeri, MD

Contents

INTRODUCTION

Platelet adhesion and ensuing thrombus formation play a central role in normal hemostasis as well as in the pathogenesis of acute coronary syndromes and thrombotic disorders. Circulating blood platelets adhere to sites of vascular injury through specific adhesion receptors despite the hemodynamic forces in flowing blood that oppose adhesion contacts. At high shear, this process is initiated by the reversible interaction between the platelet membrane glycoprotein (GP)Ib-IX-V complex and von Willebrand factor (vWF) bound to subendothelial components, following disruption of the endothelial cell lining of a blood vessel. Unique biomechanical properties of the GPIb-IX-V/vWF interaction permit the initial capture of platelets under high shear flow conditions *(1,2)*. Once tethered to the vessel wall, platelets form irreversible adhesion bonds through the interaction of platelet receptors with specific subendothelial matrix proteins and plasma proteins immobilized at the site of injury. In addition to mediating platelet adhesion, platelet receptors trigger intracellular signaling events that lead to platelet activation and the conversion of surface integrin $\alpha_{IIb}\beta_3$ into a form that is competent to bind

From: *Contemporary Cardiology:*
Platelet Function: Assessment, Diagnosis, and Treatment
Edited by: M. Quinn and D. Fitzgerald © Humana Press Inc., Totowa, NJ

soluble adhesive ligands such as plasma vWF and fibrinogen, which facilitate the crosslinking (aggregation) and further activation of platelets, providing strength and stability to the growing thrombus. The formation of a platelet plug stabilized by an insoluble fibrin network serves to prevent further blood loss from a damaged vessel.

The platelet response to areas of damaged endothelium is the same regardless of whether the injury results from a severed vessel wall, leading to a bleeding wound, or from lesions of the endothelium present in atherosclerosis. A mural thrombus can occlude a blood vessel and prevent the supply of blood to a vital organ, resulting in a life-threatening pathological condition such as a heart attack or stroke. Therapeutic strategies should therefore be aimed at preventing the initiation of pathological thrombosis without compromising hemostasis. Platelet aggregation results from the crosslinking of activated $\alpha_{IIb}\beta_3$ expressed on distinct platelets by fibrinogen and/or vWF. Exposure to pathological shear stress also induces the binding of soluble plasma vWF to the platelet GPIb-IX-V complex and $\alpha_{IIb}\beta_3$ (3–5). Although platelet adhesion and aggregation were historically viewed as distinct processes in the formation of a thrombus, it is now clear that the fundamental mechanism is similar (6), involving the interaction between platelet receptors $\alpha_{IIb}\beta_3$ and the GPIb-IX-V complex with fibrinogen and vWF in flowing blood (7–9). For example, an adherent platelet binds fibrinogen and vWF from the circulating blood, creating an ideal surface for the recruitment of further platelets. However, additional receptors such as the collagen receptors are required for the stable attachment of platelets to subendothelium structures while shear forces are generated on the platelet by the flowing blood. In this chapter we describe the molecular mechanisms of platelet adhesion and discuss the therapeutic potential of strategies designed to prevent the initiation of pathological thrombosis without excessive bleeding owing to inhibition of hemostasis.

PLATELET ADHESION RECEPTORS
The GPIb-IX-V Complex

Initially recognized as a specific vWF receptor on platelets, the GPIb-IX-V complex is now known to possess a diverse repertoire of functions in hemostasis and thrombosis. For example, the GPIb-IX-V complex mediates the interaction of nonactivated platelets with the vascular endothelium by binding to surface-expressed endothelial P-selectin (10) and with activated leukocytes through its binding to the integrin Mac-1 (11). In addition to its adhesive role, the GPIb-IX-V complex has been shown to interact with α-thrombin (12,13), high-molecular-weight kininogen *(14)*, and coagulation factors XI *(15)* and XII *(16)*. It also plays a key role in regulating the cytoskeleton of platelets *(17)*. This section will focus on the adhesive and signaling functions of the platelet GPIb-IX-V complex.

ADHESIVE FUNCTION OF THE GPIb-IX-V COMPLEX

The adhesion of circulating platelets to areas of vascular damage requires the coordinated function of multiple adhesion receptors. Under high shear flow conditions, the GPIb-IX-V complex is essential to mediate the initial adhesion of platelets to immobilized vWF exposed at sites of vascular injury *(18)*. At low shear rates, platelet adhesion can occur in a manner that is independent of GPIb-IX-V/vWF interactions and involves other adhesion receptors such as the collagen receptors *(see* The Collagen Receptors section below). Ex vivo flow studies established a key role for the platelet GPIb-IX-V complex in mediating the capture and translocation or rolling of platelets on immobilized vWF *(1,2)*. Translocation of platelets on surface-immobilized vWF leads to platelet activation *(19,20)* and the subsequent arrest of platelets through ligation of vWF with platelet $\alpha_{IIb}\beta_3$ *(1)*.

The GPIb-IX-V complex comprises four distinct transmembrane subunits, GPIbα, GPIbβ, GPIX, and GPV *(18,21–23)*. GPIbα (~135 kDa) is covalently bonded to GPIbβ (~25 kDa) via a disulfide bond near the extracellular surface of the plasma membrane. GPIbβ is noncovalently associated with GPIX (~22 kDa) to form a 1:1 complex *(24)*, whereas GPV (~82 kDa) is noncovalently associated with GPIb-IX in a 1:2 ratio *(25–27)*. Thus, the four subunits of the GPIb-IX-V complex are expressed on the platelet membrane surface with an apparent molar stoichiometry of 2:2:2:1 for GPIbα/GP Ibβ/GPIX/GPV. Approximately 25,000 copies of GPIbα, GPIbβ, and GPIX and approximately half this number for GPV are present on the surface of resting human platelets *(27,28)*. Following agonist-induced platelet activation, the number of surface-expressed GPIb-IX-V complexes may decrease owing to a cytoskeletal-mediated redistribution to membranes of the surface-connected canalicular system *(29–33)*. GPV levels are also decreased when it is cleaved from the platelet surface by proteolysis during stimulation of platelets by α-thrombin *(34)*.

The binding site for vWF has been localized to the N-terminal domain of GPIbα *(35–37)*. Two independent groups have recently reported the structure of the N-terminal domain of GPIbα *(38,39)* and of its complex with the vWF A1 domain *(39)*. The isolated GPIbα domain exhibits a generally elongated shape (Fig. 1). Eight leucine-rich repeats form the central part of the molecule, with a concave and a convex side, flanked

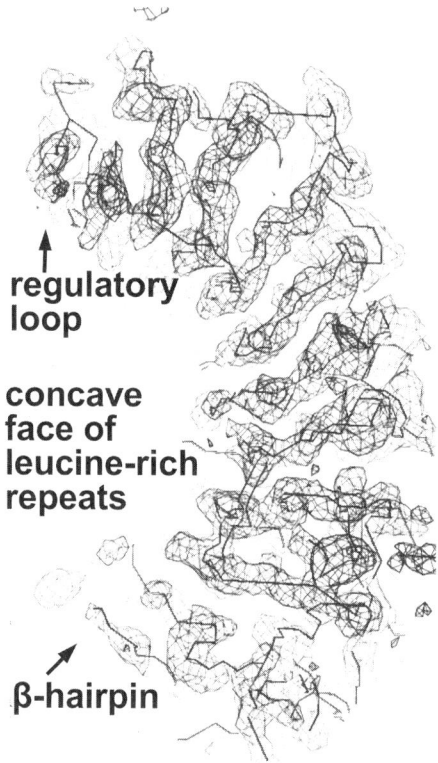

Fig. 1. Overall topology of the main portion of the GPIbα amino-terminal domain crystallized in our laboratory (by R. Celikel, K.I. Varughese, and Z.M. Ruggeri). The figure represents the electron densities of the residues from His1 to Asp269 calculated from multiwave anomalous dispersion data at an initial resolution of 3.0 Å; subsequent models were derived from data at 2.8- and 1. 8-Å resolution. The concave face of eight leucine-rich repeats, seen on the left in this orientation of the molecule, represents the main site of interaction with vWF as reported by Huizinga et al. *(39)*. The β-hairpin at the base and the regulatory loop at the top are the two structures flanking the leucine-rich repeats that contribute to vWF binding. The region of GPIbα involved in binding α-thrombin is located on top of the regulatory loop and is not seen here because it is disordered in the structure we obtained for the free receptor fragment.

at the two extremities by distinct structures. The N-terminal portion presents a finger-like β-hairpin delimited at the base by a disulfide bond between Cys4 and Cys17; the C-terminal portion contains an α-helix (residues 214–223) and a long loop (residues 227–242) with two disulfide bonds between Cys209–Cys248 and Cys211–Cys264. The loop at the C terminus and the β-hairpin at the N terminus protrude over the concave surface of the molecule and may have a regulatory function in ligand binding. The structure beyond residue 269 is not well defined in the models reported by Huizinga et al. *(39)* but is more ordered in the model reported by Uff et al. *(38)*.

This region of the molecule, rich in negatively charged Asp and Glu residues and with three Tyr residues (positions 276, 278, and 279) reported to be posttranslationally sulfated, was thought to be important in regulating vWF binding *(40)*, and we have shown that it is crucial for α-thrombin binding *(41)*. In fact, the solved 3D structure of the GPIbα A1 domain complex cannot explain any role of the receptor sulfotyrosine-containing region in vWF binding, although a function in this regard may be elicited when the interaction occurs under flow conditions. Nonetheless, the proposed contacts between the GPIbα sequence Gly271–Tyr279 and the vWF A1 domain suggested by a modeling approach *(42)* cannot be supported by the available structural data on the complex between the two molecules. On the other hand, the structure of the GPIbα fragment bound to α-thrombin that we recently solved (data to be published elsewhere) confirms that the receptor sulfotyrosine region forms contacts with the latter ligand. The work of Huizinga et al. *(39)* has defined the GPIbα residues important for the interaction with the vWF A1 domain. The main contact points involve Lys8, Ser11, His12, Glu14, and Asn16 in the β-hairpin; His37, Glu128, Lys152, Asp175, Thr176 (mislabeled as Ser in Fig. 1C of the original report), and Phe199 in the concave face of the leucine-rich repeats; and Glu225, Asn226, Tyr228, and Ser241 in the C-terminal region that includes the regulatory loop.

The cytoplasmic face of the GPIb-IX-V complex has been shown to be associated with several proteins including filamin (actin-binding protein, also known as ABP-280), which binds within the region Thr536-Leu554 of the GPIbα cytoplasmic domain *(43)*. Through this interaction, the GPIb-IX-V complex is linked to a submembrane network of F-actin structures that comprises the platelet membrane skeleton *(44)*. The cytoplasmic tail of GPIbα also contains the binding site for the dimeric signaling molecule 14-3-3ζ within the C-terminal five amino acids, Ser-Gly-His-Ser(P)-Leu *(45)*. Phosphorylation of Ser609 is essential for high-affinity binding of 14-3-3ζ *(46)*. In resting platelets, 14-3-3ζ provides a link between GPIb-IX-V and phosphoinositide 3 (PI3) kinase *(47)*. Another 14-3-3ζ binding site has been located within the cytoplasmic domain of GPIbβ following the phosphorylation of Ser166 by cyclic adenosine monophosphate (cAMP)-dependent protein kinase A (PKA) *(48,49)*. However, binding of 14-3-3ζ to GPIbβ appears to be contingent on the association of 14-3-3ζ with the C-terminal domain of GPIbα *(50)*. The cytoplasmic domain of GPIbβ also interacts with calmodulin within residues 149–167 *(51)*.

SIGNAL TRANSMISSION THROUGH GPIb-IX-V

Although no definitive evidence is presently available, signaling events leading to platelet activation are thought to be initiated by the binding of vWF or α-thrombin (and potentially Mac-1 and P-selectin) to GPIb-IX-V. These events include an elevation of cytosolic Ca^{2+} and activation of PKC and tyrosine kinases, leading ultimately to activation of integrin $\alpha_{IIb}\beta_3$ and platelet aggregation *(3,19,52,53)*. Identifying the signaling pathway(s) linking GPIb-IX-V to platelet activation may provide a means of selectively blocking the initiation of pathological thrombosis, without compromising hemostasis. Indirect evidence suggests that vWF-dependent signaling involves the crosslinking of GPIbα subunits by multivalent vWF *(54)*. For example, a monomeric proteolytic fragment of vWF containing a single A1 domain binds to the GPIb-IX-V complex and inhibits binding of native multimeric vWF but does not induce cytoskeletal rearrangement and activation of $\alpha_{IIb}\beta_3$ *(23,55)*. The observations that the GPIb-IX-V complex is associated with two immunoreceptor tyrosine-based activation motif (ITAM)-containing proteins, Fc receptor (FcR) γ-chain and FcγRIIa *(56,57)*, lends support to the crosslinking mechanism of signaling. FcγRIIa and GPIbα are proximal to within 10 nm of each other in the platelet membrane *(58)*, and both FcRγ chain and FcγRIIA coimmunoprecipitate with the GPIb-IX-V complex *(56,58)*. On crosslinking, FcRγ chain and FcγRIIA are tyrosine phosphorylated within the cytoplasmic ITAM sequence by Src family tyrosine kinases *(59)*, thereby permitting the binding and autophosphorylation of the tyrosine kinase Syk. Activated Syk initiates signaling that leads to activation of phospholipase C-γ2 (PLC-γ2) and subsequent formation of inositol triphosphate (IP_3; leading to Ca^{2+} mobilization) and diacylglycerol (DAG; leading to activation of protein kinase C [PKC]) *(56,57)*. The cytoplasmic region of GPIbα is associated with two dimeric signaling proteins, actin-binding protein and 14-3-3ζ *(43,60,61)*. These associations provide potential links to several signaling molecules, including PI3 kinase, focal adhesion kinase, Src-related tyrosine kinases (Syk, Src, Fyn Lyn, and Yes), GTPase-activating protein, and tyrosine phosphatases (PTP-1B and SHPTP10) *(21)*.

Several studies indicate that 14-3-3ζ plays a crucial role in regulating signaling through GPIb-IX-V, leading to activation of $\alpha_{IIb}\beta_3$ *(47,50,62)*. CHO cells coexpresssing GPIb-IX and $\alpha_{IIb}\beta_3$ spread on a vWF-coated surface and subsequently bound fibrinogen in an $\alpha_{IIb}\beta_3$ activation-dependent manner *(62)*. Both PI3 kinase and PKC play important roles in this process since their inhibition blocked cell spreading *(62)*. Moreover, deletion of the C-terminal 18 amino acids of GPIbα, containing the binding site for 14-3-3ζ, prevented cell spreading and fibrinogen binding to $\alpha_{IIb}\beta_3$. PI3 kinase forms a constitutive complex with both GPIb-IX-V and 14-3-3ζ in resting platelets *(47)* and may therefore play a key role in 14-3-3ζ signaling. Although dissociation of 14-3-3ζ from the GPIb-IX-V complex is seen following platelet activation *(47,50)*, it is unclear whether this is a direct effect of platelet activation, or a process that precedes activation.

The Collagen Receptors

Two major receptors for collagen are expressed on the platelet surface: the integrin $\alpha_2\beta_1$ *(63–65)*, which is also found on a wide range of other cells, and GPVI *(66,67)*, which appears to be confined to platelets and megakaryocytes. The latter receptor is a member of the Ig superfamily and plays a major role in signaling and platelet activation *(68,69)*. Both are potential targets for pharmacological control of pathological thrombosis. Under conditions of high shear blood flow, neither $\alpha_2\beta_1$ nor GPVI are capable of initiating platelet adhesion to collagen, whereas both platelet GPIb-IX-V and plasma vWF are essential for this process *(2)*. The pivotal roles of GPVI and $\alpha_2\beta_1$ in the interaction of platelets with collagen is highlighted by the impaired collagen-platelet interactions and mild bleeding disorders in patients deficient in the expression of either protein *(65,66,70,71)*. There is also evidence, albeit limited, for minor roles of other receptors such as a platelet p65, a receptor specific for type I collagen, which has been isolated, cloned, and partially characterized *(72)*. The recombinant molecule has been reported to specifically block platelet activation induced by collagen type I, but these results await confirmation. The role of another putative collagen receptor, GPIV (CD36) *(73–75)* has been more controversial. Both collagen *(75)* and thrombospondin *(73)* have been reported to be GPIV ligands, although some studies found no evidence for a role of GPIV as a collagen receptor *(76,77)*. Evidence has also been presented that GPV, a component of the GPIb-IX-V complex, binds to collagen and may be required for normal platelet responses to this agonist *(78)*. GPV is a sensitive substrate for cleavage by α-thrombin *(79)*, and ablation of the GPV gene in mice has been reported to enhance platelet activation by this agonist *(80)*, although the finding remains controversial *(81)*. A mechanism has also been proposed whereby cleavage of GPV would be a prerequisite for α-thrombin signaling through GPIbα *(53)*. During the initial stages of platelet adhesion and aggregation at sites of vascular lesion, therefore, there may be a complex interplay of events, since rapid thrombin generation and cleavage of GPV may downregulate platelet activation through collagen while favoring responses induced by thrombin bound to GPIbα.

INTEGRIN $\alpha_2\beta_1$

Integrin $\alpha_2\beta_1$ (also known as GPIa-IIa on platelets, and VLA-2 on lymphocytes) was the first major receptor recognized as mediating platelet adhesion to collagen *(82,83)*. There are on average 2000–3000 copies on the platelet surface, although expression levels can vary up to 10-fold in normal healthy individuals and are related to the incidence of cardiovascular disease *(84–86)*. This large variation in $\alpha_2\beta_1$ expression levels among normal individuals is linked to silent polymorphisms in the gene for α_2 *(87,88)*. The α_2 and β_1 subunits are noncovalently bound and have apparent molecular weights of 165 and 130 kDa, respectively. The collagen binding site has been localized to a domain in the α_2 subunit called the vWF type A domain (also known as the A-domain, or I-domain), a region comprising 200 amino acids with homology to the collagen-binding domain of vWF *(89)*. The crystal structures of both the I-domain and its complex with collagen-related peptides have been elucidated by X-ray crystallography *(90–92)*, providing valuable insights into the role of a cation binding site in modulating the collagen binding site conformation. The recognition sequence on type I collagen for α_2vWFA has been identified and contains an essential GER peptide sequence *(93)*, which coordinates with a cation (Mg^{2+} or Mn^{2+}) bound to the vWF A-domain to form a metal ion-dependent adhesion site (MIDAS) *(91,92)*. The extracellular domain of α_2 contains a sevenfold repeat segment that includes an EF hand motif with three cation binding sites, thought to optimize collagen binding to the vWF A-domain *(94)*.

Although $\alpha_2\beta_1$ is considered essential for optimal adhesion of platelets to collagen, its role as a signaling receptor has been controversial. Platelet aggregation induced by collagen in a stirred platelet suspension is impaired when $\alpha_2\beta_1$ function is blocked with an antibody *(95–98)* or snake venom-derived proteins *(99,100)*, despite the presence of GPVI on platelets. These observations suggest that $\alpha_2\beta_1$ is likely to be a significant contributor to the hemostatic process and is therefore a potential target for therapeutic inhibition of platelet activation in vivo. A two-site, two-step model of platelet activation by collagen has been proposed in which platelets first bind collagen through $\alpha_2\beta_1$ and are subsequently activated by a second receptor, now believed to be GPVI *(101–102)*. However, in GPVI-deficient platelets, collagen has been shown to stimulate protein tyrosine phosphorylation *(103,104)* and weak activation of $\alpha_{IIb}\beta_3$ *(105)*, implicating a possible role of $\alpha_2\beta_1$ in the regulation of tyrosine phosphorylation by collagen. The snake venom metalloprotease jararhagin binds to the I-domain of α_2 and cleaves the β_1-subunit, thereby preventing collagen-induced signaling *(106,107)*, including the tyrosine phosphorylation of Syk and PLC-γ2. However, these results are ambiguous since it is not clear whether the observed downregulation of tyrosine phosphorylation is owing to a decrease in platelet adhesion and therefore decreased signaling through GPVI, as would be predicted by the two-site, two-step model.

A similar argument could be made for the role of $\alpha_2\beta_1$ in the regulation of focal adhesion kinase under arterial flow conditions (108). Further insights into the role of $\alpha_2\beta_1$ in collagen-induced signaling has been obtained from studies with snake venom proteins that either inhibit $\alpha_2\beta_1$ function (99,100) or block specific $\alpha_2\beta_1$ binding sites on collagen (109). Other snake venom toxins, namely, aggretin, mucytin, and rhodocytin, have been reported to activate platelets through a pathway involving PLC that can be blocked by specific $\alpha_2\beta_1$ antibodies (110–113). Rhodocytin has been reported to induce tyrosine phosphorylation of several platelet proteins, including Syk and PLC-γ2 (112), independently of GPIb (114). However, the involvement of receptors other than $\alpha_2\beta_1$ cannot be excluded by these studies, and the question of $\alpha_2\beta_1$ specificity remains unresolved.

Under certain experimental conditions, platelet adhesion to monomeric collagen is mediated exclusively through $\alpha_2\beta_1$ (115) and is associated with platelet spreading and activation of $\alpha_{IIb}\beta_3$ but not granule secretion or thromboxane production (115). Binding of soluble collagen fragments to $\alpha_2\beta_1$ is increased following platelet activation (116), lending support to the notion that $\alpha_2\beta_1$ may exist in different functional states and that its affinity for collagen is regulated by inside-out signaling.

GLYCOPROTEIN VI

The detection of patients deficient in platelet GPVI, as well as patients with defective collagen-induced platelet responses, led to the identification of GPVI as a crucial collagen receptor (66,67,117,118). GPVI is a major transmembrane platelet glycoprotein (60–65 kDa) and is a member of the immunoglobulin superfamily (68,119), which forms a noncovalent association with the FcRγ-chain at the cell surface (120,121) that is critical for collagen-induced signal transduction. In mouse platelets, deletion of the FcRγ gene is associated with the absence of surface-expressed GPVI (122), demonstrating that the expression and function of GPVI is dependent on its association with the FcRγ-chain. The cytoplasmic domain of the FcRγ-chain contains an ITAM, which is believed to play a crucial role in collagen-induced signaling (123). The association with the FcRγ-chain enables GPVI to activate protein tyrosine kinase-mediated signaling pathways. Platelet activation by collagen leads to an increase in tyrosine phosphorylation of several proteins, including FcRγ-chain, the protein tyrosine kinase Syk, SLP-76 (Src homology 2 domain-containing leukocyte phosphoprotein of 76 kDa) and PLC-γ2 *(124,125)*.

Signaling through GPVI is thought to involve ITAM phosphorylation by Src family tyrosine kinases (including Lyn and Fyn) following receptor clustering *(59,123)*. The kinase Syk then binds to the phosphorylated ITAM domains of the FcRγ-chain through its Src homology (SH2) domains and is subsequently phosphorylated. Activated Syk then phosphorylates PLC-γ2, recruited to the plasma membrane by phosphorylated SLP-76, leading to stimulation of PLC-γ2 *(125,126)*. Activation of PLC-γ2 results in the generation of the second messengers DAG, which activates PKC isoforms, and IP_3, which induces the release of stored calcium *(127)*. Activated PKC isoforms regulate serine/threonine phosphorylation events required for full platelet activation and modulation of $\alpha_{IIb}\beta_3$ into a form competent to bind soluble fibrinogen *(128)*.

Evidence to support this model of GPVI signaling derives from studies with knockout mice lacking either FcRγ-chain, Syk, or the adaptor protein SLP-76, in which platelet activation induced by collagen is abolished *(124–126,129)*. Mouse platelets lacking both Lyn and Fyn (members of the Src family kinases) show diminished phosphorylation of both FcRγ and Syk in response to collagen, indicating an important role for these kinases *(130)*. Other Src family kinases such as Lck, Hck, Yes, or Fgr may partly compensate for the absence of Lyn and Fyn activity in these platelets *(131)*. PI3 kinase also plays a key role in GPVI/FcRγ-chain signaling: it binds to the phosphorylated ITAM of the FcRγ-chain following engagement of GPVI by collagen or collagen-related peptides *(132,133)*. Wortmannin and LY294002, two structurally unrelated inhibitors of PI3 kinase, block platelet responses downstream of GPVI ligation *(132,134)*.

The potential role of GPVI in arterial thrombus formation has been evaluated by intravital fluorescence microscopy of injured mouse carotid arteries after endothelial denudation. In these studies, GPVI-deficient mouse platelets failed to aggregate on the damaged vessel wall, and the investigators also concluded that there was a concurrent reduction in primary adhesion *(135)*. The latter finding, however, could be the consequence of reduced platelet activation with an inability to establish irreversible attachment after a normal initial tethering, which under high flow conditions is mediated by GPIbα binding to vWF immobilized onto exposed collagen *(2)*. Recent results in GPVI-deficient mice *(136)* indicate that, indeed, the initial platelet adhesion to insoluble collagen type I fibrils is not decreased, but platelet spreading, which is associated with irreversible attachment, is abolished (Fig. 2). Although it has yet to be determined whether the cytoplasmic domain of GPVI possesses signal-

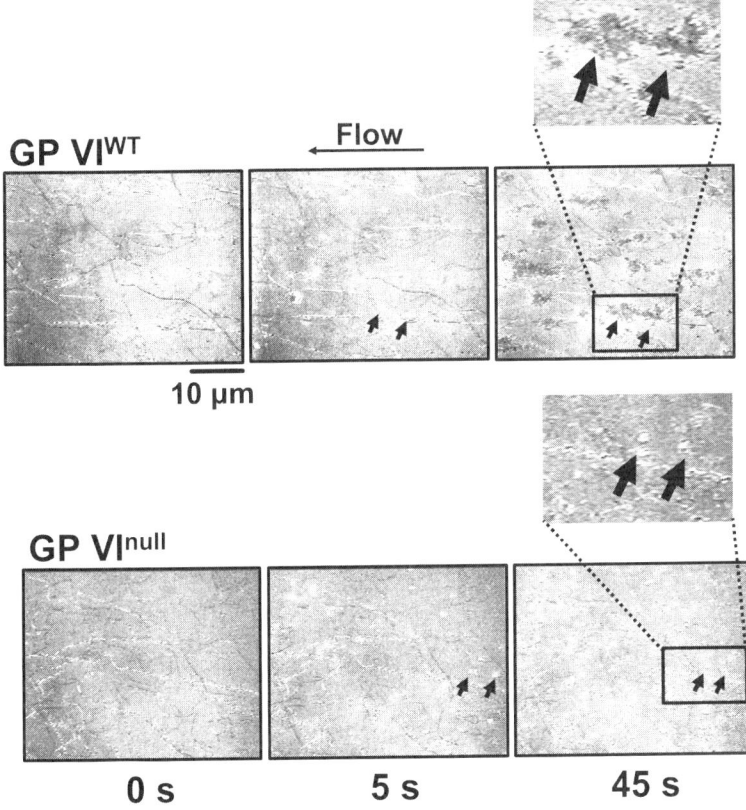

Fig. 2. Timecourse analysis of the contact interface between platelets and collagen fibrils. Blood was collected from anesthetized mice via a retroorbital puncture using 40 U/mL heparin as anticoagulant. Apyrase was added to a final concentration of 1.5 U/mL Glass cover slips were coated with insoluble fibrillar type I collagen (2.5 mg/mL) and placed in a parallel plate flow chamber. Mouse blood was perfused through the chamber at 1500/s wall shear rate. Platelets interacting with the surface were visualized with the technique of reflection interference contrast microscopy, which also allows visualization of the larger collagen fibrils immobilized on the glass bottom of the flow chamber before the beginning of blood perfusion (time 0 s). After 5 s of perfusion with either normal or GPVI[null] blood, comparable numbers of single platelets (arrow) are seen interacting with the surface. Their shape is round, indicating that spreading following activation has not yet taken place. After 45 s, in the case of normal blood perfusion, the adherent platelets have spread and occupy a larger portion of the surface; in contrast, in the case of GPVI[null] blood perfusion, platelets have the same morphology as after 5 s, indicating that they have not become activated and thus have not spread. The insets to the right present a larger magnification of the surface after 45 s of perfusion. Note that the individual boundaries of spread platelets tend to be lost. In this technique, the darker color of spread platelets compared with those that have not spread indicates a closer proximity to the collagen fibrils. (Adapted from ref. *136*.)

ing capabilities independently of its association with the FcRγ-chain, selective pharmacological modulation of the GPVI-collagen interaction or inhibition of the ensuing signaling pathways mediated by the FcRγ-chain may have therapeutic potential in alleviating the onset and progression of pathological arterial thrombosis. In this regard, mice treated with an anti-GPVI monoclonal antibody were afforded protection from a lethal thromboembolism following infusion of a mixture of collagen and epinephrine (137).

PLATELET ACTIVATION RECEPTORS

Platelet adhesion at sites of vascular lesions leads to the formation of a platelet monolayer that is insufficient, by itself, to prevent blood loss. However, following adhesion, platelet activation ensues through the pathways outlined above, leading to the local accumulation of molecules that are secreted from platelets, such as ADP, and thromboxane A_2 (TXA_2). In turn, these molecules are ligands for G protein-coupled receptors on the platelet surface that can respond rapidly to activate PLC, increase cytosolic Ca^{2+} levels, and suppress production of cAMP. In addition, tissue factor-mediated thrombin generation at the platelet surface activates platelets through their thrombin receptors and allows consolidation of the platelet thrombus by the formation of a fibrin clot. The second phase of platelet plug formation therefore involves the activation and recruitment of additional circulating platelets into the growing thrombus. This process is mediated by receptors that are well suited to respond rapidly to the locally generated agonists. The development of compounds that interfere with these receptor functions could have potential use in the pharmacological control of platelet function and in the intervention of cardiovascular and cerebrovascular disorders.

Platelet activation and inhibition responses are often mediated by receptors belonging to the seven-transmembrane receptor family (138). These receptors are coupled to G protein-linked responses and are found in a wide variety of cells, including platelets, where the ADP receptors $P2Y_1$ and $P2Y_{12}$ and the thrombin receptors (protease-activated receptors [PARs]) play key roles in platelet activation. Other seven-transmembrane receptors on platelets include the prostaglandin receptors for TXA_2 (139) and prostaglandin I_2 (PGI_2) (140), lipid receptors for platelet-activating factor (PAF) (141) and lysophosphatidic acid (142), chemokine receptors (143–145), the β-adrenergic receptor for epinephrine (146), and the serotonin receptor (147).

ADP Receptors

Although ADP by itself is a weak activator of human platelets (148), it plays a crucial role in platelet function because it potentiates the effect of other platelet agonists to amplify the platelet response *(149)*. Human platelets express at least two distinct receptors for ADP, namely, $P2Y_1$ and $P2Y_{12}$, that belong to the purinergic class of G protein-coupled receptors *(148,150–152)*. Activation of both $P2Y_1$ and $P2Y_{12}$ is required for optimal activation of platelets by ADP *(149,153)*. The Gq-coupled $P2Y_1$ receptor mediates the activation of β-isoforms of PLC, which leads to a transient rise in cytoplasmic Ca^{2+} levels, platelet shape change, and aggregation *(150,154,155)*. $P2Y_1$ is also thought to couple $G_{12/13}$ and activate platelets through the stimulation of rho kinase *(156,157)*. Platelets from knockout mice lacking either the Gαq subunit of Gq or the $P2Y_1$ receptor have an impaired aggregation response to ADP, characterized by a slowly progressive and sustained platelet aggregation, not accompanied by shape change *(158–160)*. The Gi-coupled $P2Y_{12}$ receptor downregulates adenylyl cyclase, thereby lowering cAMP levels *(153,161)*. With platelets from patients congenitally deficient in $P2Y_{12}$, ADP does not elicit the inhibition of adenylyl cyclase but induces normal shape change and a small, rapidly reversible wave of aggregation *(162–164)*. Therefore, although $P2Y_1$ is important for the initiation of platelet activation by ADP, concomitant signaling through $P2Y_{12}$ is essential for a sustained, full aggregation response. This is further illustrated by the observations that normal aggregation responses to ADP can be restored in $P2Y_{12}$-deficient platelets by adrenaline, which is coupled to Gi *(159)*, and in $P2Y_1$-deficient platelets by serotonin, which is coupled to Gq *(158,165)*.

Unlike $P2Y_1$, which is expressed in a wide range of cells, $P2Y_{12}$ has a more selective tissue distribution *(151)*, making it an important target for platelet activation inhibitors in the treatment and prevention of antithrombotic disorders. Such inhibitors currently in clinical use, or under evaluation in clinical trials, include ticlopidine *(149,166)*, clopidogrel *(149,166)*, and AR-C69951 MX *(167–169)*. Ticlopidine and clopidogrel are members of the thienopyridine family, and both have been recommended for the secondary prevention of thrombotic diseases, especially in aspirin-resistant or aspirin-intolerant patients *(170)*. It is thought that a thiol group in $P2Y_{12}$ plays a crucial role in the covalent inhibition by clopidrogrel and ticlopidine *(169)*, which is irreversible and lasts for the life of the platelet (7–10 d) *(171)*.

Thrombin Receptors

Thrombin, a serine protease, is a potent activator of platelets, which elicits signaling, at least in part, through the G protein-linked receptors known as PARs. Unlike other seven-transmembrane receptors, these receptors activate platelets through a unique mechanism involving the conversion of an extracellular proteolytic cleavage event into a transmembrane signal *(172)*. Thrombin binds to and cleaves the N-terminal extracellular domain of the PARs, thereby releasing a peptide and exposing a new N terminus, which then acts as a ligand to the receptor *(172)*. The unmasked cryptic tethered ligand is capable of activating the thrombin receptor independently of thrombin itself or further proteolytic cleavage *(172–174)*. Synthetic peptidomimetics that are homologous to the N-terminal amino acid sequences of the tethered ligands are effective activators of the receptor *(172,174,175)*. The cleaved peptide is also a strong platelet agonist, although the receptor involved has not been identified *(176)*.

The first PAR discovered was PAR-1 *(172)*, which, on human platelets, is present at about 1500–2500 copies and responds to levels of α-thrombin as low as 1.0 nM. Four distinct PARs have been identified: PAR-1 *(172–177)*, PAR-3 *(178)*, and PAR-4 *(179)* are all thrombin-sensitive receptors, whereas PAR-2 is a trypsin-activated (and thrombin-insensitive) receptor *(180,182)*. Although PAR-2 is not a thrombin receptor, its structural and functional mechanisms of activation are analogous to those of the thrombin-sensitive PARs *(183,184)*. PAR-2 is not expressed in human platelets *(185,186)*.

The response of PAR-1$^{-/-}$ knockout mouse platelets is not compromised since these platelets have functional PAR-3, with properties analogous to PAR-1 expressed on human platelets. Human platelets express PAR-1 and PAR-4 but little or no PAR-3 *(187)*, whereas mouse platelets express PAR-3 and PAR-4. On human platelets, PAR-1 and PAR-4 comprise a dual-receptor system for thrombin-induced platelet activation *(187)*. Blocking PAR-4 function with a monoclonal antibody had no effect on platelet aggregation in response to low-dose (1 nM) thrombin. However, antibody inhibition of PAR-1 completely prevented platelet activation in response to low (1 nM) thrombin, but only partially at higher (30 nM) thrombin concentrations *(187)*. Simultaneous inhibition of both PAR-1 and PAR-4 resulted in complete abrogation of platelet response to thrombin, even at a concentration of 30 nM *(187)*. Further support for the dual-receptor model has been obtained from studies of changes in cytosolic Ca^{2+} levels. Two distinct phases of thrombin receptor-dependent Ca^{2+} transients have been demonstrated during platelet activation: a very early, short-lived spike response mediated through PAR-1 activation and a delayed, more prolonged Ca^{2+} signal mediated through PAR-4 activation *(188,189)*.

Ligand binding to the PARs leads to Gq-linked responses associated with the activation of the β-isoforms of PLC, which hydrolyzes membrane-associated phosphatidylinositol 4,5-bisphosphate *(127)*. This hydrolysis produces the second messengers IP$_3$ (which contributes to

Ca^{2+} mobilization from internal stores) and DAG (which activates protein kinase C). The increase in cytosolic Ca^{2+} levels results in tyrosine phosphorylation of other downstream effector proteins such as the myosin light chain, and activation of signaling pathways linked to $\alpha_{IIb}\beta_3$ activation (127,190). The phosphorylation of myosin light chain is mediated by the calmodulin-dependent myosin light chain kinase, which regulates the myosin-based movement of actin (29). The increase in cytosolic Ca^{2+} regulates many events leading to platelet aggregation, including the p38 mitogen-activated protein kinase-dependent activation of phospholipase A2, which hydrolyzes membrane phospholipids, leading to the production of arachidonic acid and thromboxane synthesis (191).

Since PAR-1 and PAR-4 evoke distinct waves of intracellular Ca^{2+} mobilization, selective inhibition of thrombin-induced platelet activation in humans requires strategies that target both PAR-1 and PAR-4, without blocking the important fibrinogen-cleaving functions of thrombin. In this regard, antibodies directed against the cleavage sites of PAR-1 and PAR-4, block platelet responses to a wide range of thrombin concentrations (189,192). Peptide antagonists have been designed that are structurally analogous to the PAR-1 peptide sequence (193,194). A prototype PAR-1 agonist peptide selectively binds and inhibits PAR-1 activation by low, but not high levels of α-thrombin (194), raising the possibility that such compounds may be effective antithrombotic agents under conditions in which low thrombin concentrations are present. However, functional inhibition of both PAR-1 and PAR-4 may be necessary for optimal antiplatelet therapy.

Thromboxane Receptor

TXA_2, a labile product formed from arachidonic acid by way of the enzyme cyclooxygenase, is an important modulator of platelet function and serves to amplify the platelet activation signal following stimulation by primary agonists such as thrombin and ADP. Low concentrations of ADP or thrombin do not elicit a full platelet aggregation response without the presence of TXA_2. Aspirin, which blocks TXA_2 production by inhibiting cyclooxygenase activity, is an effective antithrombotic agent. However, at higher concentrations, ADP and thrombin can fully activate platelets in the absence of TXA_2. The TXA_2 receptor expressed on human platelets has a mass of 57 kDa and is coupled to several G proteins to activate phospholipase A_2 and phospholipase C. Activation of the TxA_2 receptor leads to tyrosine phosphorylation of several signaling proteins including Syk (195).

CONCLUSIONS

Characterization of signal transduction pathways mediated by platelet adhesion and activation receptors is essential for designing strategies for the pharmacological regulation of platelet-mediated pathologies. As progress is made in elucidating the molecular mechanisms of platelet adhesion and activation, targets for therapeutic intervention are being uncovered. GPIb antagonists have proven antithrombotic benefits in animal studies *(196)*, and $\alpha_{IIb}\beta_3$ antagonists have demonstrated therapeutic benefits in clinical trials of acute coronary disorders *(197)*. Genetic manipulation of the mouse genome is providing valuable insights into signaling pathways in platelets by defining structure-function relationships of specific proteins. For example, knockout mice lacking GPIbα display the phenotype associated with Bernard-Soulier syndrome, including a prolonged bleeding time and giant platelets *(198)*. However, the transgenic expression of human GPIbα on these mouse platelets reverses, or rescues, the Bernard-Soulier phenotype, demonstrating the crucial role of the GPIb-IX-V receptor in normal platelet physiology *(198)*. Gene targeting has also shed light on the importance of specific signaling proteins in platelet function, as exemplified by Gαq knockout mice, which have prolonged bleeding times and defective platelet responses to ADP, thrombin, and collagen *(160)*. Similar models have demonstrated the importance of the signaling molecules Syk *(199)* and Src *(200)* and are providing essential information about the signaling pathways utilized by adhesion receptors. Ultimately, these studies will lead to the identification of new ways of therapeutically regulating platelet adhesive functions by targeting relevant signaling proteins.

REFERENCES

1. Savage B, Saldivar E, Ruggeri ZM. Initiation of platelet adhesion by arrest onto fibrinogen or translocation on von Willebrand factor. Cell 1996;84:289–297.
2. Savage B, Almus-Jacobs F, Ruggeri ZM. Specific synergy of multiple substrate-receptor interactions in platelet thrombus formation under flow. Cell 1998; 94:657–666.
3. Kroll MH, Hellums JD, McIntire LV, Schafer AI, Moake JL. Platelets and shear stress. Blood 1996;88:1525–1541.
4. Peterson DM, Stathopoulos NA, Giorgio TD, Hellums JD, Moake JL. Shear-induced platelet aggregation requires von Willebrand factor and platelet membrane glycoproteins Ib and IIb-IIIa. Blood 1987;69:625–628.
5. Goto S, Ikeda Y, Saldivar E, Ruggeri ZM. Distinct mechanisms of platelet aggregation as a consequence of different shearing flow conditions. J Clin Invest 1998;101:479–486.
6. Ruggeri ZM. Old concepts and new developments in the study of platelet aggregation. J Clin Invest 2000;105:699–701.

7. Ruggeri ZM, Dent JA, Saldivar E. Contribution of distinct adhesive interactions to platelet aggregation in flowing blood. Blood 1999;94:172–178.

8. Wu YP, Vink T, Schiphorst M, et al. Platelet thrombus formation on collagen at high shear rates is mediated by von Willebrand factor-glycoprotein Ib interaction and inhibited by von Willebrand factor-glycoprotein IIb/IIIa interaction. Arterioscler Thromb Vasc Biol 2000;20:1661–1667.

9. Tsuji S, Sugimoto M, Miyata S, Kuwahara M, Kinoshita S, Yoshioka A. Real-time analysis of mural thrombus formation in various platelet aggregation disorders: distinct shear-dependent roles of platelet receptors and adhesive proteins under flow. Blood 1999;94:968–975.

10. Romo GM, Dong JF, Schade AJ, et al. The glycoprotein Ib-IX-V complex is a platelet counterreceptor for P-selectin. J Exp Med 1999;190:803–814.

11. Simon DI, Chen Z, Xu H, et al. Platelet glycoprotein Ibalpha is a counterreceptor for the leukocyte integrin Mac-1 (CD11b/CD18). J Exp Med 2000;192:193–204.

12. Okumura T, Jamieson GA. Platelet glycocalicin: a single receptor for platelet aggregation induced by thrombin or ristocetin. Thromb Res 1976;8:701–706.

13. Mazzucato M, De Marco L, Masotti A, Pradella P, Bahou WF, Ruggeri ZM. Characterization of the initial α-thrombin interaction with glycoprotein Ibα in relation to platelet activation. J Biol Chem 1998;273:1880–1887.

14. Bradford HN, Dela Cadena RA, Kunapuli SP, Dong J-F, Lopez JA, Colman RW. Human kininogens regulate thrombin binding to platelets through the glycoprotein Ib-IX-V complex. Blood 1997;90:1508–1515.

15. Baglia FA, Badellino KO, Li CQ, Lopez JA, Walsh PN. Factor XI binding to the platelet glycoprotein Ib-IX-V complex promotes factor XI activation by thrombin. J Biol Chem 2002;277:1662–1668.

16. Bradford HN, Pixley RA, Colman RW. Human factor XII binding to the glycoprotein Ib-IX-V complex inhibits thrombin-induced platelet aggregation. J Biol Chem 2000;275:22756–22763.

17. Jackson SP, Mistry N, Yuan Y. Platelets and the injured vessel wall—"rolling into action." Focus on glycoprotein Ib/V/IX and the platelet cytoskeleton. Trends Cardiovasc Med 2000;10:192–197.

18. Ware J. Molecular analyses of the platelet glycoprotein Ib-IX-V receptor. Thromb Haemost 1998;79:466–478.

19. Mazzucato M, Pradella P, Cozzi MR, De Marco L, Ruggeri ZM. Sequential cytoplasmic calcium signals in a two-stage platelet activation process induced by the glycoprotein Ibα mechanoreceptor. Blood 2002;100:2793–2800.

20. Yap CL, Anderson KE, Hughan SC, Dopheide SM, Salem HH, Jackson SP. Essential role for phosphoinositide 3-kinase in shear-dependent signaling between platelet glycoprotein Ib/V/IX and integrin $\alpha_{IIb}\beta_3$. Blood 2002;99:151–158.

21. Andrews RK, Shen Y, Gardiner EE, Dong J, Lopez JA, Berndt MC. The glycoprotein Ib-IX-V complex in platelet adhesion and signaling. Thromb Haemost 1999;82:357–364.

22. Berndt MC, Shen Y, Dopheide SM, Gardiner EE, Andrews RK. The vascular biology of the glycoprotein Ib-IX-V complex. Thromb Haemost 2001;86:178–188.

23. Andrews RK, Berndt MC. Adhesion-dependent signalling and the initiation of haemostasis and thrombosis. Histol Histopathol 1998;13:837–844.

24. Du X, Beutler L, Ruan C, Castaldi PA, Berndt MC. Glycoprotein Ib and glycoprotein IX are fully complexed in the intact platelet membrane. Blood 1987;69:1524–1527.

25. Breit SN, Green I. Modulation of endothelial cell synthesis of von Willebrand factor by mononuclear cell products. Haemostasis 1988;18:137–145.

26. Lopez JA. The platelet glycoprotein Ib-IX complex. Blood Coagul Fibrinolysis 1994;5:97–119.
27. Berndt MC, Gregory C, Kabral A, Zola H, Fournier D, Castaldi PA. Purification and preliminary characterization of glycoprotein Ib complex in the human platelet membrane. Eur J Biochem 1985;151:637–649.
28. Modderman PW, Admiraal LG, Sonnenberg A, Von dem Borne AE. Glycoproteins V and Ib-IX form a noncovalent complex in the platelet membrane. J Biol Chem 1992;267:364–369.
29. Kovacsovics TJ, Hartwig JH. Thrombin-induced GPIb-IX centralization on the platelet surface requires actin assembly and myosin II activation. Blood 1996;87:618–629.
30. van Zanten GH, Heijnen HFG, Wu Y, et al. A fifty percent reduction of platelet surface glycoprotein Ib does not affect platelet adhesion under flow conditions. Blood 1998;91:2353–2359.
31. Hourdille P, Heilmann E, Combrie R, Winckler J, Clemetson KJ, Nurden AT. Thrombin induces a rapid redistribution of glycoprotein Ib-IX complexes within the membrane systems of activated human platelets. Blood 1990;76:1503–1513.
32. George JN, Torres MM. Thrombin decreases von Willebrand factor binding to platelet glycoprotein Ib. Blood 1988;71:1253–1259.
33. Michelson AD, Barnard MR. Thrombin-induced changes in platelet membrane glycoproteins Ib, IX, and IIb-IIIa complex. Blood 1987;70:1673–1678.
34. Michelson AD, Benoit SE, Furman MI, Barnard MR, Nurden P, Nurden AT. The platelet surface expresssion of glycoprotein V is regulated by two independent mechanisms: proteolysis and the reversible cytoskeletal-mediated redistrbution to the surface-connected canalicular system. Blood 1996;87:1396–1408.
35. Handa M, Titani K, Holland LZ, Roberts JR, Ruggeri ZM. The von Willebrand factor-binding domain of platelet membrane glycoprotein Ib. Characterization by monoclonal antibodies and partial amino acid sequence analysis of proteolytic fragments. J Biol Chem 1986;261:12579–12585.
36. Vicente V, Kostel PJ, Ruggeri ZM. Isolation and functional characterization of the von Willebrand factor-binding domain located between residues His_1-Arg_{293} of the alpha-chain of glycoprotein Ib. J Biol Chem 1988;263:18473–18479.
37. Vicente V, Houghten RA, Ruggeri ZM. Identification of a site in the alpha chain of platelet glycoprotein Ib that participates in von Willebrand factor binding. J Biol Chem 1990;265:274–280.
38. Uff S, Clemetson JM, Harrison T, Clemetson KJ, Emsley J. Crystal structure of the platelet glycoprotein Ibalpha N-terminal domain reveals an unmasking mechanism for receptor activation. J Biol Chem 2002;277:35,657–35,663.
39. Huizinga EG, Tsuji S, Romijn RAP, et al. Structures of glycoprotein Ibα and its complex with von Willebrand factor A1 domain. Science 2002;297:1176–1129.
40. Dong J-F, Li CQ, Lopez JA. Tyrosine sulfation of the glycoprotein Ib-IX complex: identification of sulfated residues and effect on ligand binding. Biochemistry 1994;33:13946–13953.
41 Marchese P, Murata M, Mazzucato M, et al. Identification of three tyrosine residues of glycoprotein Ibα with distinct roles in von Willebrand factor and α-thrombin binding. J Biol Chem 1995;270:9571–9578.
42. Vasudevan S, Roberts JR, McClintock RA, et al. Modeling and functional analysis of the interaction between von Willebrand factor A1 domain and glycoprotein Iba. J Biol Chem 2000;275:12763–12768.
43. Andrews RK, Fox JEB. Identification of a region in the cytoplasmic domain of the platelet membrane glycoprotein Ib-IX complex that binds to purified actin-binding protein. J Biol Chem 1992;267:18605–18611.

44. Fox JE, Boyles JK, Berndt MC, Steffen PK, Anderson LK. Identification of a membrane skeleton in platelets. J Cell Biol 1988;106:1525–1538.

45. Du X, Fox JE, Pei S. Identification of a binding sequence for the 14-3-3 protein within the cytoplasmic domain of the adhesion receptor, platelet glycoprotein Iba. J Biol Chem 1996;271:7362–7367.

46. Bodnar RJ, Gu M, Li Z, Englund GD, Du X. The cytoplasmic domain of the platelet glycoprotein Ibα is phosphorylated at serine 609. J Biol Chem 1999; 274:33474–33479.

47. Munday AD, Berndt MC, Mitchell CA. Phosphoinositide 3-kinase forms a complex with platelet membrane glycoprotein Ib-IX-V complex and 14-3-3zeta. Blood 2000;96:577–584.

48. Calverley DC, Kavanaugh J, Rogh GJ. Human signaling protein 14-3-3ζ interacts with platelet glycoprotein Ib subunits Ibα and Ibβ. Blood 1998;91:1295–1303.

49. Andrews RK, Harris SJ, McNally T, Berndt MC. Binding of purified 14-3-3 ζ signaling protein to discrete amino acid sequences within the cytoplasmic domain of the platelet membrane glycoprotein Ib-IX-V complex. Biochemistry 1998;37:638–647.

50. Feng S, Christodoulides N, Resendiz JC, Berndt MC, Kroll MH. Cytoplasmic domains of GpIbalpha and GpIbbeta regulate 14-3-3zeta binding to GpIb/IX/V. Blood 2000;95:551–557.

51. Andrews RK, Munday AD, Mitchell CA, Berndt MC. Interaction of calmodulin with cytoplasmic domain of the platelet membrane glycoprotein Ib-IX-V complex. Blood 2001;98:681–687.

52. Kroll MH, Harris TS, Moake JL, Handin RI, Schafer AI. von Willebrand Factor binding to platelet GPIb initiates signals for platelet activation. J Clin Invest 1991;88:1568–1573.

53. Ramakrishnan V, DeGuzman F, Bao M, Hall SW, Leung LL, Phillips DR. A thrombin receptor function for platelet glycoprotein Ib-IX unmasked by cleavage of glycoprotein V. Proc Natl Acad Sci USA 2001;98:1823–1828.

54. Kasirer-Friede A, Ware J, Leng L, Marchese P, Ruggeri ZM, Shattil SJ. Lateral clustering of platelet GP Ib-IX complexes leads to up-regulation of the adhesive function of integrin $\alpha_{IIb}\beta_3$. J Biol Chem 2002;277:11949–11956.

55. Satoh K, Asazuma N, Yatomi Y, et al. Activation of protein-tyrosine kinase pathways in human platelets stimulated with the A1 domain of von Willebrand factor. Platelets 2000;11:171–176.

56. Falati S, Edmead CE, Poole AW. Glycoprotein Ib-V-IX, a receptor for von Willebrand factor, couples physically and functionally to the Fc receptor gamma-chain, Fyn, and Lyn to activate human platelets. Blood 1999;94:1648–1656.

57. Torti M, Bertoni A, Canobbio I, Sinigaglia F, Lapetina EG, Balduini C. Rap 1B and Rap2B translocation to the cytoskeleton by von Willebrand factor involves FcgammaII receptor-mediated protein tyrosine physphorylation. J Biol Chem 1999;274:13690–13697.

58. Sullam PM, Hyun WC, Szollosi J, Dong J, Foss WM, López JA. Physical proximity and functional interplay of the glycoprotein Ib-IX-V complex and the Fc receptor FcgammaRIIA on the platelet plasma membrane. J Biol Chem 1998; 273:5331–5336.

59. Watson SP, Asazuma N, Atkinson B, et al. The role of ITAM- and ITIM-coupled receptors in platelet activation by collagen. Thromb Haemost 2001;86:276–288.

60. Cunningham JG, Meyer SC, Fox JEB. The cytoplasmic domain of the α-subunit of glycoprotein (GP) Ib mediates attachment of the entire GP Ib-IX complex to the cytoskeleton and regulates von Willebrand factor-induced changes in cell morphology. J Biol Chem 1996;271:11581–11587.

61. Du X, Harris SJ, Tetaz TJ, Ginsberg MH, Berndt MC. Association of a phospholipase A_2 (14-3-3 protein) with the platelet glycoprotein Ib-IX complex. J Biol Chem 1994;269:18287–18290.
62. Gu M, Xi X, Englund GD, Berndt MC, Du X. Analysis of the roles of 14-3-3 in the platelet glycoprotein Ib-IX-mediated activation of integrin alpha (IIB)beta(3) using a reconstituted mammalian cell expression model. J Cell Biol 1999;147:1085–1096.
63. Santoro SA. Identification of a 160,000 dalton platelet membrane protein that mediates the initial divalent cation-dependent adhesion of platelets to collagen. Cell 1986;46:913–920.
64. Kunicki TJ, Nugent DJ, Staats SJ, Orchekowski RP, Wayner EA, Carter WG. The human fibroblast class II extracellular matrix receptor mediates platelet adhesion to collagen and is identical to the platelet glycoprotein Ia-IIa complex. J Biol Chem 1988;263:4516–4519.
65. Nieuwenhuis HK, Akkerman JWN, Houdijk WPM, Sixma JJ. Human blood platelets showing no response to collagen fail to express surface glycoprotein Ia. Nature 1985;318:470–472.
66. Moroi M, Jung SM, Okuma M, Shinmyozu K. A patient with platelets deficient in glycoprotein VI that lack both collagen-induced aggregation and adhesion. J Clin Invest 1989;84:1440–1445.
67. Moroi M, Jung SM, Shinmyozu K, Tomiyama Y, Ordinas A, Diaz-Ricart M. Analysis of platelet adhesion to a collagen-coated surface under flow conditions: involvement of glycoprotein VI in the platelet adhesion. Blood 1996;88:2081–2092.
68. Clemetson JM, Polgar J, Magnenat E, Wells TN, Clemetson KJ. The platelet collagen receptor glycoprotein VI is a member of the immunoglobulin superfamily closely related to FcαR and the natural killer receptors. J Biol Chem 1999;274:29019–29024.
69. Clemetson KJ, Clemetson JM. Platelet collagen receptors. Thromb Haemost 2001;86:189–197.
70. Arai M, Yamamoto N, Moroi M, Akamatsu N, Fukutake K, Tanoue K. Platelets with 10% of the normal amount of glycoprotein VI have an impaired response to collagen that results in a mild bleeding tendency. Br J Haematol 1995; 89:124–130.
71. Kehrel B, Balleisen L, Kokott R, et al. Deficiency of intact thrombospondin and membrane glycoprotein Ia in platelets with defective collagen-induced aggregation and spontaneous loss of disorder. Blood 1988;71:1074–1078.
72. Chiang TM, Rinaldy A, Kang AH. Cloning, characterization, and functional studies of a nonintegrin platelet receptor for type I collagen. J Clin Invest 1997;100:514–529.
73. Asch AS, Liu I, Briccetti FM, et al. Analysis of CD36 binding domains: ligand specificity controlled by dephosphorylation of an ectodomain. Science 1993;262:1436–1440.
74. Tandon NN, Kralisz U, Jamieson GA. Identification of glycoprotein IV (CD36) as a primary receptor for platelet-collagen adhesion. J Biol Chem 1989;264:7576–7583.
75. Diaz-Ricart M, Tandon NN, Carretero M, Ordinas A, Bastida E, Jamieson GA. Platelets lacking functional CD36 (glycoprotein IV) show reduced adhesion to collagen in flowing whole blood. Blood 1993;82:491–496.
76. Kehrel B, Kronenberg A, Rauterberg J, et al. Platelets deficient in glycoprotein IIIb aggregate normally to collagens type I and III but not to collagen type V. Blood 1993;82:3364–3370.
77. Daniel JL, Dangelnaier C, Strouse R, Smith JB. Collagen induces normal signal transduction in platelets deficient in CD36 (platelet glycoprotein IV). Thromb Haemost 1994;72:353–356.
78. Sylvie M, Mangin P, Lenain N, et al. Platelet glycoprotein V binds to collagen and participates in platelet adhesion and aggregation. Blood 2001;98:1038–1046.

79. Phillips DR, Poh-Agin P. Platelet plasma membrane glycoproteins. Identification of a proteolytic substrate for thrombin. Biochem Biophys Res Commun 1977;75:940–947.

80. Ramakrishnan V, Reeves PS, DeGuzman F, et al. Increased thrombin responsiveness in platelets from mice lacking glycoprotein V. Proc Natl Acad Sci USA 1999;96:13336–13341.

81. Kahn ML, Diacovo TG, Bainton DF, Lanza F, Trejo J, Coughlin SR. Glycoprotein V-deficient platelets have undiminished thrombin responsiveness and do not exhibit a Bernard-Soulier phenotype. Blood 1999;94:4112–4121.

82. Staatz WD, Rajpara SM, Wayner EA, William GC, Santoro SA. The membrane glycoprotein Ia-IIa (VLA-2) complex mediates the Mg++-dependent adhesion of platelets to collagen. J Cell Biol 1989;108:1917–1924.

83. Pischel KD, Bluestein HG, Woods VL. Platelet glycoprotein Ia,Ic, and IIa are physicochemically indistinguishable from the very late activation antigens adhesion-related proteins of lymphocytes and other cell types. J Clin Invest 1988;81:505–513.

84. Kunicki TJ. The role of platelet collagen receptor (glycoprotein Ia/IIa; integrin $\alpha_2\beta_1$) polymorphisms in thrombotic disease. Curr Opin Haematol 2001;8:227–281.

85. Moshfegh K, Wuillemin WA, Redondo M. Association of two silent polymorphisms of platelet glycoprotein Ia/IIa receptor with risk of myocardial infarction: a case-control study. Lancet 1999;353:351–354.

86. Santoso S, Kunicki TJ, Kroll H, Haberbosch W, Gardemann A. Association of the platelet glyroprotein Ia C807T gene polymophism with nonfatal myocardial infarction in younger patients. Blood 1999;93:2449–2453.

87. Kunicki TJ, Kritzik M, Annis DS, Nugent DJ. Hereditary variation in platelet integrin $\alpha_2\beta_1$ density is associated with two silent polymorphisms in the α_2 gene coding sequence. Blood 1997;89:1939–1943.

88. Kritzik M, Savage B, Nugent DJ, Santoso S, Ruggeri ZM, Kunicki TJ. Nucleotide polymorphisms in the α_2 gene define multiple alleles which are associated with differences in platelet $\alpha_2\beta_1$ density. Blood 1998;92:2382–2388.

89. Takada Y, Hemler ME. The primary structure of the VLA-2/collagen receptor a2 subunit (platelet GPIa): Homology to other integrins and the presence of a possible collagen-binding domain. J Cell Biol 1989;109:397–407.

90. Emsley J, King SL, Bergelson JM, Liddington RC. Crystal structure of the I domain from integrin $\alpha_2\beta_1$. J Biol Chem 1997;272:28512–28517.

91. Emsley J, Cruz M, Handin R, Liddington R. Crystal structure of the von Willebrand factor A1 domain and implications for the binding of platelet glycoprotein Ib. J Biol Chem 1998;273:10396–10401.

92. Emsley J, Knight CG, Farndale RW, Barnes MJ, Liddington RC. Structural basis of collagen recognition by integrin $\alpha_2\beta_1$. Cell 2000;100:47–51.

93. Knight CG, Morton LF, Onley DJ, et al. Identification in collagen type I of an integrin $\alpha_2\beta_1$-binding site containing an essential GER sequence. J Biol Chem 1998;273:33287–33294.

94. Dickeson SK, Walsh JJ, Santoro SA. Contributions of the I and EF hand domains to the divalent cation-dependent collagen binding activity of the $\alpha_2\beta_1$ integrin. J Biol Chem 1997;272:7661–7668.

95. Coller BS, Beer JH, Scudder LE, Steinberg MH. Collagen-platelet interactions: evidence for a direct interaction of collagen with platelet GPIa/IIa and an indirect interaction with platelet GPIIb/IIIa mediated by adhesive proteins. Blood 1989;74:182–192.

96. Keely PJ, Parise LV. The $\alpha_2\beta_1$ integrin is a necessary co-receptor for collagen-induced activation of syk and subsequent phosphorylation of phospholipase Cy2 in platelets. J Biol Chem 1996;271:26668–26676.

97. Savage B, Ginsberg MH, Ruggeri ZM. Influence of fibrillar collagen structure on the mechanisms of platelet thrombus formation under flow. Blood 1999;94:2704–2715.

98. Verkleij MW, Morton LF, Knight CG, de Groot PG, Barnes MJ, Sixma JJ. Simple collagen-like peptides support platelet adhesion under static but not under flow conditions: interaction via $\alpha_2\beta_1$ von Willebrand factor with specific sequences in native collagen is a requirement to resist shear forces. Blood 1998;91:3808–3816.

99. Wang R, Kini RM, Chung MC. Rhodocetin, a novel platelet aggregation inhibitor from the venom of *Calloselasma rhodostoma* (Malayan pit viper): synergistic and noncovalent interaction between its subunits. Biochemistry 1999;38:7584–7593.

100. Marcinkiewicz C, Lobb RR, Marcinkiewicz MM, et al. Isolation and characterization of EMS16, a C-lectin type protein from *Echis multisquamatus* venom, a potent and selective inhibitor of the $\alpha_2\beta_1$ integrin. Biochemistry 2000;39:9859–9867.

101. Santoro SA, Walsh JJ, Staatz WD, Baranski KJ. Distinct determinants on collagen support $\alpha_2\beta_1$ integrin mediated platelet adhesion and platelet activation. Cell Regul 1991;2:905–913.

102. Morton LF, Peachey AR, Barnes MJ. Platelet-reactive sites in collagens type I and type III. Evidence for separate adhesion and aggregatory sites. Biochem J 1989;258:157–163.

103. Ichinohe T, Takayama H, Ezumi Y, et al. Collagen-stimulated activation of Syk but not c-Src is severely compromised in human platelets lacking membrane glycoprotein VI. J Biol Chem 1997;272:63–68.

104. Ichinohe T, Takayama H, Ezumi Y, Yanagi S, Yamamura H, Okuma M. Cyclic AMP-insensitive action of c-Src and Syk protein-tyrosine kinases through platelet membrane of glycoprotein VI. J Biol Chem 1995;270:28029–28036.

105. Kehrel B, Wierwille S, Clemetson KJ, et al. Glycoprotein VI is a major collagen receptor for platelet activation: it recognizes the platelet-activating quaternary structure of collagen, whereas CD36, glycoprotein IIB/IIIa, and von Willebrand factor do not. Blood 1998;91:491–499.

106. Kamiguti AS, Hay CR, Zuzel M. Inhibition of collagen-induced platelet aggregation as the result of cleavage of $\alpha_2\beta_1$-integrin by the snake venom metalloproteinase jararhagin. Biochem J 1996;320:635–641.

107. Kamiguti AS, Theakson RD, Watson SP, Bon C, Laing GD, Zuzel M. Distinct contributions of glycoprotein VI and $\alpha_2\beta_1$ integrin to the induction of platelet protein tyrosine phosphorylation and aggregation. Arch Biochem Biophys 2000;374:356–362.

108. Polanowska-Grabowska R, Geanacopoulos M, Gear ARL. Platelet adhesion to collagen via the $\alpha_2\beta_1$ integrin under flow conditions causes rapid tyrosine phosphorylation of pp125[FAK]. Biochem J 1993;296:543–547.

109. Zhou Q, Danglemaier C, Smith JB. The hemorrhagin catrocollastin inhibits collagen-induced platelet aggregation by binding to collagen via its disintegrin-like domain. Biochem Biophys Res Commun 1996;219:720–726.

110. Huang T-F, Liu C-Z, Yang S-H. Aggretin, a novel platelet-aggregation inducer from snake *Calloselasma rhodostoma* venom, activates phospholipase C by acting as a glycoprotein Ia/IIa agonist. Biochem J 1995;309:1021–1027.

111. Teng CM, Ko FN, Tsai IH, Hung ML, Huang TF. Trimucytin: a collagen-like aggregating inducer isolated from *Trimeresurus mucrosquamatus* snake venom. Thromb Haemost 1993;69:286–292.

112. Inoue K, Ozaki Y, Satoh K, et al. Signal transduction pathways mediated by glycoprotein Ia/IIa in human platelets: comparison with those of glycoprotein VI. Biochem Biophys Res Commun 1999;246:114–120.

113. Chung CH, Au LC, Huang TF. Molecular cloning and sequence analysis of aggretin, a collagen-like platelet aggregation inducer. Biochem Biophys Res Commun 1999;263:723–727.
114. Shin Y, Morita T. Rhodocytin, a functional novel platelet agonist belonging to the htreodimeric C-type lectin family, induces platelet aggregation independently of glycoprotein Ib. Biochem Biophys Res Commun 1998;245:741–745.
115. Nakamura T, Kambayashi J, Okuma M, Tandon NN. Activation of the GP IIb-IIIa complex induced by platelet adhesion to collagen is mediated by both $\alpha_2\beta_1$ integrin and GP VI. J Biol Chem 1999;274:11897–11903.
116. Jung SM, Moroi M. Platelets interact with soluble and insoluble collagens through characteristically different reactions. J Biol Chem 1998;273:14827–14837.
117. Sugiyama T, Okuma M, Ushikubi F, Sensaki S, Kanaji K, Uchino H. A novel platelet aggregating factor found in a patient with defective collagen-induced platelet aggregation and autoimmune thrombocytopenia. Blood 1987;69:1712–1720.
118. Moroi M, Okuma M, Jung SM. Platelet adhesion to collagen-coated wells: analysis of this complex process and a comparison with the adhesion to matrigel-coated wells. Biochim Biophys Acta Mol Cell Res 1992;1137:1–9.
119. Jandrot-Perrus M, Busfield S, Lagrue A-H, et al. Cloning, characterization, and functional studies of human and mouse glycoprotein VI: a platelet-specific collagen receptor from the immunoglobulin superfamily. Blood 2000;96:1798–1807.
120. Gibbins JM, Okuma M, Farndale R, Barnes M, Watson SP. Glycoprotein VI is the collagen receptor in platelets which underlies tyrosine phosphorylation of the Fc receptor gamma-chain. FEBS Lett 1997;413:255–259.
121. Tsuji M, Ezumi Y, Arai M, Takayama H. A novel association of Fc receptor γ-chain with glycoprotein VI and their co-expression as a collagen receptor in human platelets. J Biol Chem 1997;272:23528–23531.
122. Nieswandt B, Schulte V, Bergmeiser W, et al. Expression and function of the mouse collagen receptor glycoprotein VI is strictly dependent on its association with the FcRgamma chain. J Biol Chem 2000;275:23998–24002.
123. Gibbins JM, Asselin J, Farndale R, Barnes M, Law CL, Watson SP. Tyrosine physphorylation of the Rc receptor γ-chain in collagen-stimulated platelets. J Biol Chem 1996;271:18095–18099.
124. Poole A, Gibbins JM, Turner M, et al. The Fc receptor gamma-chain and the tyrosine kinase Syk are essential for activation of mouse platelets by collagen. EMBO J 1997;16:2333–2341.
125. Gross BS, Lee JR, Clements JL, et al. Tyrosine phosphorylation of SLP-76 is downstream of Syk following stimulation of the collagen receptor in platelets. J Biol Chem 1999;274:5963–5971.
126. Clements JL, Lee JR, Gross B, et al. Fetal hemorrhage and platelet dysfunction in SLP-76-deficient mice. J Clin Invest 1999;103:19–25.
127. Berridge MJ. Inositol trisphostphate and calcium signalling. Nature 1993;361:315–325.
128. Shattil SJ, Brass LF. Induction of the fibrinogen receptor on human platelets by intracellular mediators. J Biol Chem 1987;262:992–1000.
129. Falet H, Barkalow KL, Pivniouk VI, Barnes MJ, Geha RS, Hartwig JH. Roles of SLP-76 phosphoinositide 3-kinase, and gelsolin in the platelet shape change initiated by the collagen receptor GPVI/FcRγ-chain complex. Blood 2000;96:3786–3792.
130. Quek LS, Pasquet JM, Hers I, et al. Fyn and Lyn phosphorylate the Fc receptor γchain downstream of glycoprotein VI in murine platelets, and Lyn regulates a novel feedback pathway. Blood 2000;96:4246–4253.
131. Judd BA, Koretzky GA. The role of the adaptor molecule SLP-76 in platelet function. Oncogene 2001;20:6291–6299.

132. Pasquet J-M, Bobe R, Gross B, et al. A collagen related peptide regulates phospholipase Cγ2 via phosphatidylinositol 3-kinase in human platelets. Biochemistry 1999;342:171–177.

133. Gibbins JM, Briddon S, Shutes A, et al. The p85 subunit of phosphatidylinositol 3-kinase associates with the Fc receptor γ-chain and linker for activator T cells (LAT) in platelets stimulated by collagen and convulxin. J Biol Chem 1998;273:34437–34443.

134. Lagrue AH, Francischetti IM, Guimarães JA, Jandrot-Perrus M. Phosphatidylinositol 3'-kinase and tyrosine-phosphatase activation positively modulates convulxin-induced platelet activation: comparison with collagen. FEBS Lett 1999;448:95–100.

135. Massberg S, Gawaz M, Gruner S, et al. A crucial role of glycoprotein VI for platelet recruitment to the injured arterial wall in vivo. J Exp Med 2003;197:41–49.

136. Kato K, Kanaji T, Russell S, et al. The contribution of glycoprotein VI to stable platelet adhesion and thrombus formation illustrated by targeted gene deletion. Blood 2003;102:1701–1707.

137. Nieswandt B, Schulte V, Bergmeier W, et al. Long-term antithrombotic protection by in vivo depletion of platelet glycoprotein VI in mice. J Exp Med 2001;193:459–470.

138. Dohlman HG, Thorner J, Caron MG, Kefkowitz RJ. Model systems for the study of seven-transmembrane-segment receptors. Annu Rev Biochem 1991;60:653–688.

139. Hirata M, Hayashi Y, Ushikubi F, et al. Cloning and expression of cDNA for a human thromboxane A2 receptor. Nature 1991;349:617–620.

140. Katsuyama M, Sugimoto Y, Namba T, et al. Cloning and expression of a cDNA for the human prostaglandin receptor. FEBS Lett 1994;344:74–78.

141. Burgers JA, Akkerman JW. Regulation of the receptor for platelet-activating factor on human platelets. Biochem J 1993;291:157–161.

142. Bandoh K, Aoki J, Hosono H, et al. Molecular cloning and characterization of a novel human G-protein-coupled receptor, EDG7, for lysophosophatidic acid. J Biol Chem 1999;274:27776–27785.

143. Abi-Younes S, Sauty A, Mach F, Sukhova GK, Libby P, Luster AD. The stromal cell-derived factor-1 chemokine is a potent platelet agonist highly expressed in atherosclerotic plaques. Circ Res 2000;86:131–138.

144. Clemetson KJ, Clemetson JM, Proudfoot AE, Power CA, Baggiolini M, Wells TN. Functional expression of CCR1, CCR3, CCR4, and CXCR4 chemokine receptors on human platelets. Blood 2000;96:50–57.

145. Kowalska MA, Ratajczak MZ, Majka M, J et al. Stromal cell-derived factor 1 and macrophage-derived chemokine: 2 chemokines that activate platelets. Blood 2000;96:50–57.

146. Caron MG, Kobilka BK, Frielle T, Bolanowski MA, Benovic JL, Lefkowitz RJ. Cloning of the cNDA and genes for the hamster and human β$_2$-adrenergic receptors. J Recept Res 2000;8:7–21.

147. Kagaya A, Mikuni M, Yamamoto H, Muraoka S, Yamawaki S, Takahashi K. Heterologous supersensitization between serotonin2 and a2-adenergic receptor-mediated intracellular calcium mobilization in human platelets. J Neural Transm 1992;88:25–36.

148. Daniel JL, Dangelmaier C, Jin J, Ashby B, Smith JB, Kunapuli SP. Molecular basis for ADP-induced platelet activation. I. Evidence for three distinct ADP receptors on human platelets. J Biol Chem 1998;273:2024–2029.

149. Cattaneo M, Gachet C. ADP receptors and clinical bleeding disorders. Arterioscler Thromb Vasc Biol 1999;19:2281–2285.

150. Jin J, Daniel JL, Kunapuli SP. Molecular basis for ADP-induced platelet activation. II. The P2Y1 receptor mediates ADP-induced intracellular calcium mobilization and shape change in platelets. J Biol Chem 1998;273:2030–2034.

151. Hollopeter G, Jantzen H-M, Vincent D, et al. Identification of the platelet ADP receptor targeted by antithrombotic drugs. Nature 2001;409:202–206.

152. Zhang FL, Luo L, Gustafson E, et al. ADP is the cognate ligand for the orphan G-protein coupled receptor SP1999. J Biol Chem 2001;276:8608–8615.

153. Jin J, Kunapuli SP. Coactivation of two different G protein-coupled receptors is essential for ADP-induced platelet aggregation. Proc Natl Acad Sci USA 1998;95:8070–8074.

154. Hechler B, Léon C, Vial C, et al. The $P2Y_1$ receptor is necessary for adenosine 5'-diphosphate-induced platelet aggregation. Blood 1998;92:152–159.

155. Savi P, Beauverger P, Labouret C, et al. Role of P2Y1 purinoceptor in ADP-induced platelet activation. FEBS Lett 1998;422:291–295.

156. Bauer M, Retzer M, Wilde JI, et al. Dichotomous regulation of myosin phospho-rylation and shape change by Rho-kinase and calcium in intact human platelets. Blood 1999;94:1665–1672.

157. Wilde JI, Retzer M, Seiss W, Watson SP. ADP-induced platelet shape change: an investigation of the signalling pathways involved and their dependence on the method of platelet preparation. Platelets 2000;11:286–295.

158. Fabre J-E, Nguyen M, Latour A, et al. Decreased platelet aggregation, increased bleeding time and resistance to thromboembolism in $P2Y_1$-deficient mice. Nat Med 1999;5:1199–1202.

159. Léon C, Vial C, Gachet C, et al. The $P2Y_1$ receptor is normal in a patient presenting a severe deficiency of ADP-induced platelet aggregation. Further evidence for a distinct P2 receptor responsible for adenylyl cyclase inhibition. Thromb Haemost 1999;81:775–781.

160. Offermanns S, Toombs CF, Hu Y-H, Simon MI. Defective platelet activation in $G\alpha_q$-deficient mice. Nature 1997;389:183–186.

161. Gachet C. ADP receptors of platelets and their inhibitors. Thromb Haemost 2001;86:222–232.

162. Cattaneo M, Lecchi A, Randi AM, McGregor JL, Mannucci PM. Identification of a new congenital defect of platelet function characterized by severe impairment of platelet responses to adenosine diphosphate. Blood 1992;80:2787–2796.

163. Cattaneo M, Lecchi A, Lombardi R, Gachet C, Zighetti ML. Platelets from a patient heterozygous for the defect of $P2_{CYC}$ receptors have a secretion defect despite normal thromboxane A_2 production and normal granule stores. Arterioscler Thromb Vasc Biol 2000;20:e101–e106.

164. Nurden P, Savi P, Heilmann E, et al. An inherited bleeding disorder linked to a defective interaction between ADP and its receptor on platelets. J Clin Invest 1995;95:1612–1622.

165. Léon C, Hechler B, Freund M, et al. Defective platelet aggregation and increased resistance to thrombosis in purinergic $P2Y_1$ receptor-null mice. J Clin Invest 1999;104:1731–1737.

166. Savi P, Herbert JM. Pharmacology of ticlopidine and clopidogrel. Haematologica 2000;85:73–77.

167. Ingall AH, Dixon J, Bailey A, et al. Antagonists of the platelet P2T receptor: a novel approach to anti-thrombotic therapy. J Med Chem 1999;42:213–220.

168. Humphries RG. Pharmacology of AR-C69931MX and related compounds: from pharmacological tools to clinical trials. Haematologica 2000;85:66–72.

169. Savi P, Labouret C, Delesque N, Guette F, Lupker J, Herbert JM. P2y(12), a new platelet ADP receptor, target of clopidogrel. Biochem Biophys Res Commun 2001;283:379–383.

170. Daniel NG, Goulet J, Bergeron M, Paquin R, Landry P-E. Antiplatelet drugs: is there a surgical risk? J Can Dental Assoc 2002;68:683–687.

171. Sharis PJ, Cannon CP, Loscalzo J. The antiplatelet effects of ticlopidine and clopidogrel. Ann Intern Med 1998;129:394–405.
172. Vu T-KH, Hung DT, Wheaton VI, Coughlin SR. Molecular cloning of a functional thrombin receptor reveals a novel proteolytic mechanism of receptor activation. Cell 1991;64:1057–1068.
173. Vu T-KH, Wheaton VI, Hung DT, Coughlin SR. Domains specifying thrombin-receptor interaction. Nature 1991;353:674–677.
174. Chen J, Ishii M, Wang L, Ishii K, Coughlin SR. Thrombin receptor activation: confirmation of the intramolecular tethered liganding hypothesis and discovery of an alternative intermolecular liganding mode. J Biol Chem 1994;269:16041–16045.
175. Faruqi TR, Weiss EJ, Shapiro MJ, Huang W, Coughlin SR. Structure-function analysis of protease-activated receptor 4 tethered ligand peptides. Determinants of specificity and utility in assays of receptor function. J Biol Chem 2000; 275:19728–19734.
176. Furman MI, Liu L, Benoit SE, Becker RC, Barnard MR, Michelson AD. The cleaved peptide of the thrombin receptor is a strong platelet agonist. Proc Natl Acad Sci USA 1998;95:3082–3087.
177. Rasmussen UB, Vouret-Craviari V, Jallet S, et al. CDNA clonging and expression of a hamster α-thrombin receptor coupled to Ca^{2+} mobilization. FEBS Lett 1991;288:123–128.
178. Ishihara H, Connolly AJ, Zeng D, et al. Protease-activated receptor 3 is a second thrombin receptor in humans. Nature 1997;386:502–506.
179. Xu W-F, Andersen H, Whitmore TE, et al. Cloning and characterization of human protease-activated receptor 4. Proc Natl Acad Sci USA 1998;95:6642–6646.
180. Nystedt S, Emilsson K, Wahlestedt C, Sundelin J. Molecular cloning of a potential proteinase activated receptor. Proc Natl Acad Sci 1994;91:9208–9212.
181. Molino M, Barnathan ES, Numerof R, et al. Interactions of mast cell tryptase with thrombin receptors and PAR-2. J Biol Chem 1997;272:4043–4049.
182. Camerer E, Huang W, Coughlin SR. Tissue factor- and factor X-dependent activation of PAR2 by factor VIIa. Proc Natl Acad Sci USA 2000;97:5255–5260.
183. Nystedt S, Emilsson K, Larsson AK, Strombeck B, Sundelin J. Molecular cloning and functional expression of the gene encoding the human proteinase-activated receptor 2. Eur J Biochem 1995;232:84–89.
184. Mirza H, Schmidt V, Derian C, Jesty J, Bahou WF. Mitogenic responses mediated through the proteinase activated receptor 2 are induced by mast cell α- and β-tryptases. Blood 1997;90:3914–3922.
185. Cupit LD, Schmidt VA, Bahou WF. Proteolytically activated receptor-3. A member of an emerging gene family of protease receptors expressed on vascular endothelial cells and platelets. Trends Cardiovasc Med 1999;9:42–48.
186 Steinhoff M, Vergnolle N, Young S, et al. Agonists of proteinase-activated receptor 2 induce inflammation by a neurogenic mechanism. Nat Med 2000;6:151–158.
187. Kahn ML, Nakanishi-Matsui M, Shapiro MJ, Ishihara H, Coughlin SR. Protease-activated receptors 1 and 4 mediate activation of human platelets by thrombin. J Clin Invest 1999;103:879–887.
188. Covic L, gresser al, kuliopulos a. Biphasic kinetics of activation and signaling for PAR1 and PAR4 thrombin receptors in platelets. Biochemistry 2000;39:5458–5467.
189. Bahou WF, Coller BS, Potter CL, Norton KJ, Kutok JL, Goligorsky MS. The thrombin receptor extracellular domain contains sites crucial for peptide ligand-induced activation. J Clin Invest 1993;91:1405–1413.
190. Brass LF, Manning DR, Cichowski K, Abrams C. Signaling through G proteins in platelets to the integrins and beyond. Thromb Haemost 1997;78:582–589.

191. Kramer RM, Roberts EF, Um SL, et al. p38 mitogen-activated protein kinase phosphorylates cytosolic phospholipase A_2 (cPLA$_2$) in thrombin-stimulated platelets. Evidence that proline-directed phosphorylation is not required for mobilization of arachidonic acid by cPLA$_2$. J Biol Chem 1996;271:27723–27729.

192. O'Brien PJ, Prevost N, Molino M, et al. Thrombin responses in human endothelial cells. Contributions from receptors other than PAR1 include the transactivation of PAR2 by thrombin-cleaved PAR1. J Biol Chem 2000;275:13502–13509.

193. Bernatowicz M, Klimas C, Hartl K, Peluso M, Alegretto N, Seiler SM. Development of potent thrombin receptor antagonist peptides. J Med Chem 1996;39:4879–4887.

194. Andrade-Gordon P, Maryanoff BE, Derian CK, et al. Design, synthesis, and biological characterization of a peptide-mimetic antagonist for a tethered-ligand receptor. Proc Natl Acad Sci USA 1999; 96:12257–12262.

195. Maeda H, Inazu T, Nagau K, Maruyama S, Nakagawara G, Yamamura H. Possible involvement of protein-tyrosine kinases such as p72[SYK] in the disc-sphere change response of porcine platelets. J Biochem 1995;17:1201–1208.

196 Yamamoto H, Vreys I, Stassen JM, Yoshimoto R, Vermylen J, Hoylaerts MF. Antagonism of vWF inhibits both injury induced arterial and venous thrombosis in the hamster. Thromb Haemost 1998;79:202–210.

197. Scarborough RM, Kleiman NS, Philips DR. Platelet glycoprotein IIb/IIa antagonists. What are the relevant issues concerning their pharmacology and clinical use? Circulation 1999;100:437–444.

198. Ware J, Russell S, Ruggeri ZM. Generation and rescue of a murine model of platelet dysfunction: the Bernard-Soulier Syndrome. Proc Natl Acad Sci USA 2000;97:2803–2808.

199. Law DA, Nannizzi-Alaimo L, Ministri K, et al. Genetic and pharmacologic analyses of Syk function in $\alpha_{IIb}\beta_3$ signaling in platelets. Blood 1999;93:2645–2652.

200. Soriano P, Montgomery C, Geske R, Bradley A. Targeted disruption of the c-src proto-oncogene leads to osteopetrosis in mice. Cell 1991;64:693–702.

4 Structure–Function of the Platelet Cytoskeleton

Elaine L. Bearer, MD, PhD

INTRODUCTION

Platelet activation results in a rapid series of reproducible morphological events that transform the nonsticky, discoid circulating platelet into a sticky, spikey glue. This morphological transformation depends on actin and is a common feature of all cell-based clotting systems across evolution. An exciting recent discovery is the identification of the protein complex that mediates the actin polymerization underlying this event, Arp2/3 *(1)*. This chapter presents the background for this discovery by first reviewing the morphology of resting and activated platelets. Then examples of other proteins involved in stabilizing and reorganizing the platelet actin cytoskeleton are described, and the findings that place Arp2/3 at the center of these events are presented. Finally, a model integrating the various activities of these proteins with the morphologi-

From: *Contemporary Cardiology:*
Platelet Function: Assessment, Diagnosis, and Treatment
Edited by: M. Quinn and D. Fitzgerald © Humana Press Inc., Totowa, NJ

Table 1
Complexity Factors in Platelet Actin Dynamics

Time	Changes occur at different rates depending on external and internal factors
Number of components	>100 actin binding proteins in platelets
Redundancy	More than one protein performing the same physiological function
Multitasking	The same protein performing multiple functions at the same time—bundling and stabilizing
Modular functionality	The same biochemical activity at the molecular level contributing to different functions at the cellular level
Partnering	Different proteins working in groups Group membership not static
Activity of individual proteins affected by	ADP–ATP actin ratio, filament-to-monomer ratio Abundance-relative concentrations of each partner to actin Posttranslational modification Isoform effects
Individual platelet variations	Age of platelet in circulation Composition of platelet when formed
Donor variability	Allelic variation of each protein

cal changes of activation is proposed. The chapter focuses on the actin cytoskeleton, although platelets also have microtubules *(2)* and a vimentin-like intermediate filament protein *(3)*.

The Actin Cytoskeleton

The actin cytoskeleton is complex at many levels (Table 1). In the time dimension, it is continuously changing, and the rate of change differs at different points in the activation process and between different parts within the same platelet. In all cells and in vitro, actin filaments are in a slow dynamic equilibrium with actin monomers. Even in quiescent cells and resting platelets, actin filaments constantly turn over. Within seconds of activation by agonists, the rate of turnover dramatically increases as actin filaments are rapidly severed and recreated. This rapid rate of filament turnover gradually subsides and is replaced by the slower process of organizing these new filaments into multifilament assemblies. Organization of filamentous structures continues at progressively slower rates for hours to days as the thrombus matures, contracts, and resolves. The large number of proteins involved and the many different ways their activity is influenced increase this complexity. Over 100 different cytoskeletal or cytoskeleton-related proteins have been identified in platelets (4). Each of these proteins can play multiple roles in various cellular processes.

Analysis of the interactions between these many proteins over time requires strategies similar to those of new computational systems biology now at the forefront of biological inquiry (5,6). Over many years, biochemists working to identify and study each of these proteins in platelets in isolation, in combination, and inside the cell have developed experimental strategies and analytical approaches comparable to dynamic systems theory. Their original work is well worth reading, although only some of it can be summarized here.

Actin is highly abundant in platelets (estimated at 14–20% of the total protein [7,8]), and other actin-binding and regulating proteins are also expected to be in platelets. Since actin is highly conserved across eukaryotes, it also is expected that these regulatory and binding proteins will be conserved. Thus proteins discovered in human platelets are likely to have homologs with similar functions across species. In addition, the platelet is a fragment of the cortical cytoplasm of the bone marrow megakaryocyte. Thus, it is already a semipurified subcellular particle, naturally devoid of the nucleus and other cellular structures that contaminate subcellular fractionations performed in vitro from nucleated culture or tissue cells. Particularly valuable for biochemical analysis is the ability to activate simultaneously large numbers of platelets to polymerize actin experimentally in the test tube, thus acquiring a population undergoing similar biochemical events synchronously.

Experimental Techniques

There are significant challenges to experimentation aimed at defining the platelet cytoskeleton. First, platelets are anucleate, which makes DNA transfections impossible. Second, platelets have yet to be produced in vitro—there is no culture system that reliably produces human platelets in numbers sufficient for molecular study. Third, blood platelets from human donors commonly used for investigation are "wild type," which has both advantages and disadvantages. The advantage is that any process common among platelets from different donors is a reliable indication that it is important for platelet function and not an artifact of inbreeding or culture systems.

Conversely, however, the complement of proteins in platelets from individual donors may differ. Because the platelet is so tiny, small variations can mean big differences. Not only are there differences between donors, there are also differences between individual platelets from any one donor, owing to differences in the age of each platelet and in inequalities arising during formation in the bone marrow. Finally, human platelets are very small, 3.1 ± 0.3 mm in diameter, with an average thickness of 1.0 ± 0.2 μm and a calculated volume of only 7 fL *(9,10)*. Mouse platelets are even smaller. This small size means that even though there may be 150,000 platelets/dL of blood, the total volume of platelets is low. Therefore the total amount of protein, even for a protein relatively abundant within the platelet itself, is also low compared with that of red blood cells or most plasma proteins. Variations in protein content, size, and age of any individual platelet, together with its small size, can be impediments to the application of morphological techniques and must be kept in mind when one is interpreting biochemical results from populations of platelets or morphological results from small numbers of platelets.

Most satisfying would be an experimental system that can reveal the function of specific proteins during platelet thrombus formation in the whole animal. However, generating mice homozygous for a deletion in platelet proteins has been hampered by the late stage of differentiation of the platelet. In order to observe specific platelet defects, the gene must not be required for embryogenesis, nor for the differentiation of megakaryocytes from bone marrow precursors. Furthermore, some coagulation is required for successful birthing. Mice deficient in platelet function have coagulopathies causing death during birthing. It is of note that even for actin itself, we still do not know whether polymerization and consequent shape change are required for adequate coagulation.

For a few genes suspected to be involved in shape change, knockouts have been successfully generated, including gelsolin *(11)*, vasodilator-stimulated phosphoprotein (VASP) *(12–14)*, spectrin *(15)*, and μ-calpain *(16)*. For profilin I, however, homozygous knockouts are embryonic lethal, and hetrozygotes also have limited embryonic survival *(17)*. Thus, for many platelet proteins it has been necessary to develop other clever strategies to manipulate proteins inside the mature platelet in order to determine their function. Such experimental strategies include (1) permeabilization of the platelet to allow entry of labeled molecules or specific inhibitors *(1,18,19)*, and (2) tagging proteins with cell-permeable octapeptides, such as the signal sequence from Kaposi's fibroblast growth factor, for delivery across the cell membrane *(20)*.

Because of these limitations to experimental manipulation, direct correlations between activity of a protein in vitro and its role in platelet function have been achieved in only a few cases. Thus a large amount of knowledge remains to be discovered about how the platelet enacts its vital coagulative function in the body.

MORPHOLOGY OF PLATELET ACTIVATION

Platelets circulating in the blood are discoid. Within seconds of exposure to an agonist, such as activated factor II (thrombin), morphological changes begin, as evidenced by quick-freeze capture within 2 s of thrombin stimulation on a helium-cooled copper block *(21)*. The first detectable event is a change in the structure of the membrane skeleton and the filaments associated with it. A flip in the anionic phospholipids of the membrane bilayer accompanies this change, together with an opening of the surface-connected canalicular system. This is followed by large-scale morphological changes, including rounding, protrusion of filopodia, and spreading. Some morphological changes that occur in platelets in suspension may be different from those occurring during spreading on a flat surface *(22)*. This difference may be a consequence of the type of structure to which the platelet is adhering. Flat surfaces induce different organization of the integrin adhesion receptors than do long fibrin fibrils. The morphological changes during spreading on glass are well documented. Exposure of platelets to glass has proved to be a powerful way to observe events of shape change during spreading on a flat surface.

Video microscopy demonstrates that, when exposed to glass, platelets in plasma undergo a reproducible sequence of morphological events: first rounding, followed by the projection of filopodia, then spreading, and finally contraction (Fig. 1) *(23)*. Early events in shape change may be reversible, although protruding structures would be expected to affect the ability of platelets to circulate through the microvasculature. Because this sequence of morphological changes is reproducible from one platelet to the next, the stage in activation of any individual platelet after fixation can be reliably determined. Thus, the morphology of the platelet fixed during spreading on glass has become a reliable indicator of whether a particular event in the process of shape change has been disturbed or preserved under various experimental treatment conditions *(1,18,20,24)*. Staining of filamentous actin with fluorescently labeled phalloidin provides a rapid method to detect effects on actin polymerization and filament organization *(24)*. This approach is potentially useful for high-throughput analysis of the effect of drugs on platelet activation. Proteins involved in regulating these events are now being discovered by their effect on this series of events *(1)*.

Different agonists and different matrix proteins produce different morphological results, possibly by stimulating different downstream regulatory proteins. In vivo, it is most likely that circulating platelets encounter many different agonists simultaneously, and this is also true for studies performed in plasma.

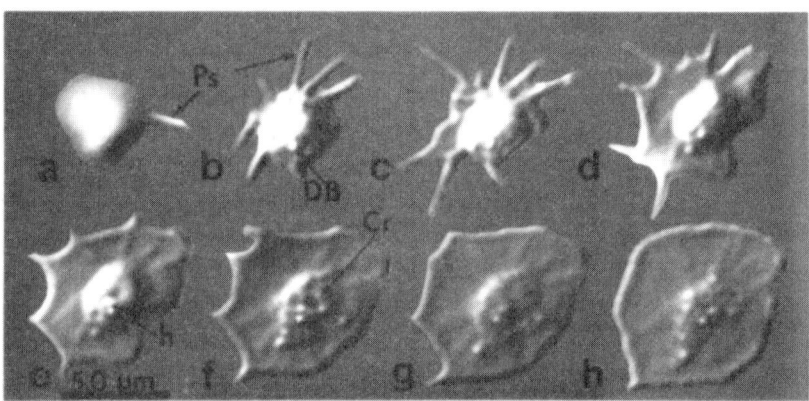

Fig. 1. Video imaging of platelets spreading on glass. **(a–d)** Frames from a video sequence of a single platelet taken at 0, 1, 2, 3, 4, 7, 8, and 13 min during contact with substrate in plasma showing the events in the transformation from spherical (a) to spread (H). The central core of cytoplasm contracts (b) as multiple filopodia project in the space of 1 min. Subsequently, elongation of filopodia is accompanied by spreading of the interfilopodial lateral membrane. DB, -dense body; h, -hyalomere; and Cr, -crater. (Reproduced from ref. *23*, with permission.)

ACTIN REORGANIZATIONS IN PLATELET ACTIVATION

Actin reorganization parallels the morphological changes during activation and spreading. In the fully spread platelet, actin filaments are organized into four morphologically and functionally distinct structures: the contractile ring, a correlate of rounding; filopodia; lamellipodia; and stress-like fibers (Fig. 2) *(24)*. These structures are readily imaged by fluorescent microscopy after staining with fluorescently labeled phalloidin. These structures correlate with those observed by Nomarski optics in video sequences of platelets adhering in plasma to glass. They can form within the first 1–2 min of exposure to glass, and most platelets display them after 10 min. The formation of these structures occurs sequentially. During rounding, the contractile ring begins to separate from the membrane skeleton. Next, filopodia protrude. As adhesion begins, lamellipodia spread out while stress-like bundles of actin filaments coalesce internally. Lamellipodia can form between filopodia or *de novo* from the edge of the platelet. As adhesion matures over 30–60 min, first adhesion plaques are consolidated, as can be visualized with antibody staining for vinculin *(25)* or VASP *(26–29)*, and then stress-like fibers rearrange into parallel bundles in preparation for the contractile events that underlie clot retraction.

Actin polymerization, filament reorganizations, and contractions of the filament network are regulated by a complicated series of biochemi-

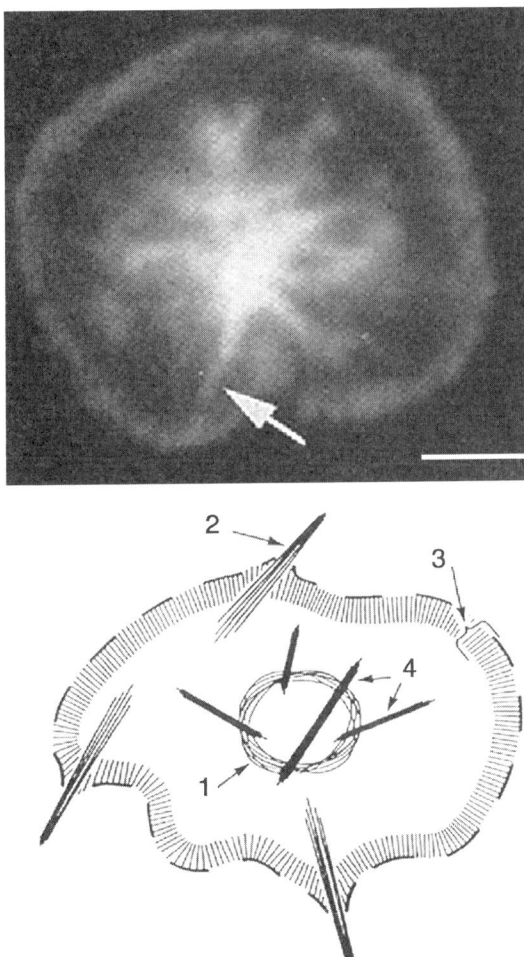

Fig. 2. F-actin distribution in a spread platelet. Fluorescent phalloidin staining of representative spread platelet **(top)** reveals distinct actin-rich areas. These can be classified **(bottom)** in order of appearance: contractile ring (1), filopodia (2); lamellipodia (3), and stress-like fibers (4). The contractile ring is on a different focal plane than the lamellipodia and is not imaged in this example (A). Bar = 5 μm in A. (Reproduced from ref. *24*, with permission.)

cal interactions within the platelet. These begin with an external signal that is transmitted across the membrane, producing a cascade of protein interaction culminating in an effect on the actin structures. This cascade involves many different signaling pathways that also produce other downstream effects. One event in this cascade is a change in the integrin receptor such that it becomes "sticky," i.e., enzymatic activity inside the platelet changes its surface properties on the outside. This has been termed *inside-out signaling (30)*. The precise signaling pathway that activates actin reorganizations in platelets is not known but by analogy to other cells is thought to involve the rho family of small GTPases, including rhoA, rac1 and -2, and cdc42 *(31)*. Different agonists probably activate different upstream signaling events, all of which must culminate via a convergent pathway on Arp2/3. This pathway in platelets remains an area of intense investigation.

A major question is how the timed formation of these different structures out of the same essential building block, actin, is achieved. One attractive idea was that each structure might be induced and organized by a different set of actin-associated proteins, but, as we shall see, this turned out to be incorrect.

THE PROTEINS OF THE ACTIN CYTOSKELETON

ACTIN

Actin has long been recognized as a key contributor to the initial events in platelet activation. Actin is a globular protein, 42.5 kDa in molecular weight. The human genome contains three actin isoforms, α, β, and γ. Platelets contain primarily β and γ isoforms *(32,33)*, at very high concentrations (0.5 mM, estimated 15–20% of the total protein) *(7,8)*. Inside the platelet (as in most eukaryotic cells), actin is found in both monomeric and filamentous polymer states *(34)*. In the unstimulated platelet, 40–50% of this actin is polymerized, whereas within 20 s of activation, this increases to 70% *(35)*. It is estimated that there are approx 2000 filaments in each platelet, with an average length of 1.1 μm *(19)*. During the various stages of platelet function, the distribution and organization of the actin filaments within the platelet change. Each new structure appears to be initiated by a different sequence of signaling events, performs a unique function, and is associated with a different complement of proteins *(24)*. Molecules associated with the actin structures are either involved in the behavior of the actin or are stabilized by their association with actin in order to perform other functions.

The key step in platelet shape change is actin polymerization. Whether this process is a result of elongation of short severed filaments or *de novo* polymerization of actin monomers is still not clear, although recent evidence, summarized below, shows that Arp2/3 nucleation is required. How actin polymerizes has been the subject of many studies over a number of years. Purified actin polymerizes on its own in the test tube. This polymerization has long been the focus of biochemical investigation, and it is not possible to describe all of the details here. For more details, readers should consult cell biology text books. Key features of the actin polymerization process relevant to this discussion are the following. Actin polymerization occurs in two steps: formation of a trimer, which nucleates filament formation, and elongation of trimers or other actin polymers to create longer filaments. The critical step in filament formation is thought to be stabilization of the trimer, which is thermodynamically unstable. Once stabilized, elongation by monomer addition occurs rapidly from the barbed or fast growing end, and 10 times more slowly from the other, pointed, end *(36–38)*. Actin monomers bind either ATP or ADP and a divalent cation, either Ca^{2+} or Mg^{2+}. ATP-charged actin has high affinity for the barbed end, whereas ADP actin binds to both ends equally. Thus, when actin monomers are recharged to polymerize by exchanging ADP for ATP, they polymerize more rapidly at the barbed end. Profilin, a small 14-kDa protein formerly thought to sequester actin and inhibit polymerization, has more recently been shown to catalyze this ADP-ATP exchange *(39,40)*, recharging actin monomers for rapid barbed end elongation.

During shape change, different proteins must interact directly with actin to cause a profound reorganization of the platelet cytoskeleton. In order to mediate the precision of these events in shape change, the proteins that disassemble and reassemble actin filaments, bundle and orient them, attach the filaments to surface adhesions, and mediate the contractile event must be tightly choreographed. The full complement of proteins involved in these many activities and how their activities are coordinated to produce four different actin filament-rich structures within the 1–10 min of platelet shape change and adhesion are still unknown.

Proteomics Approach to the Actin Cytoskeleton

To identify all the platelet proteins that bind to actin in a single step, we used filamentous (F)-actin affinity chromatography (Fig. 3) *(24)*. Resting and ADP-activated platelets are solubilized by detergent and sonicated to depolymerize existing filaments. After clarification by centrifugation, parallel aliquots of the lysate are passed over either an F-actin or a control column, coupled to monomeric (G) actin, insulin, or bovine serum albumin. The eluted proteins can be separated by sodium dodecyl sulfate-polyacrylamide gel electrophoresis (SDS-PAGE) and those eluting uniquely from the F-actin column subjected to further study. Using this technique, 33 different protein bands are obtained in sufficient abundance for biochemical analysis. This large number of different proteins poses a logistical question: how to select those of most physiologic significance.

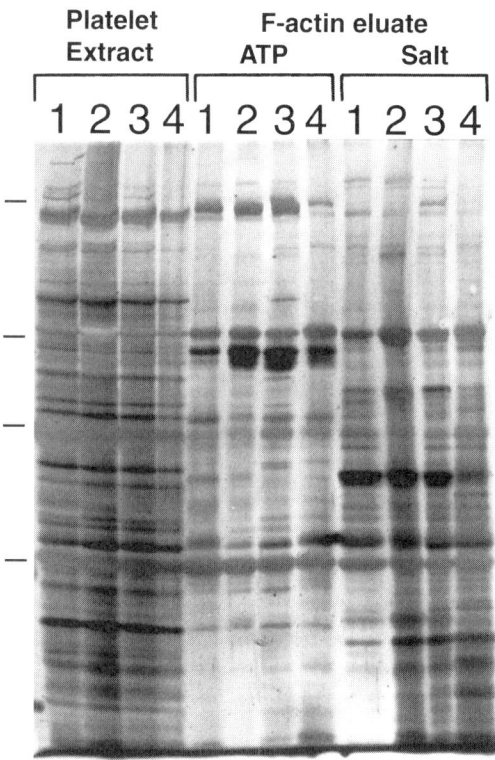

Fig. 3. Biochemical analysis of platelet actin-binding proteins by F-actin affinity columns. Extracts of ADP-activated human platelets from four different donors (lanes 1–4) were loaded onto four different filamentous actin affinity columns. After washing with column buffer, proteins bound to actin were sequentially eluted first with 5 mM ATP and then with 1 M KCl (salt). Extracts and eluates were electrophoresed in parallel on 10% SDS-PAGE. Each band represents a different protein species. The pattern of proteins from different donors reveals some variability, although the more abundant protein species are enriched across all donors. Molecular weight markers indicated to the left, from the top, are: 200, 98, 68, and 43 kDa. (Reproduced from ref. *24*, with permission.)

Our strategy to identify physiologically significant proteins from among the 33-actin binding proteins is to raise antibodies specific to each novel protein and use the antibodies as probes to obtain clues about their function. The unknown protein bands are cut from preparative curtain gels of F-actin eluates and used to generate polyclonal antisera in mice. The resultant antiserum provides tools to localize each protein in the spread platelet by immunofluorescence, to detect the protein in Western blots, to follow it through purification protocols, and to clone it from expression libraries and thereby derive the sequences.

Using antibodies against 14 of these proteins, we found that each distinct actin-rich structure of the spread platelet was also biochemically distinct—each actin structure contained a different complement of these actin-binding proteins (Fig. 4). Some proteins were present in all actin structures, and some were restricted to one or the other of the structures forming in the first 10 minutes of spreading on glass—the filopodia, lamellipodia, contractile ring, or stress fibers.

The 14 unknown proteins fell into nine categories, including two for polymerization, according to their location in spread platelets, human skeletal muscle and chick fibroblasts (Table 2). Some proteins were found in all actin structures, and, some in only one or the other. Most were also found in fibroblasts in similar structures as in platelets, whereas a few were expressed in skeletal muscle.

Each actin-rich structure appears at a different time and develops at a different rate. Filopodia appear first and elongate rapidly, whereas lamellipodia begin next, with a quick start, slower progression, and termination by 10 min. The contractile ring also begins quickly but then moves slowly inward throughout spreading. Stress fibers develop even more slowly, connecting surface adhesions across the platelet, and are sometimes not detected until 30 min or more after exposure to glass. Thus, a major question is: how do proteins interact with actin and each other to produce the timed formation of these structures and their corresponding functions within the 1–10 min of shape change?

Polymerization underlies all of these events. Since the protein(s) involved in actin polymerization in platelets were not known, we decided to focus on polymerization to see whether this comprehensive F-actin affinity approach might identify the protein(s) responsible *(24,41)*. We therefore looked for proteins whose staining pattern correlated with sites where actin filaments were expected to form during spreading, using location as a clue of function. Proteins were assigned numbers for identification according to their order in SDS-PAGE gels of actin column eluates and classified into nine groups according to molecular weights and staining patterns in platelets, fibroblasts, and muscle. At this point, the working hypothesis was that each structure is nucleated by a different protein. Nucleation would initiate the difference between structures. We therefore selected three proteins, found in each structure, i.e., along filopodia, at the tips of stress-like fibers, and at the outer edge of the lamellipodia, to search for these nucleators: 2E4/kaptin, Arp2, and VASP. At the time we cloned them, all three of these proteins were novel, although subsequently two, Arp2 and VASP, were studied and named by other groups. This leaves six groups of novel proteins, 11 proteins in all, which remain to be characterized.

ANTIBODY   **ACTIN**

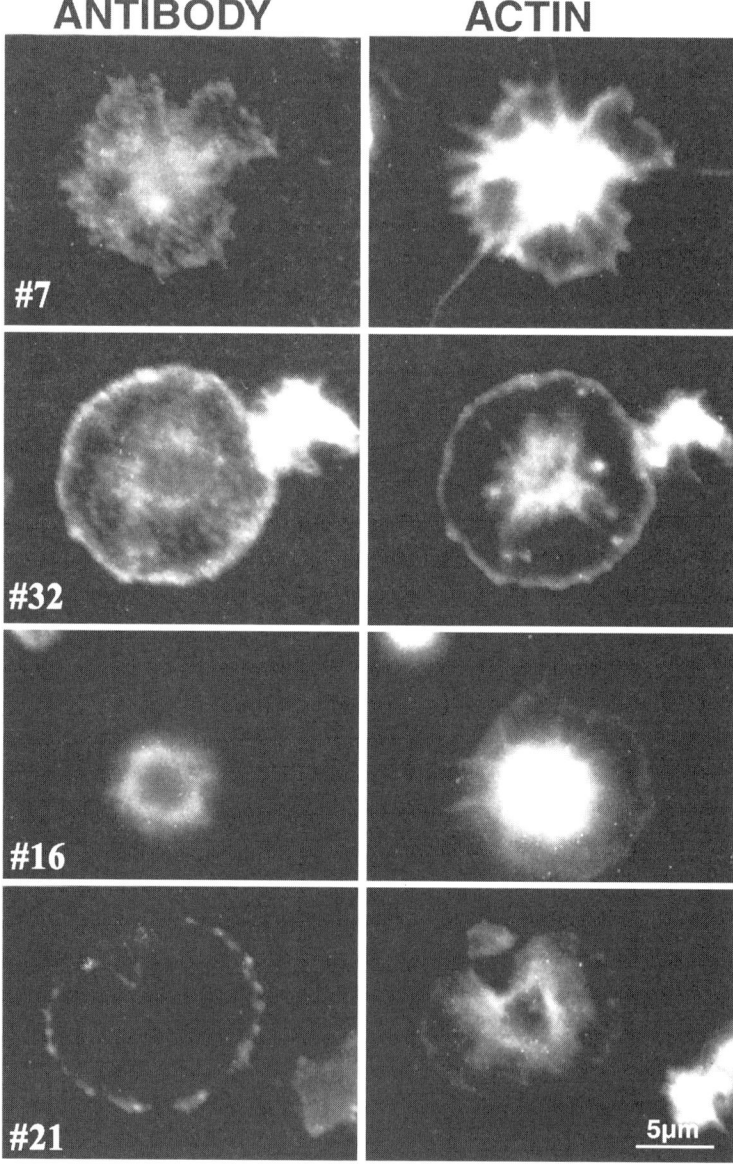

Fig. 4. Location of various actin-binding proteins in spread platelets. Antibodies were raised against proteins eluting from the F-actin columns and used to label spread platelets by immunofluorescence (left panels) with fluorescent phalloidin used as a counterstain for actin filaments (right panels). Shown are four examples of different staining patterns. This indicates that different actin structures contain a different complement of proteins. Proteins associated with particular structures could mediate either their formation, their maintenance, or their function. (Reproduced from ref. *24*, with permission.)

Table 2
Examples of Actin Binding Proteins in Platelets

Structure/function	Protein	Approximate size (kDa)
Membrane skeleton	Spectrin	220/240
	Adducin ($\alpha\,\gamma$)	103/84
	ABP	260/280
Monomer binding	Thymosin $\beta 4$	5
	Profilin 1	14
	Profilin 2	14
Barbed end capping	CapZ, capping protein	32/34
	Gelsolin	82
Side binding	α-Actinin	110
	Tropomyosin	34
Severing	Cofilin	16-18
	Gelsolin	82
Contractile ring	Myosin IIA	210
Polymerization		
Pointed end binding/nucleation	Arp2/3 complex	47, 44, 40, 36, 21, 18, 13
Protecting barbed ends	VASP	55/57
	Kaptin/2E4	45
Higher order structures	ABP	260/280
	VASP	55/57
	α-Actinin	110
	Fascin	58

The immediate effectors of actin filament dynamics are the proteins directly interacting with actin. Upstream of these proteins are enzymatic signaling events that regulate their activity, which is a hot area of investigation in which little is yet defined and will not be discussed further here. Actin-binding proteins can be subdivided into those that affect actin structures and those that use actin to be localized in a particular place in the cytoplasm in order to perform some other function. Those proteins that affect actin structures can be further subdivided into three types: (1) those that regulate actin dynamics, such as nucleators, monomer-binding proteins, capping proteins, and severing factors; (2) those that stabilize filaments and/or organize filaments into higher order structures, such as bundles or orthogonal networks; and (3) those that use actin tracks as supports for transport or contraction, i.e., motors. All these proteins must work in concert to coordinate cell shape changes. Each of these activities plays specific roles in a particular event during platelet shape change.

ACTIN DYNAMICS IN RESTING PLATELETS

Two aspects of actin behavior in resting platelets have received the most attention: the biochemical basis of stability of actin filaments in the presence of high monomer concentrations and the morphology of the actin-rich structures that contribute to discoid shape.

Biochemical Basis of Filament Stability in Resting Platelets

In resting platelets, actin filaments are stable, and the monomer pool is high (300–350 μM) *(42,43)*, hundreds of times greater than the critical concentration for polymerization in vitro (0.2–1.0 μM) *(36)*. Several factors contribute to this paradox. First, monomer binding proteins sequester actin so that it is not available to polymerize. Second, side-binding proteins stabilize filaments such that they cannot depolymerize. Finally, barbed end capping proteins block elongation of existing filaments. In addition, the rigidity of the intact membrane skeleton probably also mechanically interferes with protrusive activity that might otherwise cause deviation from the discoid shape optimal for free circulation in the microvasculature.

Different proteins perform each of these functions. Monomer sequestration is performed by thymosin β4 (Tβ4). Most of the soluble actin in the platelet is found in a 1:1 complex with Tβ4 *(44)*. Tβ4 is a 5-kDa protein that binds only to actin monomers. Its only function detected so far inside cells is actin monomer binding *(45)*. When actin monomer is bound to Tβ4, it cannot polymerize. Tβ4 has a Kd for monomeric actin of 0.4–0.7 μM, and is present in platelets at approx 560 μM. Mathematical calculations that assume most (95%) of the barbed ends in platelets are capped, and based on these in vitro binding constants, predict that most of the monomeric actin in platelets is sequestered in the form of Tβ4-actin dimers.

Capping the barbed ends of filaments in resting platelets may be primarily performed by CapZ/capping protein, a heterodimer *(46,47)*. There are 2–5 μM of capping protein in platelets. The behavior of this protein in resting compared with thrombin-activated platelets is complicated. In one report, 75–80% of the total capping protein in resting platelets sediments under conditions that pellet filaments of both the central core and the membrane skeleton *(46)*. After thrombin stimulation (10 s), 15% of this capping protein leaves the high-speed pellet and becomes soluble. Conversely, in another report *(47)*, 35% of the capping protein in resting platelets is found in the low-speed Triton-insoluble pellet, which contains only the central core filaments and not the membrane skeleton. After thrombin stimulation (20 s), capping protein increases to 60% in this pellet, but so do many other structures including most of the membrane skeleton. Thus, whereas some capping protein dissociates from actin altogether in the early stages of thrombin stimulation, that associated with the low-speed pellet increases. This increase in the low-speed pellet probably represents a tighter association between the filaments of the core and those in the membrane, possibly as a consequence of the contractile events occurring during rounding, which is the morphological correlate of this time point. Indeed, immunomicroscopy by both studies localizes capping protein to the membrane of the lamellipodia after spreading.

Taken together, these two studies suggest that most of the capping protein is associated with the membrane-bound filaments in the resting platelet, since these are soluble at low g-force after Triton extraction and would not be found in the low-speed pellet. After thrombin, the membrane skeleton is not solubilized and becomes more firmly attached to the core filaments, which results in the appearance of membrane-associated proteins such as capping protein in the low-speed pellet. Variability of detection of capping protein in the supernatant probably reflects a dynamic equilibrium during the process of polymerization, when capping protein comes on and off filaments too rapidly to capture by these biochemical techniques. Capping protein may play its most crucial role in platelet physiology during polymerization after agonist activation.

Uncapping of the barbed ends by capping protein has been postulated to accompany activation and be responsible for the rapid polymerization of filaments (8,18,48–50). Capping protein shifts from an insoluble filament-associated state to a soluble unattached state after stimulation in a reversible dynamic fashion with capping and uncapping of growing filaments throughout the process of shape change. Capping of some filaments focuses elongation on those particular filaments that are not capped (51). The formation of complex multifilament networks such as those formed during platelet spreading probably involves continuous rounds of polymerization, severing, and capping, with individual filaments growing at different rates to different lengths.

In addition to inhibition of polymerization by monomer sequestration and capping, actin in the resting platelet is also stabilized in filaments by side-binding proteins. Stabilization of filaments in the resting platelet is likely to be mediated by many different side-binding proteins, chief among which are the tropomyosins (52).

TROPOMYOSINS

Little recent information has been added to the understanding or function of tropomyosins in platelets (53–55). There are nine isoforms, some generated by alternative splicing (56). Known as components of the contractile apparatus in muscle, tropomyosins bind in the groove along the length of actin filaments, protecting them from small depolymerizing factors such as cofilin but not from severing by gelsolin. They can regulate myosin-based movements by permitting or blocking myosin's access to the filament, and thus play a role in clot retraction. Different isoforms may block access to different myosins, thus controlling the type of motility occurring on specific filaments *(57)*. In addition, tropomyosins block cofilin depolymerization, thus regulating the stability of filaments *(58)*. In platelets, tropomyosins are likely to stabilize filaments in the resting state as well as throughout all stages of thrombus formation. Tropomyosin-stabilized filaments may serve as a nidus for the rapid burst of polymerization that follows agonist activation, both for barbed end elongation and for docking sites of Arp2/3 activation off the sides *(59,60)*.

VASP

Another protein that binds the sides of filaments and stabilizes them is VASP (Fig. 5) *(29)*. Recent information presents a complex picture of VASP's role in actin dynamics. VASP was first discovered as a major substrate of protein kinase A activated by vasoactive substances such as nitroprusside *(61)*. VASP binds filaments and blocks severing by gelsolin *(29)* but also bundles filaments in vitro *(62)* and induces polymerization *(29,63,64)*. VASP forms tetramers *(65)*, which may explain its in vitro bundling properties. VASP may compete with capping protein or gelsolin for the barbed ends of filaments and thereby be permissive for barbed end elongation *(29,63,66,67)*. The combination of uncapping and bundling of the tips of nascent filaments may produce sites for localized filament elongation, such as that producing filopodia.

VASP is phosphorylated on three sites by cyclic nucleotide-activated protein kinase A, and phosphorylation correlates with suppression of platelet activation *(68–70)*. By corollary, dephosphorylation is associated with activation *(71)*. This directly links VASP with the signal trans-

---

Fig. 5. *(opposite page)* VASP bundles filaments, stabilizing them against severing by gelsolin, and accelerates polymerization. (**A**) Direct observation of severing of phalloidin-labeled filaments occurs in the presence of gelsolin and calcium. In the presence of VASP, actin filaments are bundled (**B**) and do not sever when gelsolin and calcium are added (**C**). Bundling by VASP may be cooperative, since bundles appear even at low VASP concentrations. (**D**) VASP also induces polymerization of monomeric actin in the pyrene-actin assay. (**E**) VASP blocks the depolymerization of actin filaments normally caused by gelsolin in a dose-dependent manner, even though gelsolin binds to the filaments, as shown in sedimentation assays followed by gel and Western blot analysis. (Reproduced from refs. *29* and *31*, with permission.)

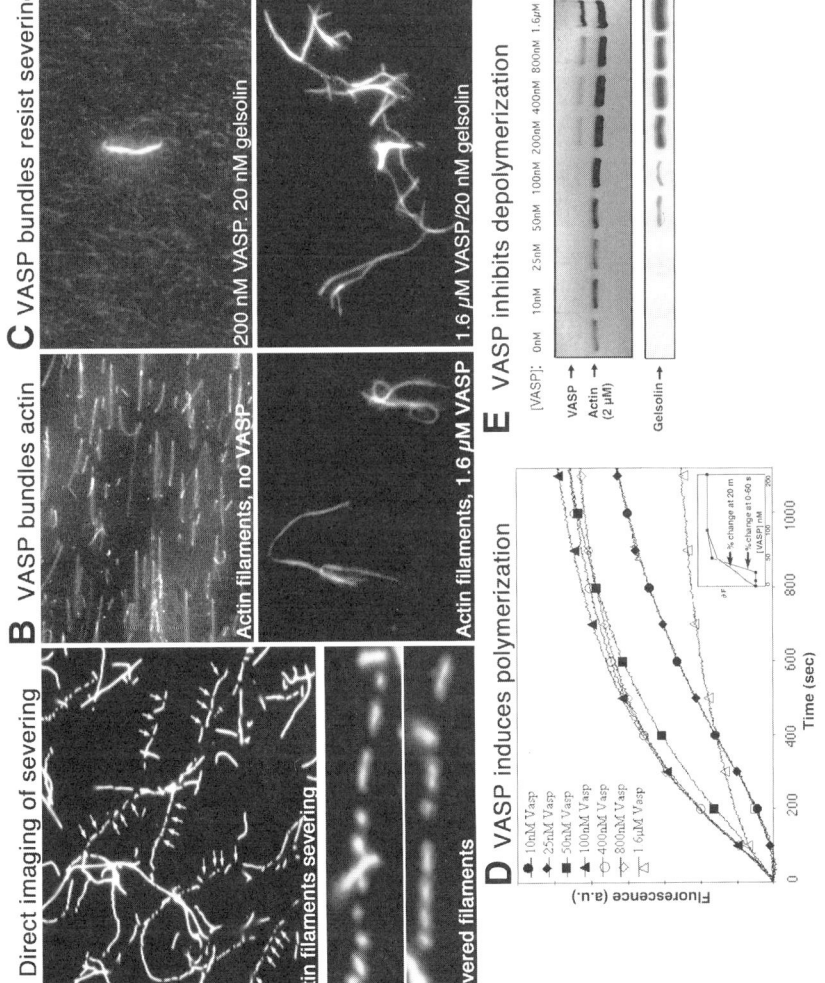

A Direct imaging of severing

Actin filaments severing

Severed filaments

B VASP bundles actin

Actin filaments, no VASP

Actin filaments, 1.6 µM VASP

C VASP bundles resist severing

200 nM VASP, 20 nM gelsolin

1.6 µM VASP/20 nM gelsolin

D VASP induces polymerization

- ● 10nM Vasp
- ◆ 25nM Vasp
- ■ 50nM Vasp
- ▲ 100nM Vasp
- ○ 400nM Vasp
- ▽ 800nM Vasp
- △ 1.6µM Vasp

Fluorescence (a.u.)

Time (sec)

%-change at 20 m

%-change at 0-60 s

[VASP] nM

E VASP inhibits depolymerization

[VASP]: 0nM 10nM 25nM 50nM 100nM 200nM 400nM 800nM 1.6µM

VASP →
Actin → (2 µM)

Gelsolin →

87

duction pathway that inhibits platelet activation. Thus VASP is a potential target for therapeutic intervention of coagulation disorders.

VASP knockout mice have also been generated with minimal phenotypic effects. These platelets demonstrate slightly increased adhesion *(12,13,72)*, increased spreading *(72)*, and a slight decrease in RGD binding in response to the cyclic nucleotides that activate protein kinase A and inhibit platelet shape change. A *Drosophila* homolog of VASP, Ena, was discovered in a genetic screen for genes that suppressed the effect of mutations in the abl oncogene homolog *(73)*, and subsequently a third VASP-like protein, Evl, was identified *(74)*. All three of these proteins share three domains, EVH1, polyproline-rich, and EVH2. These domains are also found in several other proteins in both *Drosophila* and humans, including one expressed during eye development in flies *(75)*. Humans have all three VASP-like proteins, VASP, Ena, and Evl, and probably other proteins with homologies in one or the other of the three main VASP domains. The finding that VASP knockouts have minor effects suggests the presence of other VASP homologs or proteins with redundant functions to VASP.

VASP's activity inside cells is variable. In different circumstances, VASP seems to play alternative roles of either accelerating actin polymerization or decreasing it. For example, platelet extracts support the motility of several intracellular bacteria, including *Listeria monocytogenes (62,76,77)*. This motility is dependent on bacterial stimulation of actin polymerization by the recruitment of a "polymerization machine," which includes VASP *(27,78–82)*. However, in Ena/VASP/ knockout cells, bacterial motility is slower, but cellular motility is faster than in parent wild-type cells *(78)*. Expression of VASP has the reciprocal effect of increasing bacterial motility and decreasing cellular locomotion.

This paradoxical effect suggests that under some conditions, probably in conjunction with one set of actin-binding proteins, VASP potentiates polymerization, whereas under other conditions with a different set of proteins, VASP slows polymerization. We explained this paradox by showing that VASP stabilizes filaments (Fig. 5A, B, and D) *(29)*. Stabilization of nascent filaments slows cell movements, which require constant remodeling of short filaments, but promotes bacterial movements by increasing the stability of the actin tails. In vitro VASP blocks gelsolin-induced severing, which would stabilize filaments in the platelet *(29)*. This would explain defects in platelet shape change in VASP knockouts *(12,14)*. In addition, VASP colocalizes with gelsolin at the leading edge, where actin filament turnover is rapid, but not in adhesion plaques and stress fibers, where actin filament turnover is much slower

(Fig. 6) *(29)*. Thus overexpression of VASP would be expected to increase filament stability, whereas loss of VASP would result in higher filament turnover. Our results have been confirmed in cultured cells *(63)*. This balance of polymerization vs stabilization is likely to depend on the local ratio of VASP-to-actin concentrations and the amount and type of other actin-regulating proteins.

VASP thus exemplifies four of the complexity principles listed in Table 1: (1) redundancy: several homologs, Ena, EvP, and VASP; (2) multitasking: both bundling and nucleating; (3) modular activity: blocks polymerization in the resting cell, and promotes it after activation; and (4) posttranslational modifications affect functions, and phosphorylated residues regulate actin affinity.

Cells in culture from double VASP/Ena knockout mice can be used as substrate to test what part of the VASP protein is required to rescue each aspect of the phenotype—*Listeria* motility, cell adhesion, and cell motility *(83)*. Overexpression of deletion mutants or short domains of Ena in Ena/VASP knockout cells is a test for functional complementation of individual domains within the protein. Two domains are essential to restore normal cellular behavior: the cyclic nucleotide-dependent phosphorylation sites and the actin-binding domain. Expression of the EVH2 domain from the C terminus, which contains a focal adhesion/actin-binding localization domain, is sufficient to restore the rate of random cell locomotion of wild-type cells.

MORPHOLOGY AND BIOCHEMISTRY OF THE MEMBRANE CYTOSKELETON IN THE RESTING PLATELET

The resting platelet has three distinct actin-rich structures that can be identified morphologically: the membrane skeleton, the radiating filaments from the central core, and the cage of filaments in the cortex deep to the membrane skeleton. The location and distribution of monomer binding, severing, and side-binding proteins among these structures is poorly understood. Thus, the precise role of these proteins is inferred from their in vitro activities and the phenotypes of mutants.

The Membrane Skeleton

The membrane skeleton of the resting platelet acts as a physical restraint to surface protrusions and thereby maintains the discoid shape and nonadhesive properties in circulation. The membrane skeleton is composed of a meshwork of filaments, as observed by electron microscopy (Fig. 7) *(21,84,85)*. Biochemical analysis, performed by sedimenting the Triton-soluble material with high-speed centrifugation, demonstrates the presence of actin-binding protein (ABP), a 260–280-kDa protein *(86–88)* originally discovered in macrophages and by sequence a close relative of filamin *(89)*. In vitro, ABP organizes actin into an orthogonal network *(90,91)*. Also found in the high-speed "membrane skeleton" pellet are GPIb, the von Willebrand factor (vWF) receptor, and spectrin *(22,88,92–94)*. The structure of the detergent-extracted membrane skeleton was elegantly demonstrated by electron microscopy of platinum replicas of detergent-extracted resting platelets spun down onto cover slips and critical-point-dried *(93)*. Immunogold decoration of these fixed membrane shells confirmed that the filamentous meshwork observed in platelets captured live by quick-freezing and imaged by fracture-etching and thin-section microscopy *(21,84)* was composed of spectrin, as predicted, as well as myosin, ABP, and adducin.

Recent genetic evidence demonstrates a critical role for spectrin in maintaining platelets in the quiescent state. Hereditary spherocytosis in mice and humans can be a consequence of mutations in either the α- or

---

Fig. 6. *(opposite page)* Location of VASP and gelsolin in spreading platelets. VASP (green) is enriched in stress-like fibers and is also present in lesser amounts at the leading edge, Gelsolin (red) is more abundant at the edge and is not present in the adhesion plaques and stress-like fibers. In some instances, VASP is found at the tips of filopodial projections (bottom inset) and in others not (top right inset). (Reproduced from ref. *29*, with permission.)

Fig. 7. *(opposite page)* Changes in membrane skeleton captured by quick-freeze of living platelets within seconds of thrombin stimulation. **(A)** This section electron microscopy of platelets captured within seconds of exposure to thrombin reveals the presence of a regular array of filaments (arrows) lying just beneath the plasma membrane. **(A')** At higher magnifications, tiny connections between these filaments and between the filaments and the membrane are detected (arrow). **(B,C)** After freeze-fracture, etching, and platinum shadowing, this regular array appears as a sheet of aligned filaments lining the inner surface of the plasma membrane (arrows). Granules (G) and the cytoplasmic (P) face of the plasma membrane (PF) have less organized textures. (Reproduced from ref. *21*, with permission.)

Fig. 8. *(opposite page)* The contractile ring contains Arp2/3 and may be analogous to the "actin-regulating wave" of cultured cells. **(A)** The contractile ring is easily imaged with the F-actin stain phalloidin. **(B)** In platelets double labeled for Arp2 (red) and F-actin (green), a large amount of Arp2 can be seen in this ring, with only small amounts at the site of polymerization at the outermost edge. **(C)** Phase contrast microscopy overlay with the red Arp2 stain further confirms that the "wave" is apparently moving inward from the edge of the cell. (Reproduced from refs. *1* and *24*, with permission.)

Figure 6

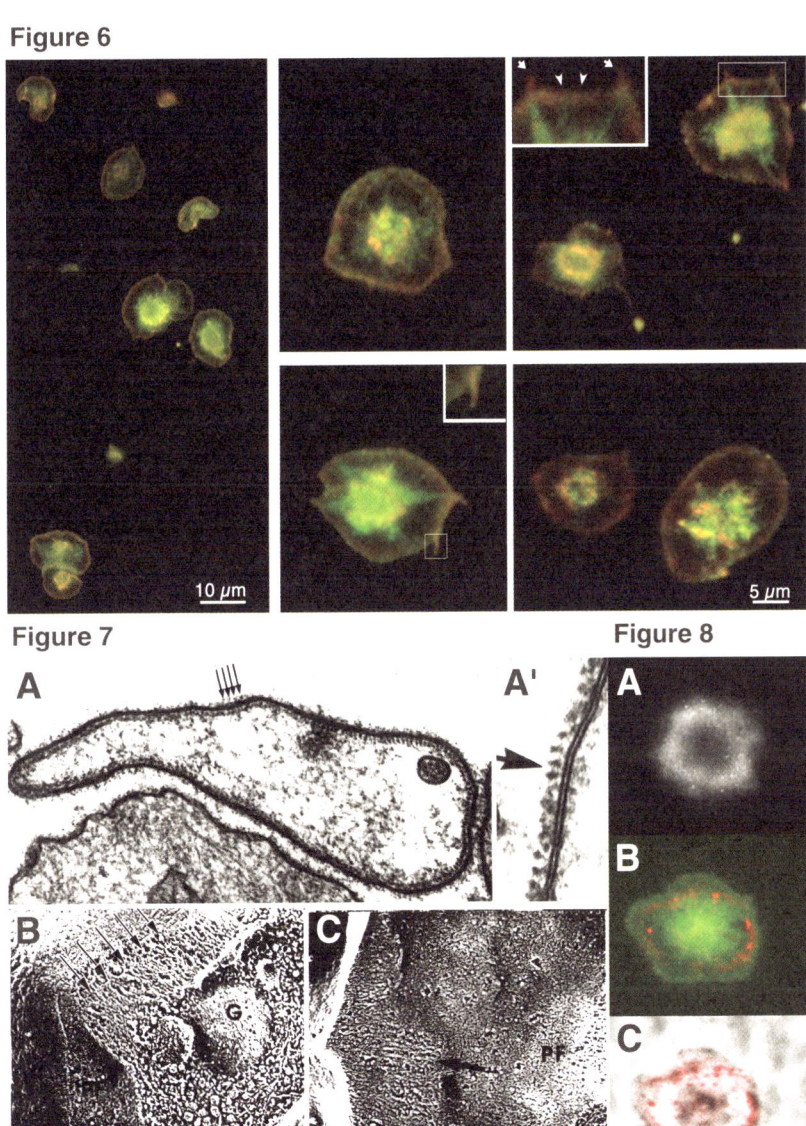

Figure 7

Figure 8

the β-spectrin gene and is associated with hemolytic anemia *(15)*. Life-threatening thrombotic events accompany this disease. The basis for this increased thrombosis is probably the spectrin deficiency in the platelets, since platelets from spectrin-deficient mice display increased thrombosis transplanted into bone marrow-ablated hosts or hosts with genetic stem cell deficiency without hemolytic anemia. Thus, platelets are hyperactive in the absence of spectrin, which argues for a role of spectrin in suppressing activation.

The membrane skeleton is also a target of cold-activated shape change, possibly via calcium influx that activates proteases and initiates other enzymatic cascades. When subjected to cold, platelets round and polymerize actin (95). After cold storage, transfused platelets are rapidly cleared from the circulation. However, this clearance appears to be owing to an irreversible clustering of the vWF receptor, GP1b, which is glycosylated and then becomes a receptor for phagocytosis by macrophages (96,97). The irreversibility of clustering is likely to be a consequence of changes in the membrane skeleton that tethers GPIb across the membrane. Clustering does not affect the in vitro response of the platelet to agonists, including its ability to undergo all the morphological events of shape change.

Filamentous Core

In addition to the membrane skeleton, resting platelets also have a core of filaments that radiate out like a pinwheel from the center to the surface membrane (85). These radiating filaments would be expected to act as a tension device (98,99), probably in order to provide 3D elasticity to the discoid shape. Although biophysical measurements of such elasticity have not been performed, it seems likely that such tension would allow the platelet to rebound easily after deformation without compromising its ability to be buffeted or squeezed during passage through narrow blood vessels.

At the platelet surface, radiating actin bundles separate into individual filaments and curve to lie parallel to the membrane. Thin section of living platelets frozen within seconds of thrombin activation reveals an array of 6–9-nm filaments, spaced at 10–15 nm intervals lying parallel to the membrane (Fig. 7) (100). These filaments lie 7–10 nm inside the electron-dense fuzz of the membrane skeleton and attach to it by short perpendicular spikes (21,84). This regular array of filaments is like a cage, which contracts during the rounding stage of activation induced restructuring of the membrane skeleton and changes in its relationship to the radiating filaments from the central core. It accompanies the first, rounding, stage of activation, as will be described in the next section.

ACTIN DYNAMICS DURING ACTIVATION
AND SHAPE CHANGE

Rounding and the Contractile Ring

The first stage of platelet activation is rounding. At least three biochemical events underlie rounding: disassembly of the membrane skeleton, formation of a contractile ring, and severing and depolymerization of existing filaments.

Disassembly of the Membrane Skeleton

Disassembly of the membrane skeleton involves posttranslational modifications of its protein components. The enzymatic pathways that lead to these modifications are as yet poorly understood. Proteolysis is thought to be mediated by calcium-dependent proteases, possibly μ-calpain. Platelets from mice deficient in μ-calpain have abnormal clotting *(16)*, and inhibition of μ-calpain caused defects in secretion, thrombin-induced aggregation, and spreading *(20)*. An early target of proteolysis is spectrin. Spectrin is proteolyzed upon activation in a Ca^{2+}-dependent manner and then released from the membrane skeleton *(101,102)*. In addition to proteolysis, many phosphorylation and dephosphorylation events occur. Myosin light chain is dephosphorylated and shifts from the high- to the low-speed pellet of Triton-extracted platelets, indicating binding to the core actin bundles *(103)*. In addition, phosphorylation of the βIII cytoplasmic domain of the platelet integrin receptor recruits myosin II *(104–106)*. Platelets from mice deficient in the ICY phosphorylation site in this integrin receptor have defective aggregation and fail to retract clots, demonstrating a key role for myosin-integrin interactions in these two stages of platelet function.

Adducin

Another target in the membrane skeleton of both phosphorylation and proteolysis is adducin. Adducin, originally identified as a component of the red blood cell membrane skeleton *(107)*, is also found in the platelet membrane skeleton *(108)*. The adducins are a family of proteins encoded by three genes in human that express three different proteins, α (103 kDa), β (97 kDa), and γ (84–86 kDa). Adducin forms heterodimers and tetramers α, β in red cells and α, γ in platelets and other cells. Domains in all three adducins include a globular head, a neck, and a 22-amino acid tail domain with protein kinase C (PKC) phosphorylation sites and myristylated alanine-rich C-kinase substrate (MARCKS) homology. In the red cell membrane, adducin links the barbed ends of actin filaments to spectrin. In platelets, adducin is equivalent in abundance to capping protein, 6 m*M*. It is also found in the membrane skeleton, and after activation adducin undergoes PKC-dependent phosphorylation in the MARCKS domain at Ser726 and is also proteolyzed, probably by calpain *(109)*. Inhibition of PKC seems to prevent proteolysis of adducin, suggesting that phosphorylation regulates proteolysis. Degradation of these components of the membrane skeleton permits subsequent shape change.

Formation of the Contractile Ring

Released from its membrane tether and pulled by contractions toward the center of the platelet, some components of the membrane skeleton separate from the membrane and form a ring that tightens in toward the center of the platelet, the *contractile ring* (Fig. 2,8) *(24,110)*. Depolymerization of the cortical actin by gelsolin, separation of the lateral membrane from the underlying membrane skeleton by proteolysis of some of its components, and contraction of the core filaments that pulls the skeleton inward all contribute to the morphology of *rounding*. In platelets spread on glass, this centralizing ring is still apparent during filopodial extension and spreading but gradually dissipates as adhesion plaques and stress-like fibers mature. The centralization includes spectrin, any remaining adducin *(111)*, and the GPIb-vWF receptor, which requires myosin II *(92)*. That GPIb, a transmembrane protein, also centralizes with the contractile ring, suggests that this structure remains associated with the central membrane while decoupled from the lateral, spreading membrane.

MYOSIN IIA

The centralization of components of the membrane skeleton is most likely mediated by myosin IIA, the predominant myosin in platelets. Other unconventional myosins are also likely to be found in platelets. ATP elution from F-actin affinity chromatography releases other ATP-sensitive actin-binding proteins *(24,41)* migrating at 110–130 kDa (myosin I), 160 kDa (myosin VI), and 190 kDa (myosin V) (Fig. 3). At least 18 different types of myosins have been identified in many other cells *(112–115)*.

Myosin IIA, the predominant form of myosin II in platelets, plays significant roles in platelet formation, activation, and contraction, as evidenced by human genetic deficiencies in the *MYH9* gene encoding this myosin *(116–118)*. Significantly, these mutations also affect the expression levels and function of GPIb *(117)*.

Thus, myosin II exemplifies the modular functionality of complexity: one protein for many different cellular behaviors.

Behavior of the Contractile Ring During Activation

The contractile ring in the platelet may be analogous to the wave observed in fibroblasts in response to the mitogenic growth factor, platelet-derived growth factor (PDGF) *(119)*. In fibroblasts after stimulation green fluorescent protein (GFP)-tagged dynamin forms a large noose, looping from the cell surface to the nuclear region, and tightening rapidly over the dorsal aspect of the cell, moving like a circular wave inward toward the nucleus over a period of 15 min. The wave is dense enough to be visible by phase microscopy. By immunofluorescence, it contains dynamin, cortactin, neural isoform of Wiskott-Aldrich syndrome protein (N-WASP), and the Arp2/3 complex as well as short actin filaments, but not rac, rho, or arf6. Thus this dorsal wave differs from the cortical ruffles that appear at the leading edge. Organized actin structures such as stress fibers are lost as the wave moves inward, suggesting that the wave may also contain actin-depolymerizing agents.

The location of Arp2/3 in nonpermeabilized platelets during spreading (Fig. 8) (1) is evidence supporting the notion that the contractile ring represents a similar "actin-reorganizing wave." In the resting cell, Arp2/3 is found at the cortex. During platelet spreading on glass, a ring of Arp2/3 is found enclosing the granules, while the lateral lamellipodia advance. This ring can only be observed in platelets fixed without detergent, indicating it is membrane associated or soluble. Other components of the "actin-reorganizing wave" are also found in platelets. Platelets are known to contain cortactin (120), but its location is not known. Although platelets do not contain appreciable amounts of N-WASP (121), they do have all three of the other WASP family members, WAVE 1, 2, and 3 (verprolin family of proteins with homolog to WASP, VASP), any one of which might replace N-WASP activity in the ring (A. Oda, personal communication). Thus whether the contractile ring is analogous to these dorsal waves in cultured fibroblasts at the molecular level needs to be explored. The depolymerization of existing filaments is a crucial step in platelet shape change, and the sweep of an actin-reorganizing complex of proteins may well be the mechanism that coordinates the many activities required for the initial morphological transformation of the platelet cytoskeleton.

Depolymerization of Filaments

The first step in rebuilding a new dynamic cytoskeleton is disassembly of the stable filaments in the resting platelet. Rapid response requires that demolition be quick. The disassembly involves three separate reactions: (1) release of stabilizing proteins from filaments, (2) severing and depolymerization of these filaments, and (3) increase in polymerizable monomers, either by catalyzed ATP exchange, release from sequestration, or the depolymerization of old filaments. Possibly because this process is so critical, platelets seem to have many different proteins that can serve each of these functions. A number of proteins have been implicated in these processes: VASP dissociation releases filaments for severing and depolymerization (29), gelsolin severs them (8,90), and cofilin accelerates depolymerization (51,122,123). Profilin catalyzes ADP-ATP exchange (39,40). Capping protein releases capped barbed ends (47), and Tβ4 must also release sequestered monomer, although the mechanisms regulating these events are less well understood. Coordination of all of these activities produces a large pool of actin monomers charged with ATP for rapid polymerization.

Recently, new and important details about the activity of some of these proteins have emerged. VASP binds to the sides of actin filaments and prevents severing, as described above (29). Thus, VASP must be released from these filaments before they can be disassembled. This release could be mediated by agonist-activated dephosphorylation of VASP, since the phosphorylation state influences its actin-binding activity (124–127). Indeed, for VASP to rescue the Ena/VASP-deficient phenotype, both the actin-binding domain and the phosphorylation sites are required (71,74,79,80,83). Other proteins are also likely to be released from the stable actin filaments during the first phase of activation, including ABP, tropomyosin, and α-actinin.

Once released from stabilization, filaments are free to be severed or to depolymerize from the pointed end, facilitated by depolymerizing factors like cofilin. Probably the best known and most intensely studied protein involved in severing is gelsolin.

Gelsolin

Gelsolin was noted more than 20 years ago for its ability to solvate actin filament gels (128). Gelsolin severs filaments, caps their barbed ends, and binds to monomers (47,50,129–131). Direct observation of gelsolin's interaction with actin by video microscopy shows that gelsolin binds to the sides of filaments and breaks them after exposure to calcium. Gelsolin remains attached to one of the severed ends (131). Biochemical studies show that this attachment is to the barbed end, which blocks elongation of the severed fragments, an interaction referred to as *capping (129,130)*. Capping has the effect of promoting depolymerization, as monomers are lost from the pointed end without reciprocal addition to the barbed end. Normally balanced depolymerization from one end and addition to the other, known as *treadmilling*, maintains filaments inside quiescent cells (132). If filaments are capped at the barbed end, they unravel from their pointed ends unless they are otherwise stabilized. Cofilin, also abundant in platelets (123), potentiates unraveling by destabilizing links between actin monomers along the filament.

Gelsolin knockout mice were successfully generated but have no significant platelet defects except for a failure to round in the first step of shape change (11). This disappointing result led to the conclusion that there might be other proteins in platelets whose activity could replace that of gelsolin. Gelsolin may also be important for clot removal. The circulating form of gelsolin, brevin, disassembles leftover actin filaments from platelets in old clots. However, gelsolin activity appears to be upstream of the polymerization induced by Arp2/3, and the combined effects of severing and uncapping potentiate Arp2/3 nucleation.

COFILIN/ACTIN-DEPOLYMERIZING FACTOR/ACTOPHORIN

Cofilin/actin-depolymerizing factor (ADF) was first identified in resting platelets in a 47-kDa complex that is dephosphorylated upon thrombin stimulation *(133)*. This phosphorylated subunit was later identified as the 18–19-kDa cofilin *(123)*. Cofilin is in high concentration in platelets, 50 μ*M*—there is one cofilin for every 10 actin monomers. In resting platelets, phosphorylation is exclusively on the serine 3 at the N terminus. Dephosphorylation is activated by calcium, independent of PKC and is increased by GTPγS, which activates G-proteins. Cofilin's interaction with actin is inhibited by phosphorylation. ADP and thrombin induce dephosphorylation of cofilin/ADF, and this is inhibitied by 1-napthylphosphate but not by okadaic acid. Phosphatases mediating cofilin dephosphorylation are not known in platelets but may include a human homolog of the fly gene Slingshot *(134)*.

Cofilin/ADF in vitro acts as a depolymerizing factor that increases the rate of treadmilling 25-fold, via increasing monomer loss from the pointed end *(51)*. Cofilin coats actin filaments, possibly preferentially to ADP-actin subunits, and destabilizes them *(135)*. Cofilin binding changes the twist of actin filaments, which may contribute to the dissociation of monomer *(136,137)*. In cultured cells, anticofilin antibodies block actin polymerization in response to growth factors *(138)*. Cofilin/ADF is phosphorylated by the LIM kinase family (seronine–threonine kinase in the casein–kinase family) *(139,140)*, and overexpression of the kinase domain of LIM1 results in near total phosphorylation of cofilin and inhibits barbed end exposure in response to growth factor *(141)*. Even though cofilin destabilizes filaments in vitro, it is one of only a small set of proteins required to reproduce actin polymerization of *Listeria* motility in vitro *(142)* and for lamellipodial formation and motility in *Drosophila* S2 cells *(143)*. More information about cofilin's role in platelets will be useful both for elucidating platelet activation and for understanding cofilin's role in the universal process of actin polymerization and the dynamics of cell shape.

Outreach: The Formation of Filopodia and Lamellipodia

Coupled to depolymerization is the explosive repolymerizaton of released monomers into new filaments. New filaments are organized into multifilamentous structures. These two steps, polymerization and organization, occur sequentially and involve different sets of proteins.

THE POLYMERIZATION MACHINE, ARP2/3

Perhaps the most exciting recent discovery about the actin cytoskeleton of platelets is the identification of the Arp2/3 complex as the required polymerization machine for all actin polymerization involved in shape change and platelet spreading *(1)*. Arp2/3 is a seven-subunit protein complex. The Arp2 subunit was first discovered in platelets using F-actin affinity columns as a 44-kDa protein eluting with ATP *(24,41)*. Subsequently a complex was identified from *Acanthamoeba* by profilin affinity columns containing Arp2 as well as six other proteins *(144)*. This Arp2/3 complex was then isolated from human platelets as the factor that polymerized actin on the surfaces of Listeria bacteria *(77)*.

Many intracellular microbes induce polymerization of actin to propel themselves through the cytoplasm and thereby avoid the immune system *(145)*. However outside the cell, bacteria cannot nucleate polymerization of purified actin—thus some other cellular factor is required *(146)*. Bacteria will induce actin polymerization in platelet extracts *(76)*, which must contain the missing cellular factors. Arp2/3 complex was isolated by testing biochemically separated proteins from platelet extracts for polymerization activity on *Listeria* bacteria *(77,147)*. Covalent labeling of actin monomers with rhodamine allows imaging of filaments by fluorescence microscopy *(148)*.

The Arp2/3 complex includes two members of the actin-related protein (Arp) family and five other subunits (Table 3). All seven of the proteins are highly conserved across species, from soil amoeba, to plants, to humans *(149)*. Arp2/3 effects on actin have been studied extensively in vitro: it binds the pointed ends and stimulates barbed end elongation *(147,150)*. Arp2/3 also binds the sides of filaments *(60,151)*, where it induces a new filament to grow at a 70° angle to the first *(150,152)*. Arp2/3 is located in the lamellipodia of migrating cultured cells *(147)*.

Arp2/3 is the first actin filament nucleator to be identified as involved in the formation of actin filaments during platelet spreading (Fig. 9) *(1)*. In these studies we permeabilized platelets by either brief sonication or detergent and loaded them with various antibodies and pyrene-labeled actin monomer. Arp2/3 was inhibited with an inhibitory antibody raised against recombinant full-length Arp2. Upon stimulation with either thrombin receptor agonist peptide (TRAP) or glass, platelet shape change was monitored after loading either with the anti-Arp2 antibody or with a control antibody. Actin polymerization was assayed in the pyrene actin assay in permeabilized platelets in suspension, or with phalloidin staining of permeabilized platelets spread on glass. In the latter case, quantitative data were obtained by morphometric analysis of blood samples from 50 different donors, with more than 1000 platelets counted per experiment.

Inhibition of Arp2/3 froze platelets at the rounded initial stage of shape change and inhibited TRAP-stimulated actin polymerization (Fig. 9) (1). Both of these effects were dependent on the dose of inhibitory anti-Arp2 antibody. In contrast, platelets spread normally after perme-abilization in the absence of the antibody. Actin polymerization increased fivefold after TRAP stimulation with or without control antibody treatment. In contrast, anti-Arp2 treatment blocked this process, maintaining actin polymerization at resting levels even after TRAP stimulation. These effects were observed with whole anti-Arp2 antibody or with Fab fragments but not with any other antibody. Arp2 inhibition had little effect on the low level of polymerization activity present in resting platelets.

These results show (1) that Arp2/3 is required for actin polymerization during shape change and (2) that all actin structures are dependent on this polymerization. Thus each of the three actin filament structures formed during spreading—filopodia, lamellipodia, and stress-like fibers—are all nucleated by Arp2/3 and subsequently reorganized by other proteins into higher order structures. What are these other proteins, and how are they sorted or activated in one structure and not in another? Is the presence or absence of any one particular protein key to formation of each specific type of structure?

POLYMERIZATION ASSISTANTS, KAPTIN/2E4

Another novel actin-binding protein identified by F-actin affinity chromatography is kaptin/2E4, an approx 43-kDa ATP-sensitive end-binding protein *(24,153,154)*. In spread platelets, kaptin is located in the outer 1 μm of the outer edge of the lamellipodia, whereas in fibroblasts, antibodies to kaptin label the outermost two-thirds of filopodia as well. Kaptin elutes from F-actin columns with ATP and is extracted with ATP from both detergent-extracted fibroblast and platelet cytoskeletons. Kaptin binds the ends of actin filaments in vitro but instead of inhibiting polymerization as other capping proteins do, it potentiates it. Kaptin is upregulated in the mesoderm of embryos just prior to gastrulation, suggesting a role in cell motility *(155)*.

Kaptin's uniform location at the outermost edge and its in vitro binding to actin filaments suggest it may be involved in regulating barbed end growth *(153,154)*. The electron-dense fuzz at the tips of actin-rich processes has long been proposed to contain proteins that regulate the length of filaments *(156)*. Keptin was found in this complex in stereocilia of the inner ear *(154,163)*. Recent evidence has identified other members of this complex and suggested that this tip complex brings the barbed ends

Table 3
Arp2/3 Subunits

Protein	Protein family	Interaction with actin	Activity	Interaction with other Arp2/3 subunits	Molecular weight
Arp3	Actin related protein	Pointed end binding	Not defined	ARC2 ARC3 ARC4	47 kDa
Arp2	Actin related protein	Pointed end binding	Antibody blocks polymerization in vitro Antibody blocks platelet shape-change mor-phologically	ARC1 ARC2	44 kDa
ARC1	7 WD repeats	Filament side binding	—	Arp2 ARC2	40 kDa
ARC2	—	Branching Side binding	Antibody blocks branching in vitro Antibody blocks propulsion but not polymer-ization in cells	Arp2 Arp3 ARC1 ARC4	34 kDa
ARC3	—	—	Binds WASP/SCAR; may mediate activation of Arp2/3	Arp3 ARC4	21 kDa
ARC4	—	—	—	Arp3 ARC2 ARC3	20 kDa
ARC5	—	—	—	ARC4	16 kDa

of filaments together during filopodial formation. One of these tip com-plex proteins is VASP *(66)*. Other components of the tip complex could be a myosin, such as mysoin VI or X *(157)*. Kaptin may be at the tip owing to association with a myosin, since it elutes from F-actin columns with ATP *(24,153,154)*. Myosins have long been hypothesized to play a significant role in the formation and dynamics of filopodia *(158–160)*. Extracellular signal-related kinase (ERK) and RhoA, myosin activators, regulate protrusions in actively motile cells (161). Overexpression of exogenous myo3A, involved in polarity of the retinal rod cell, in HeLa cells produces abundant filopodial formation, with a striking accumulation of GFP-labeled myo3A at their tips (162).

Kaptin is also located at the tips of sensory cells (163). In the hair cells of the inner ear, kaptin is concentrated at the tips of the stereocilia in the electron-dense fuzz where actin monomer addition is thought to regulate sterocilia length (156). The length of each stereocilia determines the sound to which the hair cell will respond. The human gene for kaptin is located within the deafness locus, DFNA4, on chromosome 19q13.3 (163). It is not uncommon for cochlear deafness to cosegregate with platelet disorders, possibly because both hair cells and platelets rely so heavily on the actin cytoskeleton for function. Other genetic diseases with this pattern include May-Heggelin, Fechner's, and Epstein's syndromes (116,118), which are caused by mutations in the motor domain of myosin IIA.

As discussed above, capping protein, cofilin, and profilin are also required for actin polymerization initiated by Arp2/3.

As for many of the proteins discussed here, the array of cellular activities of kaptin illustrates the principle of modular functionality of ABPs. Such multiplicity of cellular functions for one biochemical activity is emerging as a common theme in the "more for less" strategies the cell uses to regulate its actin cytoskeleton. Other examples of multitasking and modular functionality are gelsolin, profiling, and VASP, each of which may mediate very different cellular outcomes depending on the timing and context of their activity.

To assume that all filopodia are created equal is probably an oversimplification. As shown in Fig. 6, VASP can only be detected at the tips of some filopodia. Arp2/3 is detected at tips and bases of some filopodia, and 2E4/kaptin is also at the tips of some filopodia. Hence, some filopodia may contain a VASP tip complex, others a myosin-kaptin complex, and still others may have both. Other tip complexes may also exist, as the principle of redundancy predicts. Furthermore, it may be misleading to rely too heavily on localization by fluorescence to assign function. As we have done for Arp 2/3, experimental manipulation of protein activity in the platelet will be necessary for a definitive determination of function of these other proteins.

Reorganization of Filaments Into Higher Order Structures

Once actin has polymerized, filaments must be organized properly to form functional structures. This organizational process requires a set of proteins that bind the sides of actin filaments and bundle or network them in various orientations. Most of the proteins displaying bundling and networking properties in vitro and in cultured cells are present in platelets, and possibly all are involved in forming the four distinct platelet actin structures. Examples of these proteins include fascin, α-actinin, and ABP.

Fascin

Recent exciting evidence from cells other than platelets suggests that fascin is key for the bundling of actin filaments in filopodia. Using an elegant combination of GFP-labeled proteins, immunofluorescence, and electron microscopy of platinum-shadowed cytoskeletons from B16F1 cells, Svitkina et al. *(66)* present evidence for a convergent elongation model of filopodial formation. In this model, Arp2/3 nucleates a loose network of branching filaments. Some filaments acquire proteins that protect them from capping, possibly VASP/Ena, although kaptin may also perform this function. The tip complex or a convergence of privileged filaments then recruits fascin, which zippers them together to form a rod-like bundle. Evidence from in vitro experiments either in brain or *Xenopus* extracts or with purified proteins validates this model *(67)*. Whether this process also occurs in platelets is not known. Our work showing an effect of VASP on gelsolin capping (Bearer, unpublished data) suggests that in platelets VASP may be more significant in blocking gelsolin effects than those of capping protein.

α-Actinin

α-Actinin, an actin bundling protein of approx 95 kDa, is involved in the muscle contractile apparatus and in adhesion plaques and stress fibers *(164)*. α-Actinin has one actin-binding site and forms homodimers in antiparallel orientation to crosslink actin filaments *(165)*. α-Actinin is also thought to bind the cytoplasmic tail of integrin receptors and tether them to actin filaments *(166)*. Interactions between α-actinin and its various binding partners are regulated by calcium, phosphatidylinositol (PIP)$_2$, and PIP$_3$ *(167,168)*. In platelets, α-actinin is phosphorylated on Y12 by focal adhesion kinase (FAK) after activation *(169,170)*. Tyrosine phosphorylation decreases α-actinin's affinity for F-actin, suggesting a role for phosphorylation of α-actinin in regulating recruitment of actin to adhesion plaques.

Activation of bundling proteins by posttranslational modification during platelet stimulation is likely to be an important part of cytoskeletal restructuring since platelets lack a nucleus and cannot increase mRNA expression. Recent evidence demonstrates the presence of stored mRNA in platelets *(171,172)*, and translation may play a role in poststimulation actin behavior at later time points. Many actin regulatory partners display different phosphorylated states in resting compared with activated platelets. For most, definitive relationship between phosphorylation and platelet function has been elusive. This is likely to be because actin polymerization is not an all-or-none phenomenon—instead, shape change is likely to involve alternating rounds of polymerization balanced with depolymerization, capping with uncapping, networks with bundles. Many different subcellular locations are likely to be at different points in this cycle at any one time.

As actin filaments form, network, and bundle, platelet adhesion also begins. Effective adhesion requires interactions between the cytoplasmic filaments and the extracellular matrix, which in coagulation is mainly fibrin and collagen. The dynamic processes within the platelet as it reorganizes its cytoskeleton must be tightly coordinated with the formation of adhesion plaques such that the final result is an integrated architecture of adhesions coupled to stress fibers that span the cytoplasm. Platelets probably exert force on the fibrin strands as they reorganize the stress fibers into the parallel arrays needed for contraction. There has been very little recent work on these events as they pertain to the cytoskeleton.

SUMMARY: A MODEL OF PLATELET ACTIN DYNAMICS

Actin is a modular building block that, once assembled into filaments, can be further organized into a variety of higher order structures. Inhibition and induction of polymerization are mediated by specific sets of cellular proteins. Organization of filaments into larger networks or bundles is driven by yet another set of proteins. Platelets contain many different proteins capable of performing each of these functions.

Changes of actin structures during spreading and the relationship to specific proteins is shown in Fig. 10. The resting platelet has four distinct actin structures: membrane skeleton, filaments of the central core, radiating filaments that connect core to membrane, and monomeric actin sequestered in the cytoplasm. More than half of the actin in resting platelets is monomeric. Each of these four types of actin plays important and distinct roles in maintaining the discoid shape of the platelet and mediating its rapid response to agonist. The membrane skeleton contains a set of filamentous interlocking proteins: spectrin, ABP, and adducin, as well as myosin IIA.

Upon activation, platelets undergo three distinct stages of morphological changes: rounding, filopodial formation, and spreading. Rounding involves the disassembly of actin filaments and formation of a contractile ring. Disassembly begins with the release of filaments from stabilizing side-binding proteins such as VASP, which allows severing by gelsolin and destabilization by cofilin. Gelsolin-capped filaments are particularly susceptible to depolymerization. The contractile ring apparently arises from the cortical cytoplasm and contains some of the membrane skeleton components as well as other proteins. The ring may be analogous to the wave of dynamin-cortactin-Arp2/3 that precedes ruffling in response to growth factor in cultured cells.

Disassembly is immediately followed by an explosive polymerization of new filaments, partly driven by the release of monomer both from sequestration by Tβ4 and from depolymerizing filaments. Profilin catalyzes ATP-ADP exchange to maintain a high level of primed monomer for barbed end elongation. Arp2/3 is activated and nucleates new filaments off the sides of short remnants of the severed old filaments as well as *de novo*. Polymerization is focused through the local activities of capping protein and cofilin. New filaments are subsequently organized

---

Fig. 9. *(opposite page)* Arp2/3 is required for platelet actin polymerization and spreading. **(A)** The effect of Arp2 inhibition on actin polymerization in permeabilized platelets. Washed platelets were briefly permeabilized with sonication to load with antibody and pyrene-labeled actin and activated with thrombin receptor agonist peptide (TRAP). Actin polymerization was measured as a function of fluorescence emission from the pyrene-actin. Anti-Arp2 antibody profoundly inhibits polymerization, and the effect is dose dependent. **(B)** Arp2 localizes at the tips of filopodia (red) and at the edges of permeabilized, spread platelets. **(C)** Permeabilized platelets round, project filopodia, and spread normally (left panel) but when treated with inhibitory Arp2 antibody, they round but fail to make filopodia or to spread (right panel). In a subset of inhibited platelets, blebbing occurs (inset, right panel) magnification bar applies to all images in C. **(D)** These effects can be quantitated and are dose dependent.

Fig. 10. *(opposite page)* Diagram of platelet cytoskeleton at different stages of activation. The discoid platelet, with a tensegral actin structure and a rigid membrane skeleton, resists deformation. Upon agonist stimulation, rounding occurs as actin filaments are severed, the membrane skeleton detaches, and activation of myosin II pulls the radial filaments inward. Actin monomers are released from sequestration. Polymerization begins with activation of the Arp2/3 complex; the contractile ring sweeps the actin regulatory wave inward, depolymerizing the radial filaments and stimulating polymerization. Filopodia project as nascent actin filaments and are organized into bundles by association with various "tip complexes" including VASP and 2E4/kaptin. Shown clockwise around the platelet at the far right are the successive steps of filopodial organization and the appearance of a branched filament network of the lamelipodium. The presence of vasodilator-stimulated phosphoprotein (VASP) at the tip may recruit adhesion plaque proteins, including adhesion receptors and other cytoskeletal regulators.

Figure 9

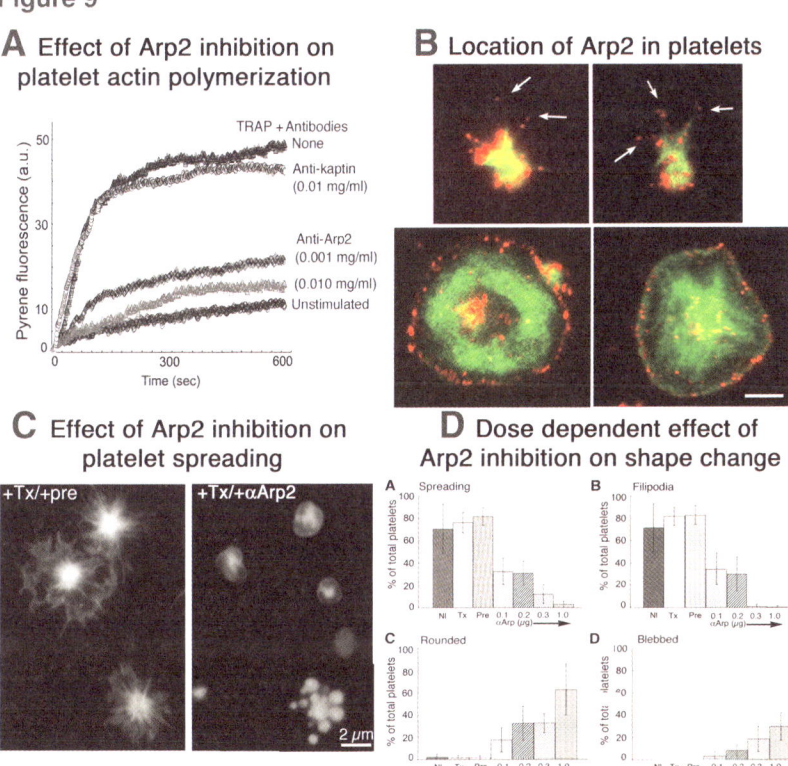

A Effect of Arp2 inhibition on platelet actin polymerization

B Location of Arp2 in platelets

C Effect of Arp2 inhibition on platelet spreading

D Dose dependent effect of Arp2 inhibition on shape change

Figure 10

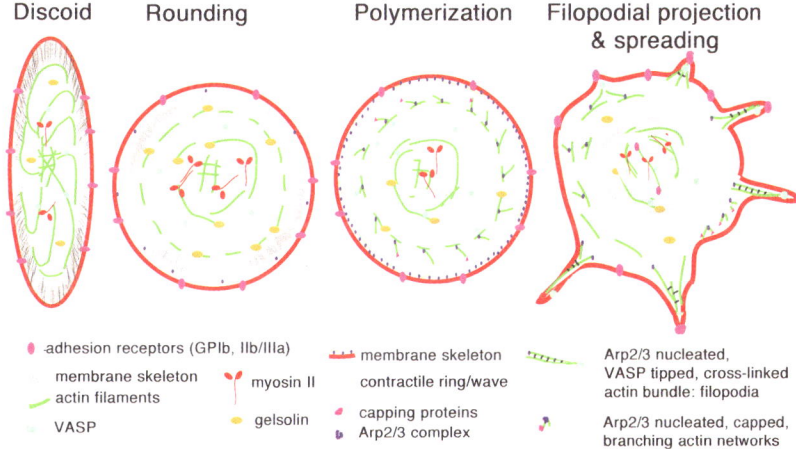

Discoid   Rounding   Polymerization   Filopodial projection & spreading

through interactions with side-binding proteins into larger structures, such as filopodia, lamellipodia, and stress-like fibers.

In conclusion, the platelet cytoskeleton is highly complex, with dynamic processes occurring over time and mediated by a large set of proteins with redundant, multitasking, and modular functions. Posttranslational modifications and contextual variables expand the repertoire of possible outcomes from any single protein's local activity. Computational and systems biology approaches together with functional proteomics and clever strategies to test function in vivo will be needed for the next steps in studying platelet biology.

ACKNOWLEDGMENTS

This work could not have been done without the vision, support, and advice of Bruce Alberts, my postdoctoral mentor who set me on the path of thinking comprehensively yet analyzing systematically. I am also grateful for the numerous contributions of Brown University students, both undergraduate and graduate, most importantly, Manoj Abraham, Eric S. Kim, Kate Matsutani, and Zhi Li, as well as postdoctoral fellow Leslie Hunter and research assistants Rob Manchester, Bob Lundsten, Judith Nutkis, and, last but not least, Jamunabai Prakash. The work was supported by grants from the American Cancer Society, a Bank of America-Gianini Award, the Salomon Award, and National Institutes of Health grant GM47638.

REFERENCES

1. Li Z, Kim ES, Bearer EL. The Arp2/3 complex is required for actin polymerization during platelet shape change. Blood 2002;99:4466–4474.
2. Haydon GB, Taylor DA. Microtubules in hamster platelets. J Cell Biol 1965; 26:673–676.
3. Tablin F, Taube D. Platelet intermediate filaments: detection of a vimentinlike protein in human and bovine platelets. Cell Motil Cytoskel 1987;8:61–67.
4. Bearer EL, Prakash JM, Li Z. Actin dynamics in platelets. Int Rev Cytol 2002;217:137–182.
5. Davidson EH, et al. A genomic regulatory network for development of genetic fine mapping of the Miyoshi myopathy locus and exclusion of eight candidate genes. Science 2002;295:1669–1678.
6. Brent R. Genomic biology. Cell 2000;100:169–183.
7. Fox JE. The platelet cytoskeleton. Thromb Haemost 1993;70:884–893.
8. Hartwig JH, Bokoch GM, et al. Platelet morphology. In Schafer JL, ed. Thrombosis and hemorrhage, 2nd ed. Williams & Wilkins, Baltimore, 1999, pp. 207–228.
9. David-Ferreira JF. The blood platelet: electron icroscopic studies. Int Rev Cytol 1974;17:99–148.
10. O'Brien JR, Woodhouse MA. Platelets. Their size, shape and stickiness in vitro: degranulation and propinquity. Exp Biol Med 1968;3:90–102.

11. Witke W, Sharpe AH, et al. Hemostatic, inflammatory, and fibroblast responses are blunted in mice lacking gelsolin. Cell 1995;81:41–51.

12. Massberg S, et al. Enhanced in vivo platelet adhesion in vasodilator-stimulated phosphoprotein (VASP)-deficient mice. Blood 2004;103:136–142.

13. Hauser W, et al. Megakaryocyte hyperplasia and enhanced agonist-induced platelet activation in vasodilator-stimulated phosphoprotein knockout mice. Proc Natl Acad Sci USA 1999;96:8120–8125.

14. Aszodi A, et al. The vasodilator-stimulated phosphoprotein (VASP) is involved in cGMP- and cAMP-mediated inhibition of agonist-induced platelet aggregation, but is dispensable for smooth muscle function. EMBO J 1999;18:37–48.

15. Wandersee NJ, et al. Hematopoietic cells from spectrin-deficient mice are sufficient to induce thrombotic events in hematopoietically ablated recipients. Blood 1998;92:4856–4863.

16. Azam M, Andrabi SS, et al. Disruption of the mouse mu-calpain gene reveals an essential role in platelet function. Mol Cell Biol 2001;21:2213–2220.

17. Witke W, et al. Profilin I is essential for cell survival and cell division in early mouse development. Proc Natl Acad Sci USA 2001;98:3832–3836.

18. Hartwig JH, Bokoch GM, et al. Thrombin receptor ligation and activatd rac uncap actin filament bared ends through phosphoinositide synthesis in permeabilized human platelets. Cell 1995;82:643–653.

19. Hartwig JH. Mechanisms of actin rearrangements mediating platelet activation. J Cell Biol 1992;118:1421–142.

20. Croce K, et al. Inhibition of calpain blocks platelet secretion, aggregation, and spreading. J Biol Chem 1999;274:36321–36327.

21. Bearer EL. Platelet membrane skeleton revealed by quick-freeze deep-etch. Anat Rec 1990;227:1–11.

22. White JG, Burris S, Escolar G. Influence of thrombin in suspension, surface activation, and high shear on platelet surface GPIb/IX distribution. J Lab Clin Med 1999;133:245–252.

23. Allen RD, Zacharski LR, et al. Transformation and motility of human platlets: details of the shape change and release reaction observed by optical and electron microscopy. J Cell Biol 1979;83:126–142.

24. Bearer EL. cytoskeletal domains in the activated platelet. Cell Motil Cytoskel 1995;30:50–66.

25. Nachmias VT, Golla R, et al. Vinculin in relation to stress fibers in spread platelets. Cell Motil Cytoskel 1991;20:190–202.

26. Reinhard M, et al. The proline-rich focal adhesion and microfilament protein VASP is a ligand for profilins. EMBO J 1995;14:1583–1589.

27. Reinhard M, et al. The 46/50 kDa phosphoprotein VASP purified from human platelets is a novel protein associated with actin filaments and focal contacts. EMBO J 1992;11:2063–2070.

28. Reinhard M, Jarchau T, Walter U. Actin-based motility: stop and go with Ena/VASP proteins. Trends Biochem Sci 2001;26:243–249.

29. Bearer EL, Prakash JM, et al. VASP protects actin filaments from gelsolin: an in vitro study with implications for platelet actin reorganizations. Cell Motil Cytoskel 2000;47:351–364.

30. Calderwood DA, Shattil SJ, Ginsberg MH. Integrins and actin filaments: reciprocal regulation of cell adhesion and signaling. J Biol Chem 2000;275:22607–22610.

31. Etienne-Manneville S, Hall A. Rho GTPases in cell biology. Nature 2002;420:629–635.

32. Kaitlina SY. Functional specificity of actin isoforms. Int Rev Cytol 2001;202:35–98.

33. Pollard TD. Genomics, the cytoskeleton and motilit. Nature 2001;409:842–843.
34. Zucker-Franklin D, et al. The actin and myosin filaments of human and bovine blood platelets. J Clin Invest 1972;51:419–430.
35. Fox JE, Phillips DR. Inhibition of actin polymerization in blood platelets by cytochalasins. Nature 1981;292:650–652.
36. Pollard TD, Cooper JA. Actin and actin-binding proteins: a critical review. Annu Rev Biochem 1986;55:987–1035.
37. Pollard TD. Rate constants for the reactions of ATP- and ADP-actin with the ends of actin filaments. J Cell Biol 1986;103:2747–2754.
38. Pollard TD, Mooseker MS. Direct measurement of actin polymerization rate constants by electron microscopy of actin filaments nucleated by isolated microvillus cores. J Cell Biol 1981;88:654–659.
39. Goldschmidt-Clermont MF, Furman MI, et al. The control of actin nucleotide exchange by thymosin β4 and profilin. A potential regulatory mechanism for actin polymerization in cells. Mol Biol Cell 1992;3:1015–1024.
40. Pantaloni D, Carlier M-F. How profilin promotes actin filament assembly in the presence of thymosin β4. Cell 1993;75:1007–1014.
41. Bearer EL, Miller K. Alberts B. Changes in platelet actin-binding-proteins with activation detected by F-actin affinity chromatography. J Cell Biol 1987;105:195a.
42. Fox JE, Phillips DR. Polymerization and organization of actin filaments within platelets. Semin Hematol 1983;20:650–652.
43. Nachmias VYT. The cytoskeleton of the blood platelet. Adv Cell Biol 1988;2:181–211.
44. Safer D, Elzinga M, et al. Thymosin beta 4 and Fx, and actin-sequestering peptide, are indistinguishable. J Biol Chem 1991;266:4029–4032.
45. Weber A, Nachmias VT, et al. Interaction of thymosin b4 with muscle and platelet actin: implications for actin sequestration in resting platelets. Biochem J 1992;31:6179–6185.
46. Nachmias VT, Golla R. Cap Z, a calcium insensitive capping protein in resting and activated platelets. FEBS Lett 1996;378:258–262.
47. Barkalow K, Witke W, et al. Coordinated regulation of platelet actin filament barbed ends by gelsolin and capping protein. J Cell Biol 1996;134:389–399.
48. Stossel TP. The machinery of cell crawling. Sci Am 1994;271:54–55, 58–63.
49. Stossel TP. Cell crawling two decades after Abercrombie. Biochem Soc Symp 1999;65:267–280.
50. Kwiatkowski DJ. Functions of gelsolin: motility, signaling, apoptosis, cancer. Curr Opin Cell Biol 1999;11:103–108.
51. Carlier M-F, Laurent V, et al. Actin depolymerizing factor (ADF/cofilin) enhances the rate of filament turnover; implication in actin-based motilit. J Cell Biol 1997;136:1307–1322.
52. Cohen I, et al. A tropomyosin-like protein from human platelets. J Mol Biol 1972;68:383–387.
53. Takubo T, et al. Localization of myosin, actin, alpha-actinin, tropomyosin and vinculin in surface-activated, spreading human platelets. Biotech Histochem 1998;73:310–315.
54. Onji T, et al. Tropomyosin-caldesmon/actomyosin systems in platelets and arterial smooth muscle: results from exchange experiments. Biochim Biophys Acta 1989;999:248–253.
55. der Terrossian E, et al. Caldesmon is present in human and pig erythrocytes. Biochem Biophys Res Commun 1989;159:395–401.

56. Pittenger MF, Kazzaz JA, Helfman DM. Functional properties of non-muscle tropomyosin isoforms. Curr Opin Cell Biol 1994;6:96–104.
57. Tang N, Ostap EM. Motor domain-dependent localization of myo1b (myr-1). Curr Biol 2001;11:1131–1135.
58. Cooper JA, et al. Actin dynamics: tropomyosin provides stability. Curr Biol 2002;12:R523–R525.
59. Blanchoin L, Pollard TD, Hitchcock-Degregori SE. Inhibition of the Arp2/3 complex-nucleated actin polymerization and branch formation by tropomyosin. Curr Biol 2001;11:1300–1304.
60. Amann KJ, Pollard TD. The Arp2/3 complex nucleates actin filament branches from the sides of pre-existing filaments. Nat Cell Biol 2001;3:306–310.
61. Halbrugge M, Walter U. Purification of a vasodilator-regulated phosphoprotein from human platelets. Eur J Biochem 1989;185:41–50.
62. Egile C, Loisel TP, et. Al. Activation of the CDC42 effector N-WASP by the *Shigella flexneri* IcsA protein promotes actin nucleation by Arp2/3 complex and bacterial actin-based motility. J Cell Biol 1999;146:1319–1332.
63. Bear JE, et al. Antagonism between Ena/VASP proteins and actin filament capping regulates fibroblast motility. Cell 2002;109:509–521.
64. Bear JE, Krause M, Gertler FB. Regulating cellular actin assembly. Curr Opin Cell Biol 2001;13:158–166.
65. Bachmann C, et al. The EVH2 domain of the vasodilator-stimulated phosphoprotein mediates tetramerization, F-actin binding, and actin bundle formation. J Biol Chem 1999;274:23549–23557.
66. Svitkina TM, et al. Mechanism of filopodia initiation by reorganization of a dendritic network. J Cell Biol 2003;160:409–421.
67. Vignjevic D, et al. Formation of filopodia-like bundles in vitro from a dendritic network. J Cell Biol 2003;160:951–962.
68. Harbeck B, Huttelmaier S, et al. Phosphorylation of the vasodilator-stimulated phosphoprotein regulates its interaction with actin. J Biol Chem 2000;275:30817–30825.
69. Horstrup K, Jablonka B, et al. Phosphorylation of focal adhesion vasodilator-stimulated phosphoprotein at Ser157 in tact human platelets correlates with fibrinogen receptor inhibition. Eur J Biochem 1994;225:21–27.
70. Lambrechts A, et al. cAMP-dependent protein kinase phosphorylation of EVL, a Mena/VASP relative, regulates its interaction with actin and SH3 domains. J Biol Chem 2000;275:36143–36151.
71. Abel K, Mieskes G, et al. Dephosphorylation of the focal adhesion protein VASP in vitro and in intact human platelets. FEBS Lett 1995;370:184–188.
72. Garcia Arguinzonis MI, et al. Increased spreading, Rac/p21-activated kinase (PAK) activity, and compromised cell motility in cells deficient in vasodilator-stimulated phosphoprotein (VASP). J Biol Chem 2002;277:45604–45610.
73. Gertler FB, Comer AR, et al. Enabled, a dosage-sensitive suppressor of utations in the Drosophila Abl tyrosine kinase, encodes an Abl substrate with SH3 domain-binding properties. Genes Dev 1995;9:521–533.
74. Kwiatkowski AV, Gertler FB, Loureiro JJ. Function and regulation of Ena/VASP proteins. Trends Cell Biol 2003;13:386–392.
75. DeMille MM, Kimmel BE, Rubin GM. A *Drosophila* gene regulated by rough and glass shows similarity to ena and VASP. Gene 1996;183:103–108.
76. Theriot JA, Rosenblatt J, et al. Involvement of profilin in the actin-based motility of *L. monocytogenes* in cells and in cell-free extracts. Cell 1994;76:505–517.

77. Welch MD, Iwamatsu A, et al. Actin polymerization is induced by Arp2/3 protein complex at the surface of *Listeria monocytogenes*. Nature 1997;385:265–269.

78. Bear JE, et al. Negative regulation of fibroblast motility by Ena/VASP proteins. Cell 2000;101:717–728.

79. Geese M, et al. Contribution of Ena/VASP proteins to intracellular motility of *Listeria* requires phosphorylation and proline-rich core but not F-actin binding or multimerization. Mol Biol Cell 2002;13:2383–2396.

80. Krause M, et al. The Ena/VASP enigma. J Cell Sci 2002;115:4721–4726.

81. Niebuhr K, Ebel F, et al. A novel proline-rich motif present in ActA of *Listeria monocytogenes* and cytoskeletal proteins is the ligand for the EVH1 domain, a protein module present in the Ena/VASP family. EMBO J 1997;16:5433–5444.

82. Laurent V, Loisel TP, et al. Role of proteins of the Ena/VASP family in actin-based motility of *Listeria monocytogenes*. J Cell Biol 1999;144:1245–1258.

83. Loureiro JJ, et al. Critical roles of phosphorylation and actin binding motifs, but not the central proline-rich region, for Ena/vasodilator-stimulated phosphoprotein (VASP) function during cell migration. Mol Biol Cell 2002;13:2533–2546.

84. Bearer EL. Anionic lipid domains in cell membranes. Thesis, Department of Biochemistry and Biophysics, University of California, San Francisco, 1983.

85. Hartwig JH, DeSisto M. The cytoskeleton of the resting human blood platelet: structure of the membrane skelton and its attachment to actin filaments. J Cell Biol 1991;112:407–425.

86. Boyles J, Fox JEB, et al. Organization of the cytoskeleton in resting, discoid platelets: reservation of actin filaments by a modified fixation that prevents osmium damage. J Cell Biol 1985;101:1463.

87. Fox JE. Identification of actin-binding protein as the protein linking the membrane skeleton to glycoproteins on platelet plasma membrane. J Biol Chem 1985;260:11970–11977.

88. Fox JE, Boyles JK, et al. Indentification of a membrane skeleton in platelets. J Cell Biol 1988;102:1748–1757.

89. Hartwig JH, Kwiatkowski D.J. Actin-binding proteins. Curr Opin Cell Biol 1991;3:87–97.

90. Hartwig JH, et al. The elegant platelet: signals controlling actin assembly. Thromb Haemost 1999;82:392–398.

91. Bertagnolli ME, Beckerle MC. Regulated membrane-cytoskeleton linkages in platelets. Ann NY Acad Sci 1994;714:8–100.

92. Kovacsovics TJ, Hartwig JH. Thrombin-induced GPIb centralization on the platelet surface requires actin actin assembly and myosin II activation. Blood 1996;87:618–629.

93. Hartwig JH, DeSisto M. The cytoskeleton of the resting human blood platelet: structure of the membrane skeleton and its attachment to actin filaments. J Cell Biol 1991;112:407–425.

94. Jennings LK, et al. Changes in the cytoskeletal structure of human platelets following thrombin activation. J Biol Chem 1981;256:6927–6932.

95. Hoffmeister KM, et al. Mechanisms of cold-induced platelet actin assembly. J Biol Chem 2001;276:24751–24759.

96. Hoffmeister KM, et al. Glycosylation restores survival of chilled blood platelets. Science 2003;301:1531–1534.

97. Hoffmeister KM, et al. The clearance mechanism of chilled blood platelets. Cell 2003;112:87–97.

98. Ingber DE. Cellular tensegrity: defining new rules of biological design that govern the cytoskeleton. J Cell Sci 1993;104:613–627.

99. Ingber DE. Tensegrity: the architectural basis of cellular mechanotransduction. Annu Rev Physiol 1997;59:575–599.
100. Stark F, Golla R, Nachmias V. Formation and contraction of a microfilamentous shell in saponin-permeabilized platelets. J Cell Biol 1991;112:903–913.
101. Fox JE, Goll DE, et al. Identification of two proteins (actin-binding protein and P235) that are hydrolyzed by endogenous Ca^{2+}-dependent protease during platelet aggregation. J Biol Chem 1985;260:1060–1066.
102. Fox JE, et al. Spectrin is associated with membrane-bound actin filaments in platelets and is hydrolyzed by the Ca^{2+}-dependent protease during platelet activation. Blood 1987;69:537–545.
103. Fox JE, Phillips DR. Role of phosphorylation in mediating the association of myosin with the cytoskeletal structures of human platelets. J Biol Chem 1982;257:4120–4126.
104. Phillips DR, et al. Integrin tyrosine phosphorylation in platelet signaling. Curr Opin Cell Biol 2001;13:546–554.
105. Phillips DR, Nannizzi-Alaimo L, Prasad KS. Beta3 tyrosine phosphorylation in alphaIIbbeta3 (platelet membrane GP IIb-IIIa) outside-in integrin signaling. Thromb Haemost 2001;86:246–258.
106. Jenkins AL, et al. Tyrosine phosphorylation of the beta3 cytoplasmic domain mediates integrin-cytoskeletal interactions. J Biol Chem 1998;273:13878–13885.
107. Gilligan DM, et al. The junctional complex of the membrane skeleton. Semin Hematol 1993;30:74–83.
108. Matsuoka Y, Li X, Bennett V. Adducin: structure, function and regulation. Cell Mol Life Sci 2000;57:884–895.
109. Gilligan DM, Sarid R, Weese J. Adducin in platelets: activation-induced phosphorylation by PKC and proteolysis by calpain. Blood 2002;99:2418–2426.
110. Stark F, Golla R, et al. Formation and contraction of a microfilamentous shell in saponin-permeabilized platelets. J Cell Biol 1991;112:903–913.
111. Barkalow KL, et al. Alpha-adducin dissociates from F-actin and spectrin during platelet activation. J Cell Biol 2003;161:557–570.
112. Kalhammer G, Bahler M. Unconventional myosins. Essays Biochem 2000;35:33–42.
113. Sellers JR. Myosins: a diverse superfamily. Biochim Biophys Acta 2000;1496:3–22.
114. Baker JP, Titus MA. Myosins: matching functions with motors. Curr Opin Cell Biol 1998;10:80–86.
115. Hasson T, Mooseker MS. The growing family of myosin motors and their role in neurons and sensory cells. Curr Opin Neurobiol 1997;7:615–623.
116. D'Apolito M, et al. Cloning of the murine non-muscle myosin heavy chain IIA gene ortholog of human MYH9 responsible for May-Hegglin, Sebastian, Fechtner, and Epstein syndromes. Gene 2002;286:215–222.
117. Di Pumpo M, et al. Defective expression of GPIb/IX/V complex in platelets from patients with May-Hegglin anomaly and Sebastian syndrome. Haematologica 2002;87:943–947.
118. Heath KE, et al. Nonmuscle myosin heavy chain IIA mutations define a spectrum of autosomal dominant macrothrombocytopenias: May-Hegglin anomaly and Fechtner, Sebastian, Epstein, and Alport-like syndromes. Am J Hum Genet 2001;69:1033–1045.
119. Krueger EW, et al. A dynamin-cortactin-Arp2/3 complex mediates actin reorganization in growth factor-stimulated cells. Mol Biol Cell 2003;14:1085–1096.
120. Vidal C, et al. Cdc42/Rac1-dependent activation of the p21-activated kinase (PAK) regulates human platelet lamellipodia spreading: implication of the cortical-actin binding protein cortactin. Blood 2002;100:4462–4469.

121. Shcherbina A, et al. WASP and N-WASP in human platelets differ in sensitivity to protease calpain. Blood 2001;98:2988–2991.

122. Blanchoin L, Pollard TD, et al. Interactions of ADF/cofilin, Arp2/3 complex, capping protein and profilin in remodeling of branched actin filament networks. Curr Biol, 2000;10:1273–1282.

123. Davidson MM, Haslan RJ. Dephosphorylation of cofilin in stimulated platelets:roles for a GTP-binding protein and Ca^{2+}. Biochem J 1994;301:41–47.

124. Harbeck B, et al. Phosphorylation of the vasodilator-stimulated phosphoprotein regulates its interaction with actin. J Biol Chem 2000;275:30817–30825.

125. Huttelmaier S, et al. Characterization of the actin binding properties of the vasodilator-stimulated phosphoprotein VASP. FEBS Lett 1999;451:68–74.

126. Huttelmaier S, et al. The interaction of the cell-contact proteins VASP and vinculin is regulated by phosphatidylinositol-4,5-bisphosphate. Curr Biol 1998;8:479–488.

127. Butt E, Abel K, et al. cAMP- and cGMP-dependent protein kinase phosphorylation sites of the focal adhesion vasodilator-stimulated phosphoprotein (VASP) in vitro and in intact human platelets. J Biol Chem 1994;269:14509–14517.

128. Yin HL, Stossel TP. Control of cytoplasmic actin gel-sol transformation by gelsolin, a calcium-dependent regulatory protein. Nature 1979;281: 583–586.

129. Sun HQ, Yamamoto M, et al. Gelsolin, a multifunctional actin regulatory protein. J Biol Chem 1999;274:33179–33182.

130. Yin HL, Hartwig JH, et al. Ca^{2+} control of actin filament length. Effects of macrophage gelsolin on actin polymerization. J Biol Chem 1981;256:9693–9697.

131. Bearer EL. Direct observation of actin filament severing by gelsolin and binding by gCap39 and CapZ. J Cell Biol 1991;115:1629–1638.

132. Wang YL. Exchange of actin subunits at the leading edge of living fibroblasts: possible role of treadmilling. J Cell Biol 1985;101:597–602.

133. Imaoka T, Lynham JA, Haslam RJ. Purification and characterization of the 47,000-dalton protein phosphorylated during degranulation of human platelets. J Biol Chem 1983;258:11404–11414.

134. Niwa R, et al. Control of actin reorganization by Slingshot, a family of phosphatases that dephosphorylate ADF/cofilin. Cell 2002;108:233–246.

135. McGough A. F-actin-binding proteins. Curr Opin Struct Biol 1998;8:166–176.

136. Bamburg JR, McGough A, Ono S. Putting a new twist on actin: ADF/cofilins modulate actin dynamics. Trends Cell Biol 1999;9:364–370.

137. McGough A, et al. Cofilin changes the twist of F-actin: implications for actin filament dynamics and cellular function. J Cell Biol 1997;138:771–781.

138. Chan AY, Bailly M, et al. Role of cofilin in epidermal growth factor-stimulated actin polymerization and lamellipod protrusion. J Cell Biol 2000;148:531–542.

139. Arber S, Barbayannis FA, et al. Regulation of actin dynamics through phosphorylation of cofilin by LIM-kinase. Nature 1998;393:805–809.

140. Yang N, Higuchi O, et al. Cofilin phosphorylation by LIM-kinase 1 and its role in Rac-mediated actin reorganization. Nature 1998;393:809–812.

141. Zebda N, et al. Phosphorylation of ADF/cofilin abolishes EGF-induced actin nucleation at the leading edge and subsequent lamellipod extension. J Cell Biol 2000;151:1119–1128.

142. Loisel TP, Boujemaa R, et al. Reconstitution of actin-based motility of *Listeria* and *Shigella* using pure proteins. Nature 1999;401:613–616.

143. Rogers SL, et al. Molecular requirements for actin-based lamella formation in *Drosophila* S2 cells. J Cell Biol 2003;162:1079–1088.

144. Machesky LM, Atkinson SJ, et al. Purification of a cortical complex containing two unconventional actins from *Acanthamoeba* by affinity chromatography on profilin-agarose. J Cell Biol 1994;127:107–115.

145. Bearer EL, Satpute-Krishnan P. The role of the cytoskeleton in the life cycle of viruses and intracellular bacteria: tracks, motors, and polymerization machines. Curr Drug Targets Infect Disord 2002;2:247–264.

146. Tilney LG, DeRosier DJ, et al. How *Listeria* exploits host cell actin to form its own cytoskeleton. II. Nucleation, actin filament polarity, filament assembly, and evidence for a pointed end capper. J Cell Biol 1992;118:83–93.

147. Welch MD, Rosenblat J, et al. Interaction of human Arp2/3 complex and the *Listeria monocytogenes* ActA protein in actin filament nucleation. Science 1998;128:105–108.

148. Bearer EL. Fluorescence microscopy of single actin filaments labeled by conjugation to rhodamine. Biol Bull 1992;115:1629–1638.

149. Higgs HN, Pollard TD. regulation of actin filament networks through the Arp2/3 complex: activation by a diverse arrray of proteins. Annu Rev Biochem 2001;70:649–676.

150. Mullins RD, Heuser JA, et al. The interaction of Arp2/3 complex with actin: nucleation, high affinity pointed end capping, and formation of branching networks of filaments. Proc Natl Acad Sci USA 1998;95:6181–6186.

151. Pantaloni D, Boujemaa R, et al. The Arp2/3 complex branches filament barbed ends: functional antagonism with capping proteins. Nat Cell Biol 2000;2:385–391.

152. Svitkina TM, Borisy GG. Arp2/3 complex and actin depolymerizing factor/cofilin in dendritic organization and readmilling of actin filament array in lamellipodia. J Cell Biol 1999;145:1009–1026.

153. Bearer EL. An actin-associated protein present in the microtubule organizing center and the growth cones. of PC-12 cells. J Neurosci 1992;12:750–761.

154. Bearer EL. 2E4(kaptin): a novel actin-associated protein from human blood platelets found in lamellipodia and the tips of the stereocilia of the inner ear. Eur J Cell Biol 1999;78:117–126.

155. Bearer EL. Actin and actin-associated proteins in *Xenopus* embryos: relationship to cytoarchitecture and gastrulation. In Pederson R, ed. Cytoskeleton in development. Academic Press, New York, 1992, p. 26.

156. Tilney LG, Tilney MS, DeRosier DJ. Actin filaments, stereocilia, and hair cells: how cells count and measure. Annu Rev Cell Biol 1992;8:257–274.

157. Berg JS, et al. Myosin-X is an unconventional myosin that undergoes intrafilopodial motility. Nat Cell Biol 2002;4:246–250.

158. Wehrle-Haller B, Imhof B. The inner lives of focal adhesions. Trends Cell Biol 2002;12:382–389.

159. Condeelis J. Life at the leading edge: the formation of cell protrusions. Annu Rev Cell Biol 1993;9:411–444.

160. Sheetz MP, et al. Extension of filopodia by motor-dependent actin assembly. Cell Motil Cytoskel 1992;22:160–169.

161. Brahmbhatt AA, et al. ERK and RhoA differentially regulate pseudopodia growth and retraction during chemotaxis. Genetic fine mapping of the Miyoshi myopathy locus and exclusion of eight candidate genes. J Biol Chem 2003;278:13016–13025.

162. Les Erickson F, et al. Localization of a class III myosin to filopodia tips in transfected HeLa cells requires an actin-binding site in its tail domain. Mol Biol Cell 2003;14:4173–4180.

163. Bearer EL, Chen AF, et al. 2E4/Kaptin (KPTN)—a candidate gene for the hearing loss locus, DFNA4. Ann Hum Genet 2000;64:189–119.

164. Lazarides E, Burridge K. Alpha-actinin: immunofluorescent localization of a muscle sructural protein in nonmuscle cells. Cell 1975;6:289–298.
165. Matsudaira P. Modular organization of actin crosslinking proteins. Trends Bichem Sci 1991;16:87–92.
166. Otey CA, Pavalko FM, et al. An interaction between α-actinin and β1 integrin subunit. J Cell Biol 1990;111:721–729.
167. Fukami K, Furuhashi K, et al. Requirements of phosphatidylinositol 4,5-bisphosphate for alpha-actinin function. Nature 1992;359:150–152.
168. Greenwood JA, Theibert AB, et al. Restructuring of focal adhesion plaques by PI-3 kinase. Regulation of PtdIns (3,4,5)-p(3) binding to alpha-actinin. J Cell Biol 2000;150:627–642.
169. Izaguirre G, Aguirre L, et al. Tyrosine phosphorylation of α-actin in activated platelets. J Biol Chem 1999;274:3712–37020.
170. Izaguirre G, Aguirre L, et al. The cytoskeltal/nonmuscle isofor of a actin is phosphorylated during degranulation of human platelets. J Biol Chem 2001; 276:28,676–28,685.
171. Maguire PB, Fitzgerald DJ. Platelet proteomics. J Thromb Haemost 2003; 1:1593–1601.
172. Lindemann S, et al. Activated platelets mediate inflammatory signaling by regulated interleukin 1beta synthesis. J Cell Biol 2001;154:485–490.

5   Platelets and Inflammation

Meinrad Gawaz, MD

INTRODUCTION

Platelets play a major physiological role in control of vascular integrity at the site of vascular lesions. However, the pathophysiological role of platelets is much broader than regulation of hemostasis and thrombosis. Platelets are critical elements in linking and modulating thrombosis, inflammation, and tissue repair. Platelets are stimulated by a variety of agonists including thrombin or ADP and also by inflammatory agents such as antibodies, complement, bacteria, and others. Platelets contribute to inflammation by interacting with inflammatory cells via adhesion and secretion of prestored proinflammatory mediators. Thus, platelets are critical elements in the pathophysiology of inflammation and modulate significantly a variety of inflammatory diseases. A profound understanding of the molecular mechanisms underlying the role of platelet in

From: *Contemporary Cardiology:*
Platelet Function: Assessment, Diagnosis, and Treatment
Edited by: M. Quinn and D. Fitzgerald © Humana Press Inc., Totowa, NJ

inflammation may result in new therapeutic strategies in acute and chronic inflammatory diseases.

THE PLATELET, THE INFLAMMATORY CELL

The fundamental role of platelets is to maintain the vascular integrity and to prevent loss of blood at sites of vascular injury. Under physiological conditions platelets circulate in the artery branch without interacting with each other or with structures of the intact vessel wall *(1)*. At the location of an endothelial disruption, subendothelial matrix proteins including collagen and von Willebrand factor (vWF) are exposed to circulating platelets that are recognized by specific platelet membrane receptors such as glycoprotein (GP)VI *(2)* or the plasma membrane complex GPIb-IX-V *(3–5)*. Once adherent to the subendothelium, platelets spread on the surface and release granule-stored components that recruit additional platelets to the arterial lesion. In addition, adhering platelets express the activated form of the fibrinogen receptor GPIIb-IIIa that mediates platelet aggregation through formation of fibrinogen bridges between two adjacent platelets *(6,7)* (Fig. 1).

Despite regulation of hemostasis, platelets are involved in thrombosis and inflammation. Hemostasis, thrombosis, and inflammation are complex mechanisms with overlapping steps and connecting pathways. Interactions between platelets and inflammatory cells (e.g., endothelium, leukocytes) take place at various stages of the inflammatory process *(8)*. They occur in the circulation as well as in extravascular inflammatory sites and are regulated through adhesion receptors and proinflammatory mediators that are released from internal stores of activated platelets. Platelets have been shown to be involved in inflammatory diseases caused by pathogens including bacteria, viruses, or parasites, leading to infectious endocarditis, sepsis, or the acquired thrombocytopenia that occurs during retroviral infections caused by the human immunodeficiency virus (HIV) and T-cell lymphotropic virus *(9)* (Table 1). In these diseases platelets participate in nonspecific immunodefense mechanisms caused by exogenous pathogens. Furthermore, platelets are involved in acute and chronic inflammation that is not directly related to infectious pathogens including diseases such as acute respiratory distress syndrome (ARDS), systemic inflammatory response syndrome, immune complex disease, allergic asthma, inflammatory bowel disease *(10)*, multiple organ failure in septic shock *(11,12)*, organ dysfunction associated with cardiopulmonary bypass *(13)*, or acute coronary syndromes *(14)* including acute myocardial infarction and reperfusion *(15,16)* (Table 1). Moreover, platelets are fundamentally involved in chronic inflammatory

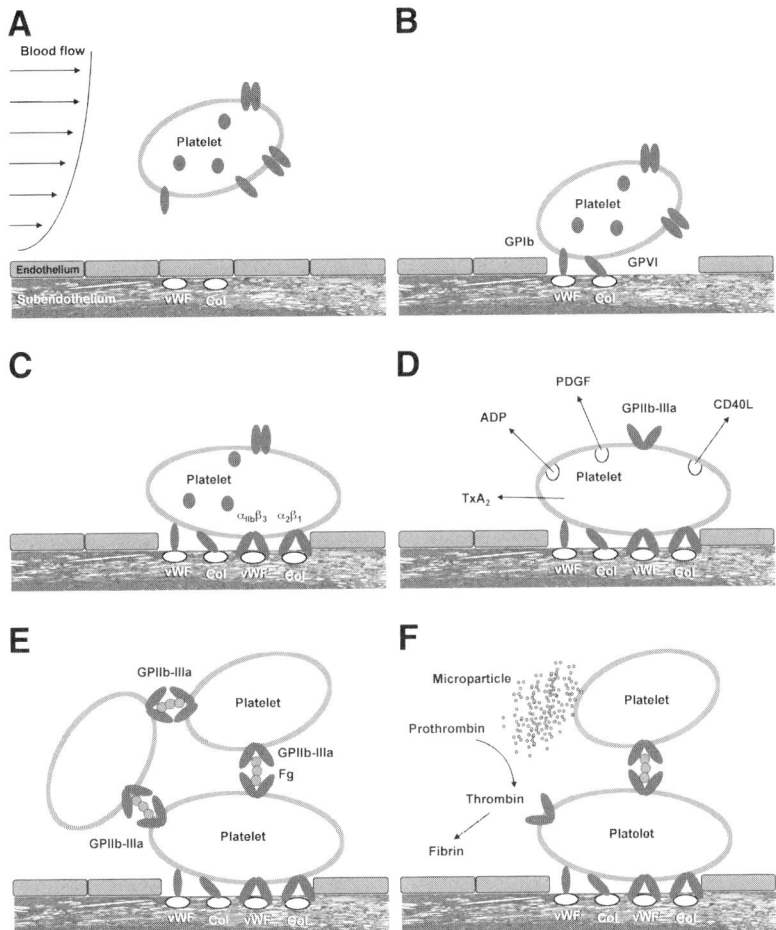

Fig. 1. (A) Platelet-dependent formation of a thrombus at an atherosclerotic plaque. Platelets do not adhere to the intact endothelial monolayer under physiological conditions. At the site of vascular lesions, extracellular matrix proteins like von Willebrand factor (vWF) and collagen (Col) are exposed to the blood. **(B)** Via the membrane adhesion receptors GPIbα and GPVI, platelets loosely adhere to the subendothelium. **(C)** This initial adhesion results in platelet activation and "opening" of the integrin receptors $\alpha_{IIb}\beta_3$ (fibrinogen receptor) and $\alpha_2\beta_1$ (collagen receptor). The interaction of $\alpha_{IIb}\beta_3$ and $\alpha_2\beta_1$ with extracellular matrix proteins stabilizes platelet adhesion (firm adhesion). **(D)** Subsequently, platelets spread and degranulate and thereby recruit additional platelets to the already adherent ones. **(E)** Platelets form microaggregates via fibrinogen "bridges" between two $\alpha_{IIb}\beta_3$ receptors. **(F)** Formation of microparticles around the platelet aggregates catalyzes thrombin generation and thus fibrin formation that stabilizes the platelet thrombus. CD40L, CD40 ligand; PDGF, platelet-derived growth factor; TXA$_2$, thromboxane A$_2$.

Table 1
Role of Platelets in Inflammation

Inflammation caused by infection
    Infectious endocarditis
    Sepsis
    Acquired idiopathic thrombocytopenia
Acute inflammation not directly related to infectious pathogens
    Acute respiratory distress syndrome (ARDS)
    Systemic inflammatory response syndrome (SIRS)
    Multiple organ failure (MOF)
    Immune complex disease
    Allergic asthma
    Cardiopulmonary bypass
    Inflammatory bowel disease
    Acute coronary syndrome (ACS)
    Myocardial infarction and reperfusion
Chronic inflammation
    Atherosclerosis
    Development of vulnerable coronary plaque
    Rheumatoid arthritis
    Periodontitis

diseases including atherosclerosis *(17,18)*, progression, and induction of vulnerable coronary plaques leading to acute coronary syndrome *(19)*, rheumatoid arthritis, or periodontitis *(10)* (Table 1). Thus, platelets are both target cell and effector in a variety of inflammatory diseases.

RECEPTORS THAT REGULATE PLATELET ADHESION TO INFLAMMATORY CELLS

The mechanisms of thrombosis and inflammation require a close interaction among platelets, endothelium, leukocytes, plasma coagulation factors, and structures of the vessel wall (extracellular matrix) *(20)*. Adhesion processes that are regulated by numerous adhesion receptors play a major role in these mechanisms. Platelets express multiple glycoproteins on their membranes that mediate the interactions with other platelets, with endothelial cells, or with leukocytes *(21,22)*. Furthermore, platelet adhesion receptors mediate platelet attachment to subendothelial matrix proteins as well as interactions with plasmatic coagulation factors. Firm contact of platelets to cells or the vascular subendothelium enables platelets to localize a procoagulatory or inflammatory response in distinct locations of the vasculature *(23)*.

Table 2
Membrane Glycoproteins Involved in Platelet Adhesion to Inflammatory Cells

Platelet membrane glycoprotein	Ligand/counterreceptor
Integrins	
$\alpha_{IIb}\beta_3$ (GPIIb-IIIa, CD41-CD61)	Fg, Fn, Vn, vWF, Ln
$\alpha_v\beta_3$ (vitronectin receptor, CD51-CD61)	Vn, Fg, Fn
$\alpha_2\beta_1$ (collagen receptor, CD49b)	Coll, Ln
$\alpha_5\beta_1$ (fibronectin receptor, CD49c)	Fn
$\alpha_6\beta_1$ (laminin receptor, CD49f)	Ln
Leucin-rich glycoproteins	
GPIb-V-IX (CD42a-b-c)	vWF, CD11b-CD18
GPIV (CD36)	TSP-1
Selectins	
P-selectin (CD62P)	PSGL-1
Immunoglobulin-like adhesion receptors	
ICAM-2	Fg, $\alpha_L\beta_2$ (LFA-1, CD11a)
PECAM-1	?
JAM-1	?
JAM-3	$\alpha_M\beta_2$ (MAC-1, CD11b)
GPVI	Coll

Abbreviations: GP, glycoprotein; Fg, fibrinogen; Vn, vitronectin; Fn, fibronectin; Coll, collagen; Ln, laminin; vWF, von Willebrand factor; TSP, thrombospondin; ICAM, intercellular adhesion molecule; PECAM, platelet-endothelial cell adhesion molecule; JAM, junctional adhesion molecule; LFA, leukocyte function-associated antigen; PSGL, P-selectin glycoprotein ligand.

Platelets express a variety of major membrane glycoproteins that are classified into four groups according to their characteristic structures: *integrins, leucine-rich glycoproteins, selectins,* and receptors of the *immunoglobulin-type (24)* (Table 2). All platelet membrane receptors have been shown to recognize a counterligand (e.g., fibrinogen) or receptor (e.g., P-selectin) on the partner cell and to mediate intercellular, heterotypic adhesion.

Integrins

Integrins are adhesion receptors that link structures of the cytoskeleton to the extracellular matrix *(25–27)*. Integrins are ubiquitous and can be found on almost all cells including platelets. In addition to platelet aggregation and adhesion, integrins participate in tissue development and differentiation as well as in the growth of atherosclerotic plaques and vascular remodeling. Integrins are noncovalently linked heterodimers consisting of α- and β-subunits. They are subdivided on the basis of the β-chain, which pairs with a specific α-chain to form a functional receptor. To date 8 β- and 14 α-subunits have been identified *(25)*. The β-subunit serves for the structural classification, and the α-subunit determines the specificity. Integrins interact with numerous glycoproteins (e.g., collagen, fibronectin, fibrinogen, laminin, thrombospondin, vitronectin, and vWF) (Table 2). These glycoproteins are components of the extracellular matrix, but they also occur in solution in plasma. The β_1- and β_3-integrins recognize the arginine-glycine-aspartate (RGD) amino acid sequence. The RGD sequence is a component of numerous extracellular matrix proteins and is also found in fibrinogen molecules. Synthetic peptides exhibiting the RGD sequence and having similar molecular structures are competitive inhibitors of ligand binding to integrins. Five different integrins have been described so far on platelets, three of the β_1-integrin class ($\alpha_2\beta_1$ [collagen receptor], $\alpha_5\beta_1$ [fibronectin receptor], and $\alpha_6\beta_1$ [laminin receptor]) and two of the β_3-integrin family ($\alpha_{IIb}\beta_3$ [fibrinogen receptor] and $\alpha_v\beta_3$ [vitronectin receptor]) *(25)* (Table 2).

GPIIb-IIIa ($\alpha_{IIb}\beta_3$) belongs to the β_3-integrins and is specific for the platelet/megakaryocyte system. GPIIb-IIIa is the most frequently occurring membrane glycoprotein of blood platelets and is constitutively expressed on the surface membrane. A substantial portion of GPIIb-IIIa is also present in intracellular stores (α-granules and the open canalicular system) and can be translocated to the plasma membrane upon activation. The main task of GPIIb-IIIa is to bind fibrinogen to the activated platelet surface, which allows platelets to aggregate (homotype intercellular adhesion). Under physiological conditions, circulating platelets carry the resting, not activated GPIIb-IIIa complex on their surface (*low-affinity state*) *(27)*. In the unactivated form, GPIIb-IIIa can only bind immobilized, but not soluble, fibrinogen. Platelet activation leads to a rapid change in the conformation of the GPIIb-IIIa complex and thereby to the exposure of high-affinity fibrinogen binding sites (*high-affinity state*) *(27)*. This allows binding of soluble fibrinogen to the platelet surface and initiates aggregation. Besides its role in platelet aggregation, GPIIb-IIIa mediates platelet adhesion to subendothelial matrix proteins (fibrinogen, vWF, vitronectin, and laminin). Additionally, the receptor interferes with endothelial cells (heterotype intercellular adhesion) via the formation of fibrinogen "bridges" between the platelet GPIIb-IIIa and the vitronectin receptor $\alpha_v\beta_3$ expressed on the luminal aspect of endothelial cells *(27)*.

Whereas GPIIb-IIIa is specific for platelets and megakaryocytes, the vitronectin receptor ($\alpha_v\beta_3$) is found on many different types of cells including platelets, endothelial cells, and smooth muscle cells *(7)*. Like GPIIb-IIIa ($\alpha_{IIb}\beta_3$), the vitronectin receptor ($\alpha_v\beta_3$) possesses the β_3-chain but this is paired with a different α-chain (α_v) *(7)*. In contrast to GPIIb-IIIa, the vitronectin receptor occurs in only very low amounts in platelets (50 receptors per platelet) and plays a very minor role in platelet function *(7)*. The vitronectin receptor also binds other RGD-containing glycoproteins such as fibrinogen, fibronectin, vWF, and thrombospondin (Table 2). $\alpha_v\beta_3$ contributes to the adhesion and migration of endothelial and smooth muscle cells to the extracellular matrix *(7)*. Like GPIIb-IIIa, $\alpha_v\beta_3$ possesses a binding site for the RGD sequence but not for the KQAGDV sequence. When $\alpha_v\beta_3$-positive cells adhere to specific matrix proteins, the receptors are enriched in the region of focal contact sites (clustering). The vitronectin receptor plays a role in angiogenesis, apoptosis, and proliferation *(7,28)*. Inhibition of $\alpha_v\beta_3$ by antagonists reduces the migration and proliferation of smooth muscle cells—mechanisms that participate in atherogenesis and intima proliferation. $\alpha_v\beta_3$ is also expressed on the luminal side of endothelial cells and mediates the adhesion of activated platelets to endothelial cells. Besides the two β_3-integrins, platelets possess three β_1-integrins that seem to regulate the primary adhesion of platelets to the subendothelial matrix of the injured vessel wall. However, the exact role of β_1-integrins in hemostasis or thrombosis remains to be determined *(7)*.

Leucine-Rich Glycoproteins

Platelets contain two membrane glycoprotein complexes, GPIb-IX-V and GPIV, which are characterized by their abundance of the amino acid leucine *(3–5)*. The GPIb-IX-V complex forms the adhesion receptor for vWF and plays a central role in primary hemostasis. The main task of GPIb-IX-V is the adhesion of circulating platelets to vWF immobilized in collagen fibrils in spite of the significant shear forces that exist in regions of arterial flow. The GPIb-IX-V complex consists of four subunits. GPIbα (150 kDa) and GPIbβ (27 kDa) are covalently linked to each other by disulfide bridges. Each GPIb molecule binds noncovalently to a GPIX molecule at a ratio of 1:1. GPV (82 kDa) is the central unit of the receptor complex and is surrounded by two GPIb and two GPIX proteins linked noncovalently with one another. All subunits of the GPIb-IX-V complex exhibit leucine-rich regions, whose functions are mostly unknown. The GPIbα subunit is very significant for the receptor function. In the region of the extracellular domain, GPIbα possesses binding sites for vWF and thrombin. The cytoplasmic domain anchors GPIbα in the cytoskeleton. Recent data indicate that GPIbα on platelets is a potential counterreceptor for Mac-1 *(29)*. Furthermore, GPIbα-associated vWF has also been proposed as a mediator of platelet-endothelium adhesion *(30)*.

Selectins

Selectins are vascular adhesion receptors that mediate the heterotype interactions of cells. The molecular structure of selectins is characterized by an extracellular lectin domain with a neighboring epidermal growth factor-like domain followed by short regions that are homologous to the regulatory complement factors *(31,32)*. Three selectins have been described *(31,32)*. E-selectin occurs on cytokine-activated endothelial cells and modulates granulocyte adhesion. Resting endothelial cells do not contain any E-selectin. L-selectin occurs constitutively on leukocytes, is shed from the leukocyte surface after activation, and participates in the adhesion of leukocytes to endothelial cells *(31,32)*. P-selectin is found in platelets and endothelial cells, where it is stored in thrombocytic α-granules and endothelial Weibel-Palade bodies, respectively. P-selectin is not expressed on the surface of resting platelets or endothelial cells. However, activation leads to the rapid release and surface expression of P-selectin on both types of cells. Both endothelial P-selectin and P-selectin exposed on activated adhering platelets at sites of endothelial disruption mediate initial tethering and rolling of leukocytes through their P-selectin glycoprotein ligand-1 (PSGL-1) *(33,34)*. P-selectin binding to leukocytes induces activation of Mac-1 and allows firm adhesion and transplatelet migration *(34)*.

Immunoglobulin-Type Receptors

Several immunoglobulin-type receptors have been described on platelets including platelet-endothelial cell adhesion molecule-1 (PECAM-1) *(6)*, intercellular adhesion molecule-2 (ICAM-2) *(35)*, and junctional adhesion molecule-1 and -3 (JAM-1 and -3) *(36–38)*. PECAM-1 occurs in platelets as well as in endothelial cells, neutrophils, and monocytes *(6)*. The receptor appears to play a part in platelet adhesion to the subendothelium and to leukocytes by binding to glycosaminoglycans on their membrane. ICAM-2 has been described on activated platelets *(35)*. The JAMs are newly discovered members of the Ig superfamily, which mediate cell-cell adhesion. Platelets contain at least two members of the JAM family including JAM-1 and JAM-3 *(36)*. Platelet JAM-1 might be involved in primary hemostasis as the crosslinking of JAM-1 with FcγRII resulted in platelet aggregation *(27)*. It is also proposed to mediate platelet adhesion to cytokine-inflamed endothelial cells *(39)*. Platelet JAM-3 has been recently shown to serve as a counterreceptor for Mac-1-mediated platelet-leukocyte interactions *(38)*.

PLATELET-DERIVED MEDIATORS THAT MODULATE FUNCTION OF INFLAMMATORY CELLS

Chemotaxis is a central mechanism to recruit inflammatory cells to a site of tissue damage or repair *(40)*. Platelets exert an important influence on the chemotaxis of other cells. During adhesion, platelets are activated and release a variety of potent chemotactic factors that are either stored in their granules or cytoplasm or synthesized after stimulation *(41,42)*. Moreover, platelets may by direct cell contact modulate the chemotactic properties of other cells including leukocytes *(43,44)* and endothelium *(45,46)*. Platelets contain three different forms of storage granules: dense bodies or dense granules, α-granules, and lysosomes. The granules are characteristic for platelets and serve as storage sites for proteins and other low-molecular-weight compounds (Table 3).

Dense Granules

The dense granules are named after their characteristic electron-optical density and contain high levels of adenine and guanine nucleotides, divalent cations, and serotonin. Thus, during the release reaction, prothrombotic constituents are liberated that recruit other platelets to adhere and aggregate. Serotonin (5-hydroxytryptamine) acts predominantly as a local vasoconstrictor and proinflammatory compound. Serotonin has been proposed to enhance the chemotactic responsiveness of human leukocytes *(47)*. Stimulation of monocytes through serotonin induces secretion of lymphocyte chemoattractant activity (interleukin-16 [IL-16]) that may promote the recruitment of T lymphocytes into an inflammatory focus *(48,49)*. Other dense-granule constituents (histamine, ATP) have been shown to support the proinflammatory reaction in the microenvironment of platelet adhesion *(41)*.

α-Granules

α-Granules represent the major granule population in size and number *(42)*. The α-granules are typical secretory vesicles that carry proteins to the cell surface to be released. Some of the released intragranular proteins adhere to the platelet surface or become integrated into the plasma membrane, and some diffuse into the extracellular fluid (Table 3). Two specific platelet proteins, β-thromboglobulin (β-TG) and platelet factor-4 (PF-4) are localized in α-granules together with proteoglycans *(50)*. The latter include a family of β-TG-antigen molecules consisting of the platelet basic protein (PBP), connective tissue-activating protein-III (CTAP-III), and neutrophil-activating protein-2 (NAP-2), which are all precursors of β-TG and PF-4. Purified PF-4 lacks

Table 3
Platelet-Derived Vasoactive, Proinflammatory, and Mitogenic Constituents

Dense granule
  Serotonin (5-HT)
  Adenine nucleotides: ATP, ADP
  Guanine nucleotides: GTP, GDP
  Histamine
α-Granule
  β-Tromboglobulin (β-TG), platelet factor-4 (PF-4)
  Platelet basic protein (PBP), connective tissue-activating protein III (CTAP-
    III), neutrophil-activating protein-2 (NAP-2)
  Epithelial neutrophil-activating protein-78 (ENA-78)
  Platelet-derived growth factor (PDGF)
  Transforming growth factor-β (TGF-β)
  Endothelial cell growth factor (ECGF)
  Epidermal growth factor (EGF)
  Vascular endothelial growth factor (VEGF)
  Insulin-like growth factor (IGF)
  Basic fibroblast growth factor (bFGF)
  Metalloproteinases 2 and 9
Lysosome
  Acid proteases
  Glycohydrolases
Cytosol
  Interleukin-1 β (IL-1 β)
  CD40 ligand (CD40L)
Lipid mediators
  Platelet-activating factor (PAF)
  Thromboxane A_2 (TXA$_2$)
  Prostaglandin E_2 (PGE$_2$)
  Lysophosphatidic acid (LPA)
  Sphingosine-1 phosphate (SP-1)
  Microparticles

chemotactic activity for leukocytes but costimulation of leukocytes with tumor necrosis factor (TNF)-α results in exocytosis of secondary granule markers or tight adhesion to different surface proteins *(51)*. PF-4 not only affects neutrophils, but it also induces the release of histamine by basophils and plays a role in eosinophil adhesion *(42)*. β-TG represents a chemokine for neutrophils, monocytes, and lymphocytes.

Epithelial neutrophil-activating protein-78 (ENA-78) is another α-granule constituent that stimulates neutrophil activation *(52)*. Among the mitogenic factors present in platelet α-granules, the specific platelet-derived growth factor (PDGF) is present together with transforming growth factor-β (TGF-β), endothelial cell growth factor (ECGF), epidermal growth factor (EGF), vascular endothelial growth factor (VEGF), vascular permeability factor (VPF), basic fibroblast growth factor (bFGF), and insulin-like growth factor (IGF) *(52)*. PDGF and TGF-β are growth factors that exert chemotactic properties on smooth muscle cells, macrophages, monocytes, and fibroblasts *(52)*. Recently, PDGF and TGF-β have been found to induce expression of VEGF in smooth muscle cells *(53)*; VEGF is an endothelial mitogen and chemokine that stimulates endothelial cell migration. Furthermore, VEGF has been shown to support transendothelial migration of monocytes and to be chemotactic for mast cells, as well as monocytes. The chemokines RANTES and macrophage inflammatory protein-1α (MIP-1α) belong to the CC chemokines and are potent chemokines for basophils, eosinophils, T lymphocytes, and monocytes *(52)*.

Lysosomes

Lysosomes contain enzymes such as acid proteases and glycohydrolases that may participate in inflammation and extravasation of leukocytes through their cytotoxic and proteolytic activity at sites of platelet accumulation at inflamed tissue *(54)* (Table 3).

Cytosol

Other important proinflammatory mediators such as IL-1β and CD40 ligand (CD40L) are present in the cytosol, are generated from mRNA, and are release upon activation *(55)*. IL-1β is a central mediator in the cytokine cascade and is a potent activator of vascular cytokine production *(55,57,58)*. CD40L is structurally related to TNF-α and translocates within seconds of activation to the platelet surface *(46,56)*. CD40L stimulates endothelium to express ICAM-1, VCAM-1 and E-selectin, thus modulating leukocyte-endothelium interaction *(46)*. Moreover, CD40L stimulates platelet secretion and stabilizes platelet aggregation by interference with GPIIb-IIIa *(59)*.

Lipid Mediators

In addition to granule- and cytoplasma-stored substances, platelets release lipid mediators upon activation including platelet-activating factor (PAF), thromboxane A_2 (TXA_2), prostaglandin E_2 (PGE_2), platelet-derived lysophosphatidic acid (LPA), and sphingosine-1-phosphate (SP-1) *(60)*. PAF is a phosphoglyceride generated from the phospholipids of cell membranes. PAF promotes leukocyte-endothelium interaction and favors diapedesis of leukocytes *(61)*. TXA_2 is another potent platelet mediator derived from the platelet membrane. Upon platelet activation TXA$_2$ is synthesized *de novo* from arachidonic acid through the action of platelet cyclooxygenase-1 (COX-1), an enzyme that is inhibited irreversibly by aspirin *(62)*. TXA$_2$ is known to induce platelet aggregation at sites of platelet activation. In addition, the arachidonic acid metabolite acts as a potent proinflammatory mediator, inducing leukocyte adhesion to and migration across activated endothelial cells *(62)*. Another rich source of proinflammatory arachidonic acid metabolites is the platelet microparticles, membrane blebs that are shed from the surface of activated platelets by membrane vesiculation *(63)*. Platelet microparticles have been shown to increase the adhesion of monocytes to endothelial cells in a time- and dose-dependent manner *(63)*. In line with this finding, microparticle-derived arachidonic acid enhanced the expression of ICAM-1 on resting endothelial cells and upregulated CD11a/CD18 as well as CD11b/CD18 on monocytes.

Another potent inflammatory mediator, which is released in high amounts by activated platelets, is the cellular phospholipid LPA *(64)*. LPA also leads to the activation of nuclear factor-κB (NF-κB) in endothelial cells, induces the upregulation of endothelial adhesion molecules, such as E-selectin and ICAM-1, and initiates the release of MCP-1 and IL-8 *(64)*. Hence, LPA released during platelet-endothelial cell interactions at sites of endothelial dysfunction could function in a paracrine manner, directly modulating inflammatory and proliferative responses in the vascular wall.

PLATELET INTERACTION WITH THE ENDOTHELIUM

The vascular endothelium is central for maintaining homeostasis. Endothelial cells produce and present molecules that define the inflammatory properties of the vessel wall. They have dynamic control over chemotaxis, adhesion, and extravasation of circulating leukocytes to areas of injury or inflammation *(65)*. Control mechanisms include the expression and release of cytokines and chemokines and cell surface presentation of adhesion molecules in response to a diverse set of environmental elements, including rheologic and oxidative stress, cytokines, hormones, and infection.

Platelet Adhesion to Endothelium

In the past, numerous studies have shown that platelets can adhere to the intact endothelial monolayer and substantially modulate endothelial cell function *(67–75)*. Thus, under certain pathophysiological circumstances, endothelial denudation and exposure of subendothelial matrix

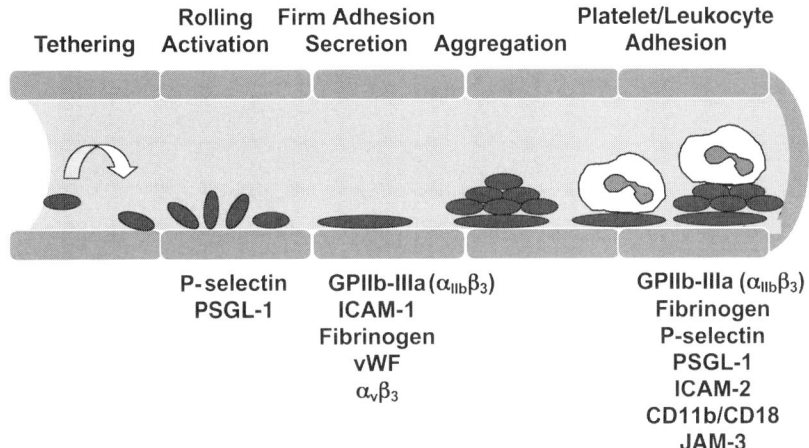

Fig. 2. Platelet adhesion to the endothelium. ICAM, intercellular adhesion molecule; JAM, junctional adhesion molecule; PSGL, P-selectin glycoprotein ligand; vWF, von Willebrand factor.

are not required for platelet adhesion to the vascular wall. Adherent platelets release a variety of proinflammatory mediators and growth hormones and have the potential to modify signaling cascades in vascular cells, inducing the expression of endothelial adhesion receptors and the release of endothelial chemoattractants. In this manner they might regulate the adhesion and infiltration of leukocytes, in particular of monocytes, into the vascular wall, a process thought to play a key role in acute and chronic inflammation. Normal "resting" endothelium represents a nonadhesive and nonthrombogenic surface that prevents extravasation of circulating blood cells *(66)*. In contrast, activated endothelial cells are proadhesive and promote the adhesion of circulating blood platelets. Adhesion of platelets to the intact but activated endothelium in the absence of previous endothelial denudation involves a surface receptor-dependent process that allows "capturing" of circulating platelets toward the vessel wall even under high shear stress. Similar to the recruitment of leukocytes *(65)*, the adhesion of platelets to the vascular endothelial surface is a multistep process, in which platelets are tethered to the vascular wall, followed by platelet rolling and subsequent firm adhesion (Fig. 2).

Whereas the adhesion receptors involved in platelet attachment to the subendothelial matrix, e.g., following rupture of an atherosclerotic plaque, have been well defined during the past decade (Fig. 1), few studies have focused on the molecular determinants that promote the interaction between platelets and the intact vascular endothelium. The initial loose contact between circulating platelets and vascular endothelium (*platelet rolling*) is mediated by selectins, present on both endothelial cells and platelets *(76–80)*. P-selectin (CD62P) is rapidly expressed on the endothelial surface in response to inflammatory stimuli by translocating from membranes of storage granules (Weibel-Palade bodies) to the plasma membrane within seconds. Endothelial P-selectin has been demonstrated to mediate platelet rolling in both arterioles and venules in acute inflammatory processes *(76,79)*. E-selectin, which is also expressed on inflamed endothelial cells, also allows a loose contact between platelets and endothelium in vivo *(80)*. In line with the concept of endothelial inflammation as a trigger for platelet accumulation, the process of platelet rolling does not require previous platelet activation, since platelets from mice lacking P- and/or E-selectin roll as efficiently as wild-type platelets *(81)*.

So far few studies have addressed the exact nature of the ligands expressed on platelets that bind to endothelial P- or E-selectin. PSGL-1, a glycoprotein that avidly associates with P-selectin, is present predominantly on myeloid cells and mediates leukocyte-endothelium interactions and leukocyte-platelet interactions in vitro and in vivo *(82,83)*.

Another sialomucin that has been identified as a potential counter-receptor for platelet P-selectin is the leucine-rich GPIb-IX-V, the vWF receptor complex. Romo et al. *(30)* have demonstrated recently that cells expressing P-selectin roll on immobilized GPIbα. Platelet rolling on activated endothelium can be inhibited by antibodies against both P-selectin and GPIbα, indicating that the vWF receptor mediates platelet adhesion both to the subendothelial matrix and to intact endothelial cells. Future studies are needed to clarify whether the association of GPIbα with P-selectin leads to platelet activation similar to GPIbα-vWF interaction.

Interactions of selectins with their counterreceptors are characterized by high on and off rates, enabling platelets to attach rapidly to the endothelial monolayer with high resistance to tensile stress, explaining why adherent platelets can oppose the drag created by the shear rates present particularly in arterioles. On the other hand, these bonds have an intrinsically high dissociation rate and thus a limited half-life, which results in detachment at the tailing edge of platelets, where the tension is greatest, resulting in forward rotational movement (*rolling*) from torque imposed by the blood flow. However, because of their biophysical characteristics, selectin-ligand interactions are not sufficient to promote firm adhesion of platelets in the blood stream. This indicates that during rotational movement, new bonds, characterized by low dissociation rates, have to be formed that promote irreversible adhesion. These tighter interactions between platelets and the vascular wall involve the interplay of platelets and endothelial integrins as well as immunoglobulin-like adhesion molecules.

Apart from leucine-rich glycoproteins, the integrins are the major group of receptors involved in mediating platelet adhesion to matrix proteins including collagen, vitronectin, fibronectin, and laminin. GPIIb-IIIa ($\alpha_{IIb}\beta_3$) is the major integrin on platelets and plays a key role in platelet accumulation on activated endothelium. In the presence of soluble fibrinogen, $\alpha_{IIb}\beta_3$ mediates heterotypic cell adhesion to $\alpha_v\beta_3$-expressing cells including endothelial cells (16,84). Moreover, platelets firmly adhere to activated endothelial cells via $\alpha_{IIb}\beta_3$, a mechanism that can be blocked by antagonists of β_3-integrins (16). In vivo, firm platelet adhesion to the endothelium can be inhibited by anti-$\alpha_{IIb}\beta_3$ monoclonal antibody and platelets defective in $\alpha_{IIb}\beta_3$ do not adhere firmly to activated endothelial cells (85). Taken together, these data indicate that, apart from mediating platelet aggregation, the platelet fibrinogen receptor is of paramount importance in mediating firm attachment of platelets to the vascular endothelium (Fig. 2).

Only a few integrins have been reported to be expressed on the luminal side of endothelial cells. Among them, the vitronectin receptor ($\alpha_v\beta_3$) appears to play a crucial role in promoting platelet adhesion. The vitronectin receptor is upregulated in response to endothelial cell activation, e.g., by IL-1β or thrombin (16,86). Inhibition of $\alpha_v\beta_3$ attenuates platelet-endothelial cell interaction (16). Hence, both platelet $\alpha_{IIb}\beta_3$ and endothelial $\alpha_v\beta_3$ are involved in mediating firm adhesion of platelets to the luminal aspect of activated endothelial cells. However, direct binding of $\alpha_{IIb}\beta_3$ to endothelial $\alpha_v\beta_3$ has not been reported so far. In fact, heterotypic cell adhesion through $\alpha_{IIb}\beta_3$ and $\alpha_v\beta_3$ requires the presence of fibrinogen, which bridges the platelet fibrinogen receptor to the endothelial vitronectin receptor (84). Recent evidence suggests that this fibrinogen-dependent bridging mechanism rather than direct receptor-ligand interactions mediates firm platelet adhesion to the endothelium both in vitro and in vivo (Fig. 3) (85). The affinity of the platelet $\alpha_{IIb}\beta_3$ for its ligand underlies strict regulation and increases with platelet activation (inside out-integrin signaling; see p.120). Although even nonactivated $\alpha_{IIb}\beta_3$ can bind to immobilized fibrinogen, platelet activation during the initial contact between platelets and endothelial cells (platelet rolling), e.g., via GPIbα-P-selectin interaction, might enhance the fibrinogen binding capacity of $\alpha_{IIb}\beta_3$ and thereby facilitate subsequent firm platelet adhesion (30).

Recently, two members of the JAM adhesion receptor family have been identified in platelets, JAM-1 and JAM-3 (36–39). Platelets constitutively express JAM-1 (F11R) and inhibit JAM-1 by blocking mono-

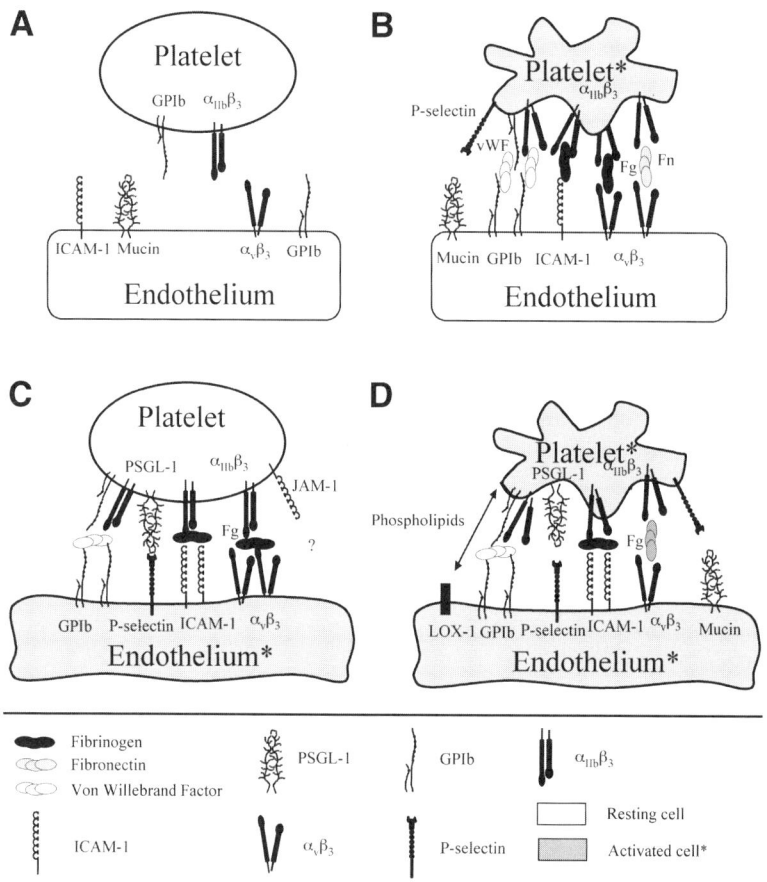

Fig. 3. Various possibilities of platelet interaction with endothelial cells. (**A**) Resting platelet and resting endothelium; (**B**) activated platelet and resting endothelium; (**C**) resting platelet and activated endothelium; (**D**) both activated platelet and endothelium. Fg, fibrinogen; Fn, fibronectin, ICAM, intercellular adhesion molecule; JAM, junctional adhesion molecule; LOX-1, lectin-like oxidized low-density lipoprotein; PSGL, P-selectin glycoprotein ligand; vWF, von Willebrand factor.

clonal antibody-reduced platelet adhesion to TNF-α-treated endothelial cells (Fig. 3).

Apart from the traditional adhesion receptors, *scavenger receptors* that bind oxidized low-density lipoprotein (oxLDL) appear to be involved in the recruitment of blood cells to the inflamed endothelial surface. The endothelial receptor for oxLDL, lectin-like oxLDL-1 (LOX-1), has been proposed to promote platelet adhesion to the endothelial cell surface *(74)*. Phosphatidylserines, exposed on the surface of activated

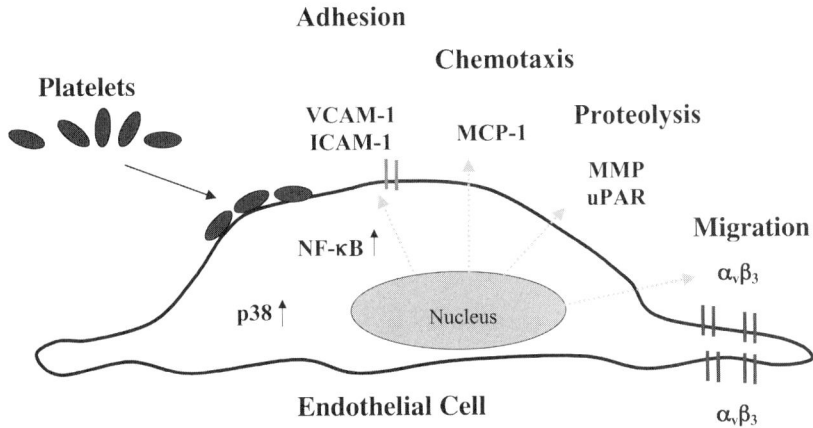

Fig. 4. Platelet induced endothelial inflammation. ICAM, intercellular adhesion molecule; MCP-1, monocyte chemoattractant protein-1; MMP, matrix metalloproteinase; NF-κB, nuclear factor-κB, uPAR, protease-activated receptor; VCAM, vascular cell adhesion molecule.

platelets, are the ligands for LOX-1. Since LOX-1 expression on endothelial cells is upregulated in vivo by hypertension and hypercholesterolinemia, the scavenger receptor might be important in initiating platelet adhesion to dysfunctional endothelium, especially in the early process of atherosclerosis (Fig. 3).

In summary, platelet-endothelial cell interactions are a multistep process, in which selectins and integrins or immunoglobin-like adhesion receptors play a predominant role. These receptor-dependent platelet-endothelial cell interactions allow transcellular communication via soluble mediators and might therefore play an important role in the initiation and progression of vascular inflammation (Fig. 3).

Platelet-Induced Endothelial Activation

During the adhesion process platelets are activated and release an arsenal of potent proinflammatory and promitogenic substances into the local microenvironment, thereby altering chemotactic, adhesive, and proteolytic properties of endothelial cells (Fig. 4). These platelet-induced alterations of the endothelial phenotype support chemotaxis, adhesion, and transmigration of monocytes to the site of inflammation. Among the various platelet-derived proinflammatory proteins, IL-1β has been identified as a major mediator of platelet-induced activation of endothelial cells *(57,58)*. The IL-1β activity expressed by platelets appears to be associated with the platelet surface *(57,58)*, and coincubation of endothelial cells with thrombin-activated platelets induces IL-1β-dependent secretion of IL-6 and IL-8 from endothelial cells. Further-more, incubation of cultured endothelial cells with thrombin-stimulated platelets significantly enhances the secretion of endothelial monocyte chemoattractant protein-1 (MCP-1) in an IL-1β-dependent manner (86,91). MCP-1 belongs to the CC family of chemokines and is thought to play a key role in the regulation of monocyte recruitment to inflamed tissue (91).

However, platelet IL-1β does not only modify endothelial release of chemotactic proteins, it also has the potential to increase endothelial expression of adhesion molecules. Surface expression of intercellular adhesion molecule-1 (ICAM-1) and $α_vβ_3$ on endothelial cells is signifi-cantly enhanced by activated platelets via IL-1β (86). Both enhanced chemokine release and upregulation of endothelial adhesion molecules through platelet-derived IL-1β act in concert and promote neutrophil and monocyte adhesion to the endothelium. IL-1β-dependent expres-sion of early inflammatory genes, such as MCP-1 or ICAM-1, involves the activation of the transcription factor NF-κB. Transient adhesion of platelets to the endothelium initiates degradation of inhibitor of κB (IκB) and supports activation of NF-κB in endothelial cells, thereby inducing NF-κB-dependent chemokine gene transcription (92,93). Parallel to this finding, transfection of "decoy" κB oligonucleotides or a dominant-negative IKB kinase (IKK) mutant attenuates platelet-induced nuclear translocation of NF-κB and MCP-1 secretion in endothelial cells (93). Likewise, platelet-induced NF-κB-activation was found to be largely reduced by IL-1β antagonists, supporting the notion that platelet IL-1β is the molecular determinant of platelet-dependent activation of the tran-scription factor.

Activation of NF-κB involves a cascade of phosphorylation processes. One family of kinases that is involved in NF-κB-dependent gene expres-sion is the mitogen-activated protein (MAP) kinases, such as p38 MAP kinase. In a manner similar to recombinant human IL-1β, activated plate-lets have the potential to induce phosphorylation of p38 MAP kinase. Correspondingly, transfection of a dominant-negative p38 mutant sig-nificantly reduced platelet-induced MCP-1 secretion in endothelial cells (94). Taken together, these data indicate that platelet-derived IL-1β ini-tiates NF-κB dependent expression of chemotactic and adhesive pro-teins in endothelial cells. In this manner, platelets promote the recruitment of both neutrophils and monocytes to the endothelial cell surface, thus inducing inflammation.

Another platelet-derived chemokine is the regulated on activation, T-cell expressed and secreted chemokine (RANTES), which has been seen to trigger monocyte arrest on inflamed and atherosclerotic endothelium

(95). Deposition of platelet RANTES induces monocyte recruitment mediated by P-selectin *(96)*. Furthermore, release of platelet-derived CD40 ligand induces inflammatory responses in endothelium. CD154 (CD40L), a 30–33-kDa protein, belongs to the TNF family of cytokines, which includes TNF-α and Fas ligand. CD40L was originally thought to be restricted to CD4+ T lymphocytes, mast cells, and basophils. Henn et al. *(46)* showed that platelets store CD40L in high amounts and release CD40L within seconds following activation in vitro. Ligation of CD40 on endothelial cells by CD40L expressed on the surface of activated platelets increased the release of IL-8 and MCP-1, the principal chemoattractants for neutrophils and monocytes *(46)*. In addition, platelet CD40L enhanced the expression of endothelial adhesion receptors including E-selectin, vascular cell adhesion molecule-1 (VCAM-1), and ICAM-1, all molecules that mediate the attachment of neutrophils, monocytes, and lymphocytes to the inflamed vessel wall. Moreover, CD40L induces endothelial tissue factor expression *(97)*. Hence, like IL-1β, CD40L expressed on platelets induces endothelial cells to release chemokines and to express adhesion molecules, thereby generating signals for the recruitment of leukocytes in the process of inflammation.

CD40 ligation on endothelial cells, smooth muscle cells, and macrophages initiates the expression and release of matrix-degrading enzymes, the matrix metalloproteinases (MMPs). These enzymes, which degrade extracellular matrix proteins, contribute significantly to the destruction and remodeling of inflamed tissue. Activated platelets release MMP-2 and MMP-9 during aggregation *(98)*. Moreover, adhesion of activated platelets to endothelial cells results in generation and secretion of MMP-9 and of the protease-activated receptor uPAR on cultured endothelium *(99)*. The endothelial release of MMP-9 was dependent on both the fibrinogen receptor GPIIb-IIIa and CD40L because inhibition of either mechanism resulted in reduction of platelet-induced matrix degradation activity of endothelial cells. Moreover, GPIIb-IIIa ligation results in substantial release of CD40L in the absence of any further platelet agonist *(100)* (Fig. 5). These results suggest that the release of platelet-derived proinflammatory mediators like CD40L is dependent on GPIIb-IIIa-mediated adhesion. This mechanism may be pathophysiologically important for the localization of platelet-induced inflammation of the endothelium at a site of platelet-endothelium adhesion.

PLATELET INTERACTION WITH LEUKOCYTES

Platelet adhesion to the endothelium or the subendothelial matrix induces platelet activation and the release of substances that are able to cause chemotaxis and migration of circulating leukocytes toward the site

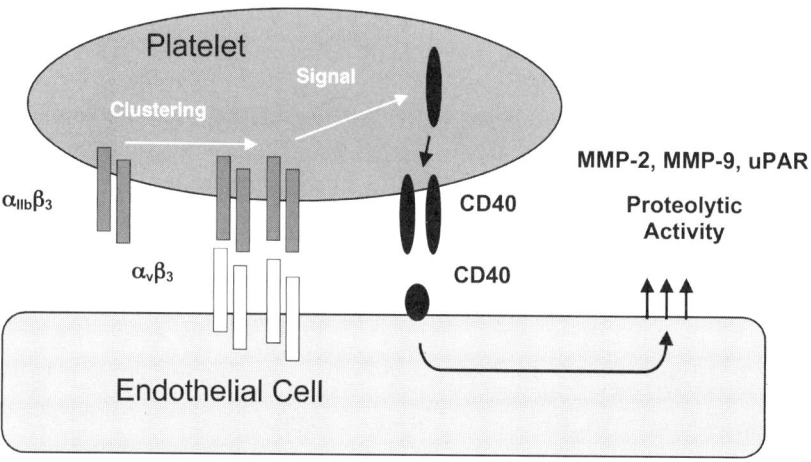

Fig. 5. GPIIb-IIIa-mediated release of CD40 ligand (CD40L) and pericellular proteolysis. MMP, matrix metalloproteinase; uPAR, protease-activated receptor.

of platelets accumulation. Platelets and leukocytes can form heterotypic conjugates, i.e., platelet-leukocyte aggregates, both in vivo and in vitro *(101)*. All leukocytes subpopulations can conjugate platelets *(102,103)*. Among them, monocytes show the greatest, and lymphocytes the least, propensity to form aggregates with platelets. Accumulating evidence indicates that close cell–cell contact mutually regulates platelet and leukocyte functions. Leukocyte-bound platelets may facilitate leukocyte rolling, adhesion, and migration on/through the vessel wall and thus enhance the accumulation of leukocytes at inflammatory sites *(104)*. For example, neutrophil adhesion to cultured endothelial cells, or neutrophil adhesion to damaged arterial segments is enhanced in the presence of platelets *(104)*. Platelet-derived microparticles may also enhance monocyte adhesion to the endothelium *(63)*. Similarly, leukocytes can enhance platelet adhesion to endothelial cells by platelet-leukocyte aggregation. Activated platelets may facilitate leukocyte recruitment into a growing thrombus; leukocytes, in turn, contribute to platelet activation and fibrin deposition *(105)*.

Mechanisms of Platelet Adhesion to Leukocytes

Like platelet adhesion to the vessel wall, leukocyte recruitment to the vascular endothelium requires multistep adhesive and signaling events including selectin-mediated rolling, leukocyte activation, and integrin-mediated firm adhesion and diapedesis *(65)* (Fig. 6). Several ligand-receptor systems have been found to be involved in platelet-leukocyte aggregation (Fig. 6). Platelet-expressed P-selectin *(106,107)* and leuko-

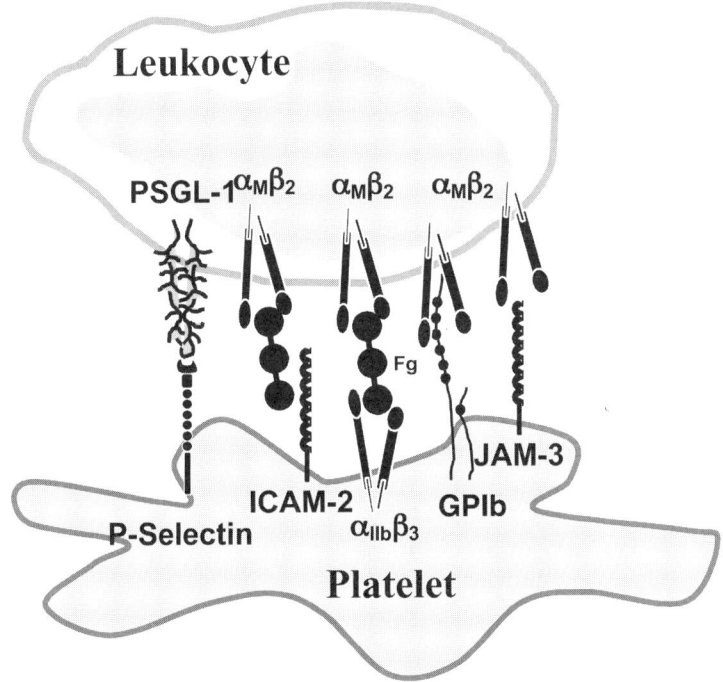

Fig. 6. Receptors that mediate platelet adhesion to leukocytes. ICAM, intercellular adhesion molecule; JAM, junctional adhesion molecule; PSGL, P-selectin glycoprotein ligand.

cyte-expressed PSGL-1/CD15 are the most important receptors for platelet-leukocyte adhesion. The bridging of platelet GPIIb-IIIa and leukocyte β_2-integrins (CD11b/CD18 and CD11c/CD18) by fibrinogen *(108)* and the ligation of CD36 (on both cell types) via thrombospondin *(109)* also contribute to platelet-leukocyte adhesion. Furthermore, CD40/CD40L *(108,109)*, ICAM-1/β_2-integrins *(87)*, GPIbα/Mac-1, and JAM-3/Mac-1 *(38)* are also involved in platelet-leukocyte adhesion. At sites of platelet adhesion to the endothelium or subendothelium, leukocyte infiltration can also occur through interactions with platelets and fibrin *(105)*.

Platelets either immobilized on a surface or activated in suspension express a complete machinery to recruit leukocytes, as follows: (1) platelet P-selectin is a mediator of the first contact (tethering); (2) interaction of platelet P-selectin with its counterreceptor PSGL-1 on leukocytes induces signaling events relevant for Mac-1 activation; and (3) the activated β_2-integrin (Mac-1) on leukocytes allows and reinforces firm platelet-leukocyte adhesion through binding to counterreceptors (ICAM-

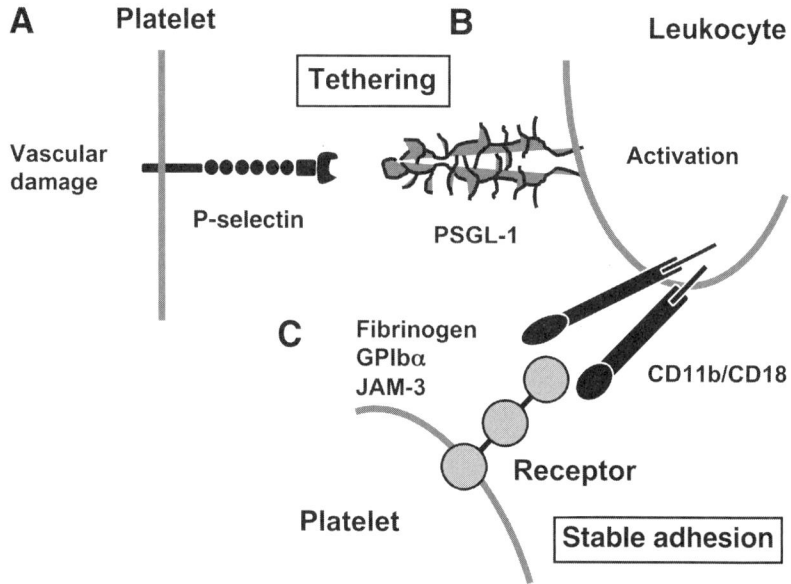

Fig. 7. Platelet-induced activation of leukocytes via P-selectin. (**A**) Platelet tethering to leukocytes via P-selectin/PSGL-1 adhesion. (**B**) P-selectin/PSGL-1-mediated leukocyte activation. (**C**) Consolidation of platelet-leukocyte adhesion via interaction of MAC-1 (CD11b/CD18) with platelet-bound fibrinogen or platelet surface-expressed GPIb or junctional adhesion molecule-3 (JAM-3). PSGL, P-selectin glycoprotein ligand.

2, fibrinogen bound to GPIIb-IIIα, GPIbα, JAM-3) present on the platelet surface (Fig. 7).

Platelet adhesion to leukocytes enhances the proinflammatory and prothrombotic activities of leukocytes *(112)*. Thus, leukocyte-bound platelets are known to enhance leukocyte adhesion molecule expression, superoxide anion generation, tissue factor expression, and cytokine synthesis *(43,44,113,114)*. These effects seem to be closely regulated by intercellular signaling via adhesion molecule ligation. PSGL-1/P-selectin ligation induces a tyrosine-kinase-dependent signal, which upregulates Mac-1 expression and enhances β_2-integrin-dependent neutrophil adhesion to ICAM-1 *(115)*. P-selectin/PSGL-1 interaction markedly enhances tissue factor activity in monocytes, and PSGL-1 blockade can inhibit tissue factor expression *(116,117)*. Furthermore, PSGL-1 engagement also mobilizes transcription factor NF-κB and induces cytokine expression in monocytes *(43)*. Signaling via β_2-integrins is necessary for neutrophil oxidative bursts, and platelets conjugating to neutrophil β_2-integrin via fibrinogen upregulate neutrophil oxidative burst activity *(118)*. β_2-integrin is also involved in the expression of β_1-

integrins ($\alpha_4\beta_1$ and $\alpha_2\beta_1$), which are important in neutrophil adhesion and migration *(119)* (Fig. 7).

Platelet-Induced Leukocyte Activation Via Soluble Mediators

Apart from direct cell-cell conjugation, leukocyte function can be influenced by platelet-derived soluble mediators. A number of proteins stored in platelet α-granules have been shown to enhance leukocyte activation (Table 2). Platelets contain large amounts of two chemokines, PF-4 and β-TG, which are stored in α-granules. PF-4 is chemotactic for neutrophils and monocytes and can induce leukocyte adhesion to endothelial cells and degranulation via activation of leukocyte function-associated antigen-1 (LFA-1) *(120)*. β-TG is the precursor of NAP-2, which stimulates neutrophil chemotaxis, adherence, calcium mobilization, and degranulation of lysosomes *(120,121)*. It is interesting to note that neutrophil-derived cathepsin G is the principal enzyme cleaving β-thromboglobulin into NAP-2, and that this product then acts on neutrophils themselves *(122–125)*. Platelet α-granules also contain PDGF, which may enhance leukocyte adhesion, degranulation, chemotaxis, phagocytosis, and tissue factor expression *(126–128)*. Moreover, platelet-released fibrinogen may induce oxidative bursts in neutrophils by bridging GPIIb-IIIa and CD11c/CD18 *(129)*.

Small molecules stored in platelet dense granules also regulate various aspects of leukocyte function. Adenine nucleotides (ATP and ADP) can induce adhesion, aggregation, and degranulation of neutrophils and monocytes. Adenine and guanine nucleotides have also been shown to evoke superoxide anion production in neutrophils *(130)*. Serotonin may enhance leukocyte rolling and adhesion by upregulating the expression of leukocyte adhesion molecules, such as Mac-1. Activated leukocytes generate PAF, which induces platelet aggregation, platelet adhesion to endothelial cells, and platelet secretion. Platelet-released chemokines, e.g., RANTES, have been reported to induce monocyte adhesion on endothelial cells *(95)*. Other soluble components released from platelet membranes may also activate leukocytes. For instance, soluble CD40L may bind to monocyte CD40 and promote tissue factor expression and cytokine/chemokine production *(97,99)*. Recombinant P-selectin has also been shown to enhance neutrophil phagocytosis by influencing β_2-integrin function *(112)*.

PLATELETS AND ATHEROSCLEROSIS

It is increasingly recognized that atherosclerosis is a chronic inflammatory condition that can be converted into an acute clinical event by atherosclerotic plaque progression, plaque rupture, and thrombosis

(131). Platelets play a major role in atherogenesis and thrombotic events in diseased arteries. Healthy endothelium maintains vascular integrity and provides a nonthrombotic inner layer of the arterial wall. Chronic endothelial injury and inflammation are key features in the pathogenesis of atherosclerosis *(131)*. Cardiovascular risk factors such as hypercholesterolemia, hypertension, smoking, and diabetes result in oxidative stress of the vascular wall, endothelial dysfunction, and platelet hyperactivity *(131)*. Atherosclerosis emerges locally and preferentially at lesion-prone sites *(132)* that are characterized by decreased shear stress because of nonlaminar, turbulent blood flow at branching vessels or curves. Normal arterial shear stress is atheroprotective, with high expression of nitric oxide synthetase and COX, whereas decreased shear stress is associated with an atherogenic endothelial phenotype, which expresses ICAM-1, MCP-1, and PDGF *(132)*. Several indications suggest that platelets significantly contribute to the inflammatory processes that promote atherosclerotic lesion formation.

Platelets play a key role in thrombotic vascular occlusion at the atherosclerotic plaque leading to acute thrombotic episodes that result in acute coronary syndrome and stroke *(1)*. After the prolonged process of silent plaque evolution, atheromas become susceptible to plaque rupture, leading to platelet adhesion and subsequent activation on the exposed, highly thrombogenic subendothelial surface, which initiates the dreaded clinical complications of thromboischemic episodes *(133,134)*. Enhanced responsiveness of the atherosclerotic plaque to platelets can be triggered, for example, by changes in the shear forces supporting platelet recruitment to the vulnerable plaque. Furthermore, biological changes in the form of chemotaxis of monocytes toward the plaque region, transmigration through the endothelial barrier, macrophage differentiation, phagocytosis, and secretion of proteolytic enzymes (plasminogen activator system, metalloproteinases) appear to contribute substantially to the instability of the plaque.

Over the past few years platelets have been recognized to play a critical role in the chemotaxis and migration of monocytes, thus promoting inflammation and progression of atherosclerosis. Experimental evidence indicates that platelets might contribute significantly to the inflammatory processes that promote atherosclerotic lesion formation. Platelets can adhere directly to the intact endothelial monolayer even in the absence of endothelial disruption *(135)*. During adhesion platelets are activated and release proinflammatory cytokines and chemoattractants (such as IL-1β, PF-4, and CD40 ligand). In vitro interactions between platelets and endothelial cells trigger the secretion of chemokines and the expression of adhesion molecules that promote the adhesion of leukocytes (Fig. 4). In this manner, the adhesion of platelets to the endothelial surface might generate signals that lead to the recruitment and extravasation of monocytes during atherosclerotic plaque progression, a process of paramount importance for atherogenesis. Moreover, platelets have been found to alter substantially the pericellular proteolytic activity of endothelial cells (activation of metalloproteinases), resulting in extracellular matrix degradation and fibrous cap thinning of a vulnerable lesion (Fig. 5) *(98)*. Thus, in areas of platelet accumulation at lesion-prone sites, an enhanced release of platelet-derived proatherogenic compounds favors atherogenetic changes within the arterial wall and the development of atherosclerotic plaques.

Recently, the occurrence of platelet-derived proatherogenic compounds like PF-4 and NAP-2 in carotid plaques has been documented *(136)*. PF-4 is a potent chemotactic factor for peripheral blood monocytes and has been found to enhance markedly the uptake of oxLDL by macrophages, an important mechanism in the development of unstable atherosclerotic plaques *(137)*. Only recently was it shown that platelet adhesion to the arterial wall is enhanced during atherogenesis *(17)*. Platelet adhesion to endothelium coincides with inflammatory gene expression and precedes atherosclerotic plaque invasion by leukocytes. Prolonged blockade of platelet adhesion in mice deficient in apolipoprotein E profoundly reduced leukocyte accumulation in the arterial intima and attenuated atherosclerotic lesion formation in the carotid artery bifurcation, the aortic sinus, and the coronary arteries (Fig. 8) *(17)*. Moreover, chronic platelet activation accelerates atherosclerosis *(18)*. Thus, platelet-induced inflammation of the vessel wall plays a major role in initiation of the atherogenetic process (Fig. 9).

CONCLUSIONS

Platelets play a critical role in acute and chronic inflammation. Major advances have been achieved in the understanding of the molecular mechanisms involved in platelet interaction with inflammatory cells. The interaction of platelets with leukocytes and endothelial cells results in substantial activation of these cell types that changes their chemotactic, adhesive and proteolytic properties significantly. Specific cell adhesion receptors such as selectins, immunoglobulin-type receptors, and integrins are involved in regulation of platelet adhesion with inflammatory cells. Therafter, release of platelet-dependent proinflammatory mediators substantially triggers the inflammatory response in the microenvironment of the site of platelet adhesion. Thus, platelet adhesion and subsequent release reaction are critical mechanisms involved in

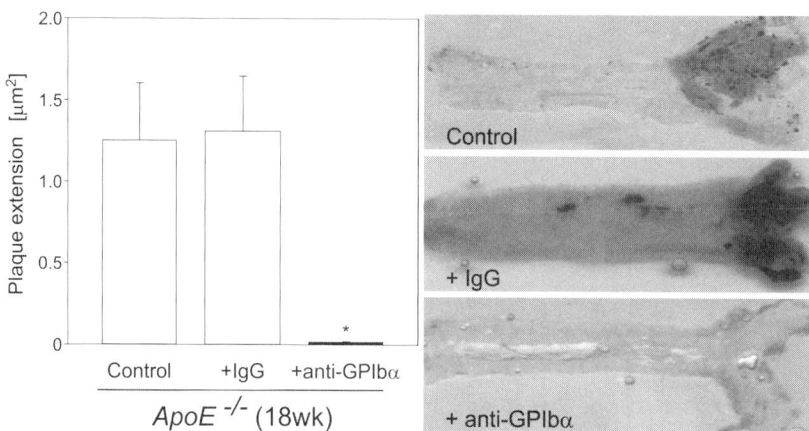

Fig. 8. Chronic GPIb inhibition of platelet-endothelium adhesion substantially inhibits atheroprogression. Plaque extension in the carotid artery in apolipoprotein E (ApoE)-deficient mice treated or not treated chronically with anti-GPIb monoclonal antibody *(17)*.

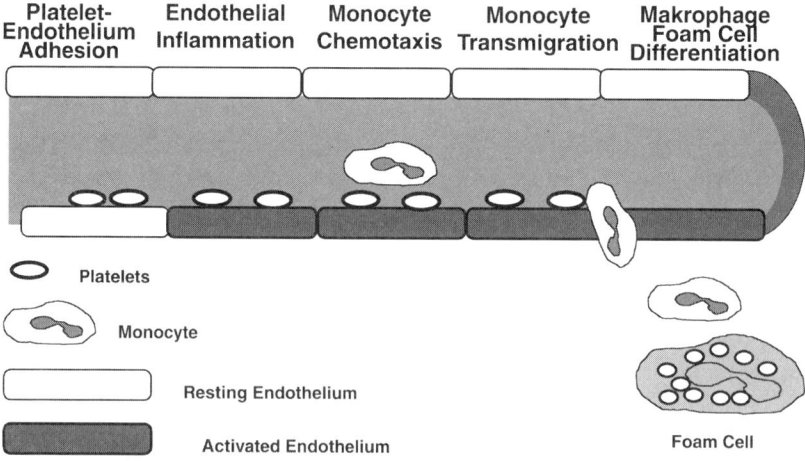

Fig. 9. Critical role of platelet adhesion in atherogenesis.

platelet-mediated inflammation and might represent targets for future therapeutic strategies in a variety of inflammatory diseases.

REFERENCES

1. Ruggeri ZM. Platelets in atherothrombosis. Nat Med 2002;11:1227–1234.
2. Nieswandt B, Watson SP. Platelet collagen interaction: is GPVI the central receptor? Blood 2003;102:449–461.

3. Ruggeri ZM. The platelet glycoprotein Ib-IX complex. Prog Hemost Thromb 1991;10:35–68.
4. Ruggeri ZM. Role of von Willebrand factor in platelet thrombus formation. Ann Med 2000;32:2–9.
5. Clemetson KJ. Platelet GPIb-V-IX complex. Thromb Haemost 1997;78:266–270.
6. Gawaz M. Platelet membrane glycoproteins. In: Gawaz M. Blood platelets. Thieme Verlag, Stuttgart, 2001, pp. 30–39.
7. Shattil SJ, Ginsberg MH. Perspectives series: cell adhesion in vascular biology. Integrin signaling in vascular biology. J Clin Invest 1997;100:1–5.
8. Wagner DD, Burger PC. Platelets in inflammation and thrombosis. Arterioscler Thromb Vasc Biol 2003;12:2131–2137.
9. Poubelle PE, Borgeat P. Platelet interactions with other cells related to inflammatory diseases. In: Gresele P, Page CP, Fuster V, Vermylen J, eds. Platelets in thrombotic and non-thrombotic disorders. Cambridge University Press, Cambridge, 2002, pp. 869–884.
10. Klinger MH, Jelkmann W. Role of blood platelets in infection and inflammation. J Interferon Cytokine Res 2002;22:913–922.
11. Gawaz M, Dickfeld T, Bogner C, Fateh-Moghadam S, Neumann FJ. Platelet function in septic multiple organ dysfunction syndrome. Intensive Care Med 1997;4:379–385.
12. Gawaz M, Fateh-Moghadam S, Pilz G, Gurland HJ, Werdan K. Severity of multiple organ failure (MOF) but not of sepsis correlates with irreversible platelet degranulation. Infection 1995;1:16–23.
13. Rinder CS, Bonan JL, Rinder HM, Mathew J, Hines R, Smith BR. Cardiopulmonary bypass induces leukocyte-platelet adhesion. Blood 1992;79:1201–1205.
14. Ott I, Neumann FJ, Gawaz M, Schmitt M, Schomig A. Increased neutrophil-platelet adhesion in patients with unstable angina. Circulation 1996;94:1239–1246.
15. Gawaz M, Neumann FJ, Ott I, Schiessler A, Schomig A. Platelet function in acute myocardial infarction treated with direct angioplasty. Circulation 1996;93:229–237.
16. Gawaz M, Neumann FJ, Dickfeld T, et al. Vitronectin receptor (alpha(v)beta3) mediates platelet adhesion to the luminal aspect of endothelial cells: implications for reperfusion in acute myocardial infarction. Circulation 1997;96:1809–1818.
17. Massberg S, Brand K, Gruner S, et al. A critical role of platelet adhesion in the initiation of atherosclerotic lesion formation. J Exp Med 2002;196:887–896.
18. Huo Y, Schober A, Forlow SB, et al. Circulating activated platelets exacerbate atherosclerosis in mice deficient in apolipoprotein E. Nat Med 2003;1:61–67.
19. Neumann FJ, Ott I, Gawaz M, Puchner G, Schomig A. Neutrophil and platelet activation at balloon-injured coronary artery plaque in patients undergoing angioplasty. J Am Coll Cardiol 1996;27:819 824.
20. McEver RP. Adhesive interactions of leukocytes, platelets, and the vessel wall during hemostasis and inflammation. Thromb Haemost 2001;86:746–756.
21. Williams MJ, Du X, Loftus JC, Ginsberg MH. Platelet adhesion receptors. Semin Cell Biol 1995;6:305–314.
22. Gawaz M. Platelet membrane glycoproteins. In: Gawaz M. Blood platelets. Thieme Verlag, Stuttgart, 2001, pp. 30–39.
23. George JN. Platelets. Lancet 2000;355:1531–1539.
24. Andrews RK, Shen Y, Gardiner EE, Berndt MC. Platelet adhesion receptors and (patho)physiological thrombus formation. Histol Histopathol 2001;16:969–980.
25. Felding-Habermann B. Integrin adhesion receptors in tumor metastasis. Clin Exp Metastasis 2003;20:203–201.

26. Liddington RC, Ginsberg MH. Integrin activation takes shape. J Cell Biol 2002;158:833–839.
27. Du X, Ginsberg MH. Integrin alpha IIb beta 3 and platelet function. Thromb Haemost 1997;78:96–100.
28. Hood JD, Cheresh DA. Role of integrins in cell invasion and migration. Nat Rev Cancer 2002;2:91–100.
29. Simon DI, Chen Z, Xu H, et al. Platelet glycoprotein Ibalpha is a counterreceptor for the leukocyte integrin Mac-1 (CD11b/CD18). J Exp Med 2000;192:193–204.
30. Romo GM, Dong JF, Schade AJ, et al. The glycoprotein Ib-IX-V complex is a platelet counterreceptor for P-selectin. J Exp Med 1999;190:803–814.
31. McEver RP. Role of selectins in leukocyte adhesion to platelets and endothelium. Ann NY Acad Sci 1994;714:185–189.
32. Furie B, Furie BC. Leukocyte crosstalk at the vascular wall. Thromb Haemost 1997;78:306–309.
33. McEver RP, Cummings RD. Perspectives series: cell adhesion in vascular biology. Role of PSGL-1 binding to selectins in leukocyte recruitment. J Clin Invest 1997;100:485–491.
34. McEver RP. Adhesive interactions of leukocytes, platelets, and the vessel wall during hemostasis and inflammation. Thromb Haemost 2001;86:746–756.
35. Diacovo TG, deFougerolles AR, Bainton DF, Springer TA. A functional integrin ligand on the surface of platelets: intercellular adhesion molecule-2. J Clin Invest 1994;94:1243–1251.
36. Chavakis T, Preissner KT, Santoso S. Leukocyte trans-endothelial migration: JAMs add new pieces to the puzzle. Thromb Haemost 2003;89:13–17.
37. Gupta SK, Pillarisetti K, Ohlstein EH. Platelet agonist F11 receptor is a member of the immunoglobulin superfamily and identical with junctional adhesion molecule (JAM): regulation of expression in human endothelial cells and macrophages. Life 2000;50:51–56.
38. Santoso S, Sachs UJ, Kroll H, et al. The junctional adhesion molecule 3 (JAM-3) on human platelets is a counterreceptor for the leukocyte integrin Mac-1. J Exp Med 2002;196:679–691.
39. Babinska A, Kedees MH, Athar H, et al. F11-receptor (F11R/JAM) mediates platelet adhesion to endothelial cells: role in inflammatory thrombosis. Thromb Haemost 2002;88:843–850.
40. Gear AR, Camerini D. Platelet chemokines and chemokine receptors: linking hemostasis, inflammation, and host defense. Microcirculation 2003;10:335–350.
41. Rendu F, Brohard-Bohn B. The platelet release reaction: granules' constituents, secretion and functions. Platelets 2001;12:261–273.
42. Harrison P, Cramer EM. Platelet alpha-granules. Blood Rev 1993;7:52–62.
43. Weyrich AS, Elstad MR, et al. Activated platelets signal chemokine synthesis by human monocytes. J Clin Invest 1996;97:1525–1534.
44. Neumann FJ, Marx N, Gawaz M, et al. Induction of cytokine expression in leukocytes by binding of thrombin-stimulated platelets. Circulation 1997;95:2387–2394.
45. Gawaz M, Neumann FJ, Dickfeld T, et al. Activated platelets induce monocyte chemotactic protein-1 secretion and surface expression of intercellular adhesion molecule-1 on endothelial cells. Circulation 1998;98:1164–1167.
46. Henn V, Slupsky JR, Grafe M, et al. CD40 ligand on activated platelets triggers an inflammatory reaction of endothelial cells. Nature 1998;391:591–594.
47. Boogaerts MA, Yamada O, Jacob HS, Moldow CF. Enhancement of granulocyte-endothelial cell adherence and granulocyte-induced cytotoxicity by platelet release products. Proc Natl Acad Sci USA 1982;79:7019–7023.

48. Laberge S, Cruikshank WW, Beer DJ, Center DM. Secretion of IL-16 (lymphocyte chemoattractant factor) from serotonin-stimulated CD8+ T cells in vitro. J Immunol 1996;156:310–315.

49. Sandler JA, Gallin JI, Vaughan M. Effects of serotonin, carbamylcholine, and ascorbic acid on leukocyte cyclic GMP and chemotaxis. J Cell Biol 1975;67:480–484.

50. Momi S, Gresele P. Platelets and chemotaxis. In: Gresele P, Page C, Fuster V, Vermylen J, eds. Platelets in thrombotic and non-thrombotic disorders. Cambridge University Press, Cambridge, 2002, pp. 393–411.

51. Brandt E, Petersen F, Ludwig A, Ehlert JE, Bock L, Flad HD. The beta-thromboglobulins and platelet factor 4: blood platelet-derived CXC chemokines with divergent roles in early neutrophil regulation. J Leukoc Biol 2000;67:471–478.

52. Power CA, Clemetson JM, Clemetson KJ, Wells TN. Chemokine and chemokine receptor mRNA expression in human platelets. Cytokine 1995;7:479–482.

53. Kronemann N, Bouloumi A, Bassus S, Kirchmaier CM, Busse R, Schini-Kerth VB. Aggregating human platelets stimulate expression of vascular endothelial growth factor in cultured vascular smooth muscle cells through a synergistic effect of transforming growth factor-beta(1) and platelet-derived growth factor(AB). Circulation 1999;100:855–856.

54. Dell'Angelica EC, Mullins C, Caplan S, Bonifacino JS. Lysosome-related organelles. FASEB J 2000;14:1265–1278.

55. Lindemann S, Tolley ND, Dixon DA, et al. Activated platelets mediate inflammatory signaling by regulated interleukin 1beta synthesis. J Cell Biol 2001;154:485–490.

56. Hermann A, Rauch BH, Braun M, Schror K, Weber AA. Platelet CD40 ligand (CD40L)-subcellular localization, regulation of expression, and inhibition by clopidogrel. Platelets 2001;12:74–78.

57. Hawrylowicz CM, Howells GL, Feldmann M. Platelet-derived interleukin 1 induces human endothelial adhesion molecule expression and cytokine production. J Exp Med 1991;174:785–790.

58. Kaplanski G, Porat R, Aiura K, Erban JK, Gelfand JA, Dinarello CA. Activated platelets induce endothelial secretion of interleukin-8 in vitro via an interleukin-1-mediated event. Blood 1993;81:2492–2495.

59. Andre P, Prasad KS, Denis CV, et al. CD40L stabilizes arterial thrombi by a beta3 integrin-dependent mechanism. Nat Med 2002;8:247–252.

60. Siess W. Athero- and thrombogenic actions of lysophosphatidic acid and sphingosine-1-phosphate. Biochim Biophys Acta 2002;1582:204–215.

61. Denizot Y. Platelet-activating factor. In: Bruchhausen FV, Authi KS, Walter U, eds. Platelets and their factors. Springer Verlag, Heidelberg, 1997, pp. 483–496.

62. Halushka PV, Pawate S, Martin ML. Thromboxane A2 and other eicosanoids. In: Bruchhausen FV, Authi KS, Walter U, eds. Platelets and their factors. Springer Verlag, Heidelberg, 1997.

63. Barry OP, FitzGerald GA. Mechanisms of cellular activation by platelet microparticles. Thromb Haemost 1999;82:794–800.

64. Palmetshofer A, Robson SC, Nehls V. Lysophosphatidic acid activates nuclear factor kappa B and induces proinflammatory gene expression in endothelial cells. Thromb Haemost 1999;82:1532–1537.

65. Springer TA. Traffic signals for lymphocyte recirculation and leukocyte emigration: the multistep paradigm. Cell 1994;76:301–314.

66. Sporn LA, Huber P. Endothelial cell biology. In: Colman RW, Hirsh J, Marder VJ, Clowes AW, George JN, eds. Hemostasis and thrombosis. Basic principles and clinical practice, 4th ed. Lippincott Williams & Wilkins, Philadelphia, 2001, pp. 615–623.

67. Venturini CM, Kaplan JE. Thrombin induces platelet adhesion to endothelial cells. Semin Thromb Hemost 1992;18:275–283.
68. Kaplan JE, Moon DG, Weston LK, et al. Platelets adhere to thrombin-treated endothelial cells in vitro. Am J Physiol 1989;257:423–433.
69. Etingin OR, Silverstein RL, Hajjar DP. von Willebrand factor mediates platelet adhesion to virally infected endothelial cells. Proc Natl Acad Sci USA 1993;90:5153–5156.
70. Itoh Y, Tomita M, Tanahashi N, Takeda H, Yokoyama M, Fukuuchi Y. Platelet adhesion to aortic endothelial cells in vitro after thrombin treatment: observation with video-enhanced contrast microscopy. Thromb Res 1998;91:15–22.
71. Reininger AJ, Korndorfer MA, Wurzinger LJ. Adhesion of ADP-activated platelets to intact endothelium under stagnation point flow in vitro is mediated by the integrin alphaIIbeta3. Thromb Haemost 1998;79:998–1003.
72. Li JM, Podolsky RS, Rohrer MJ, et al. Adhesion of activated platelets to venous endothelial cells is mediated via GPIIb/IIIa. J Surg Res 1996;61:543–548.
73. Bombeli T, Schwartz BR, Harlan JM. Adhesion of activated platelets to endothelial cells: evidence for a GPIIbIIIa-dependent bridging mechanism and novel roles for endothelial intercellular adhesion molecule 1 (ICAM-1), alphavbeta3 integrin, and GPIbalpha. J Exp Med 1998;187:329–333.
74. Kakutani M, Masaki T, Sawamura T. A platelet-endothelium interaction mediated by lectin-like oxidized low-density lipoprotein receptor-1. Proc Natl Acad Sci USA 2000;97:360–364.
75. Bombeli T, Schwartz BR, Harlan JM. Endothelial cells undergoing apoptosis become proadhesive for nonactivated platelets. Blood 1999;93:3831–3838.
76. Frenette PS, Johnson RC, Hynes RO, Wagner DD. Platelets roll on stimulated endothelium in vivo: an interaction mediated by endothelial P-selectin. Proc Natl Acad Sci USA 1995;92:7450–7454.
77. Johnson RC, Mayadas TN, Frenette PS, et al. Blood cell dynamics in P-selectin-deficient mice. Blood 1995;86:1106–1114.
78. Subramaniam M, Frenette PS, Saffaripour S, Johnson RC, Hynes RO, Wagner DD. Defects in hemostasis in P-selectin-deficient mice. Blood 1996;87:1238–1242.
79. Frenette PS, Moyna C, Hartwell DW, Lowe JB, Hynes RO, Wagner DD. Platelet-endothelial interactions in inflamed mesenteric venules. Blood 1998;91:1318–1324.
80. Frenette PS, Subbarao S, Mazo IB, von Andrian UH, Wagner DD. Endothelial selectins and vascular cell adhesion molecule-1 promote hematopoietic progenitor homing to bone marrow. Proc Natl Acad Sci USA 1998;95:14423–1448.
81. Massberg S, Enders G, Leiderer R, et al. Platelet-endothelial cell interactions during ischemia/reperfusion: the role of P-selectin. Blood 1998;92:507–515.
82. Laszik Z, Jansen PJ, Cummings RD, Tedder TF, McEver RP, Moore KL. P-selectin glycoprotein ligand-1 is broadly expressed in cells of myeloid, lymphoid, and dendritic lineage and in some nonhematopoietic cells. Blood 1996;88:3010–3012.
83. Frenette PS, Denis CV, Weiss L, et al. P-Selectin glycoprotein ligand 1 (PSGL-1) is expressed on platelets and can mediate platelet-endothelial interactions in vivo. J Exp Med 2000;191:1413–1422.
84. Gawaz MP, Loftus JC, Bajt ML, Frojmovic MM, Plow EF, Ginsberg MH. Ligand bridging mediates integrin alpha IIb beta 3 (platelet GPIIB-IIIA) dependent homotypic and heterotypic cell-cell interactions. J Clin Invest 1991;88:1128–1134.
85. Massberg S, Enders G, Matos FC, et al. Fibrinogen deposition at the postischemic vessel wall promotes platelet adhesion during ischemia-reperfusion in vivo. Blood 1999;94:3829–3838.
86. Gawaz M, Brand K, Dickfeld T, et al. Platelets induce alterations of chemotactic and adhesive properties of endothelial cells mediated through an interleukin-1-dependent mechanism. Implications for atherogenesis. Atherosclerosis 2000;148:75–85.

87. Languino LR, Duperray A, Joganic KJ, Fornaro M, Thornton GB, Altieri DC. Regulation of leukocyte-endothelium interaction and leukocyte transendothelial migration by intercellular adhesion molecule 1-fibrinogen recognition. Proc Natl Acad Sci USA 1995;92:1505–1509.

88. Altieri DC, Duperray A, Plescia J, Thornton GB, Languino LR. Structural recognition of a novel fibrinogen gamma chain sequence (117-133) by intercellular adhesion molecule-1 mediates leukocyte-endothelium interaction. J Biol Chem 1995;270:696–699.

89. Sriramarao P, Languino LR, Altieri DC. Fibrinogen mediates leukocyte-endothelium bridging in vivo at low shear forces. Blood 1996;88:3416–3423.

90. Massberg S, Vogt F, Dickfeld T, Brand K, Page S, Gawaz M. Activated platelets trigger an inflammatory response and enhance migration of aortic smooth muscle cells. Thromb Res 2003;110:187–194.

91. Lu B, Rutledge BJ, Gu L, et al. Abnormalities in monocyte recruitment and cytokine expression in monocyte chemoattractant protein 1-deficient mice. J Exp Med 1998;187:601–608.

92. Gawaz M, Page S, Massberg S, et al. Transient platelet interaction induces MCP-1 production by endothelial cells via I kappa B kinase complex activation. Thromb Haemost 2002;88:307–314.

93. Gawaz M, Neumann FJ, Dickfeld T, et al. Activated platelets induce monocyte chemotactic protein-1 secretion and surface expression of intercellular adhesion molecule-1 on endothelial cells. Circulation 1998;98:1164–1171.

94. Dickfeld T, Lengyel E, May AE, et al. Transient interaction of activated platelets with endothelial cells induces expression of monocyte-chemoattractant protein-1 via a p38 mitogen-activated protein kinase mediated pathway. Implications for atherogenesis. Cardiovasc Res 2001;41:189–199.

95. von Hundelshausen P, Weber KS, Huo Y, et al. RANTES deposition by platelets triggers monocyte arrest on inflamed and atherosclerotic endothelium. Circulation 2001;103:1772–1777.

96. Schober A, Manka D, von Hundelshausen P, et al. Deposition of platelet RANTES triggering monocyte recruitment requires P-selectin and is involved in neointima formation after arterial injury. Circulation 2002;106:1523–1529.

97. Slupsky JR, Kalbas M, Willuweit A, Henn V, Kroczek RA, Muller-Berghaus G. Activated platelets induce tissue factor expression on human umbilical vein endothelial cells by ligation of CD40. Thromb Haemost 1998;80:1008–1014.

98. Fernandez-Patron C, Martinez-Cuesta MA, Salas E, et al. Differential regulation of platelet aggregation by matrix metalloproteinases-9 and -2. Thromb Haemost 1999;82:1730–1735.

99. May AE, Kalsch T, Massberg S, Herouy Y, Schmidt R, Gawaz M. Engagement of glycoprotein IIb/IIIa (alpha(IIb)beta3) on platelets upregulates CD40L and triggers CD40L-dependent matrix degradation by endothelial cells. Circulation 2002;106:2111–2117.

100. Nannizzi-Alaimo L, Alves VL, Phillips DR. Inhibitory effects of glycoprotein IIb/IIIa antagonists and aspirin on the release of soluble CD40 ligand during platelet stimulation. Circulation 2003;107:1123–1128.

101. Bazzoni G, Dejana E, Del Maschio A. Platelet-neutrophil interactions. Possible relevance in the pathogenesis of thrombosis and inflammation. Haematologica 1991;76:491–499.

102. Rinder HM, Bonan JL, Rinder CS, Ault KA, Smith BR. Activated and unactivated platelet adhesion to monocytes and neutrophils. Blood 1991;78:1760–1769.

103. Rinder HM, Bonan JL, Rinder CS, Ault KA, Smith BR. Dynamics of leukocyte-platelet adhesion in whole blood. Blood 1991;78:1730–1737.

104. Weber C, Springer TA. Neutrophil accumulation on activated, surface-adherent platelets in flow is mediated by interaction of Mac-1 with fibrinogen bound to αIibβ3 and stimulated by platelet-activating factor. J Clin Invest 1997;100:2085–2093.

105. Palabrica T, Lobb R, Furie BC, et al. Leukocyte accumulation promoting fibrin deposition is mediated in vivo by P-selectin on adherent platelets. Nature 1992;359:848–851.

106. Larsen E, Palabrica T, Sajer S, et al. PADGEM-dependent adhesion of platelets to monocytes and neutrophils is mediated by a lineage-specific carbohydrate, LNF III (CD15). Cell 1990;63:467–474.

107. Hamburger SA, McEver RP. GMP-140 mediates adhesion of stimulated platelets to neutrophils. Blood 1990;75:550–554.

108. Konstantopoulos K, Neelamegham S, Burns AR, et al. Venous levels of shear support neutrophil-platelet adhesion and neutrophil aggregation in blood via P-selectin and beta2-integrin. Circulation 1998;98:873–882.

109. Silverstein RL, Asch AS, Nachman RL. Glycoprotein IV mediates thrombospondin-dependent platelet-monocyte and platelet-U937 cell adhesion. J Clin Invest 1989;84:546–552.

110. Alderson MR, Armitage RJ, Tough TW, Strockbine L, Fanslow WC, Spriggs MK. CD40 expression by human monocytes: regulation by cytokines and activation of monocytes by the ligand for CD40. J Exp Med 1993;178:669–674.

111. Inwald DP, McDowall A, Peters MJ, Callard RE, Klein NJ. CD40 is constitutively expressed on platelets and provides a novel mechanism for platelet activation. Circ Res 2003;92:1041–1048.

112. Blanks JE, Moll T, Eytner R, Vestweber D. Stimulation of P-selectin glycoprotein ligand-1 on mouse neutrophils activates beta 2-integrin mediated cell attachment to ICAM-1. Eur J Immunol 1998;28:433–443.

113. Nagata K, Tsuji T, Todoroki N, et al. Activated platelets induce superoxide anion release by monocytes and neutrophils through P-selectin (CD62). J Immunol 1993;151:3267–3273.

114. Østerud B. The role of platelets in decrypting monocyte tissue factor. Dis Mon 2003;49:7–13.

115. Evangelista V, Manarini S, Sideri R, et al. Platelet/polymorphonuclear leukocyte interaction: P-selectin triggers protein-tyrosine phosphorylation-dependent CD11b/CD18 adhesion: role of PSGL-1 as a signalling molecule. Blood 1999;93:876–885.

116. Celi A, Pellegrini G, Lorenzet R, et al. P-selectin induces the expression of tissue factor on monocytes. Proc Natl Acad Sci USA 1994;91:8767–8771.

117. Østerud B. Cellular interactions in tissue factor expression by blood monocytes. Blood Coagul Fibrinolysis 1995;6(suppl):S20–S25.

118. Ruf A, Patscheke H. Platelet-induced neutrophil activation: platelet-expressed fibrinogen induces the oxidative burst in neutrophils by an interaction with CD11C/CD18. Br J Haematol 1995;90:791–796.

119. Werr J, Eriksson EE, Hedqvist P, Lindbom L. Engagement of beta2 integrins induces surface expression of beta1 integrin receptors in human neutrophils. J Leuk Biol 2000;68:553–560.

120. Brandt E, Petersen F, Ludwig A, Ehlert JE, Bock L, Flad HD. The beta-thromboglobulins and platelet factor 4: blood platelet-derived CXC chemokines with divergent roles in early neutrophil regulation. J Leuk Biol 2000;67:471–478.

121. Petersen F, Bock L, Flad HD, Brandt E. Platelet factor 4-induced neutrophil-endothelial cell interaction: involvement of mechanisms and functional consequences different from those elicited by interleukin-8. Blood 1999;94:4020–4028.
122. Leonard EJ, Yoshimura T, Rot A, et al. Chemotactic activity and receptor binding of neutrophil attractant/activation protein-1 (NAP-1) and structurally related host defense cytokines: interaction of NAP-2 with the NAP-1 receptor. J Leuk Biol 1991;49:258–265.
123. Walz A, Dewald B, von Tscharner V, Baggiolini M. Effects of the neutrophil-activating peptide NAP-2, platelet basic protein, connective tissue-activating peptide III and platelet factor 4 on human neutrophils. J Exp Med 1989;170:1745–1750.
124. Walz A, Meloni F, Clark-Lewis I, von Tscharner V, Baggiolini M. [Ca^{2+}]i changes and respiratory burst in human neutrophils and monocytes induced by NAP-1/interleukin-8, NAP-2, and gro/MGSA. J Leuk Biol 1991;50:279–286.
125. Harter L, Petersen F, Flad HD, Brandt E. Connective tissue-activating peptide III desensitizes chemokine receptors on neutrophils. Requirement for proteolytic formation of the neutrophil-activating peptide 2. J Immunol 1994;153:5698–5708.
126. Shure D, Senior RM, Griffin GL, Deuel TF. PDGF AA homodimers are potent chemoattractants for fibroblasts and neutrophils, and for monocytes activated by lymphocytes or cytokines. Biochem Biophys Res Commun 1992;186:1510–1514.
127. Tzeng DY, Deuel TF, Huang JS, Baehner RL. Platelet-derived growth factor promotes human peripheral monocyte activation. Blood 1985;66:179–183.
128. Ernofsson M, Siegbahn A. Platelet-derived growth factor-BB and monocyte chemotactic protein-1 induce human peripheral blood monocytes to express tissue factor. Thromb Res 1996;83:307–320.
129. Ruf A, Schlenk RF, Maras A, Morgenstern E, Patscheke H. Contact-induced neutrophil activation by platelets in human cell suspensions and whole blood. Blood 1992;80:1238–1246.
130. Freyer DR, Boxer LA, Axtell RA, Todd RF. Stimulation of human neutrophil adhesive properties by adenine nucleotides. J Immunol 1988;141:580–586.
131. Lusis AJ. Atherosclerosis. Nature 2000;407:233–241.
132. Libby P. Inflammation in atherosclerosis. Nature 2002;420:868–874.
133. Naghavi M, Libby P, Falk E, et al. From vulnerable plaque to vulnerable patient: a call for new definitions and risk assessment strategies: Part I. Circulation 2003;108:1664–1672.
134. Corti R, Farkouh ME, Badimon JJ. The vulnerable plaque and acute coronary syndromes. Am J Med 2002;113:668–680.
135. Sachais BS. Platelet-endothelial interactions in atherosclerosis. Curr Atheroscler Rep 2001;3:412–416.
136. Pitsilos S, Hunt J, Mohler ER, et al. Platelet factor 4 localization in carotid atherosclerotic plaques: correlation with clinical parameters. Thromb Haemost 2003;90:1112–1120.
137. Nassar T, Sachais BS, Akkawi S, et al. Platelet factor 4 enhances the binding of oxidized low-density lipoprotein to vascular wall cells. J Biol Chem 2003;278:6187–6193.

6 Platelet Signal-Dependent Protein Synthesis

Stephan Lindemann, MD,
Thomas M. McIntyre, PhD,
Stephen M. Prescott, MD,
Guy A. Zimmerman, MD,
and Andrew S. Weyrich, PhD

PRIMARY FUNCTIONS OF PLATELETS

Platelets as Immediate Effectors of Hemostasis

Our understanding of platelet functions has been in evolution since their discovery. Blood platelets were initially observed in the middle of the 19th century by many investigators including Zimmermann in 1860, Schultze in 1865, Osler in 1874, and Hayem in 1878 *(1)*. Studies by

From: *Contemporary Cardiology:*
Platelet Function: Assessment, Diagnosis, and Treatment
Edited by: M. Quinn and D. Fitzgerald © Humana Press Inc., Totowa, NJ

Bizzozero *(2,3)* were the first to recognize the adhesive qualities of platelets, their participation in thrombosis and leukocyte recruitment, and their role in blood coagulation. These monumental findings, which have withstood the test of time, have expanded at a remarkable rate and continue to be the primary focus of investigative research in the platelet arena *(4)*.

Studies of platelet function are typically divided into four main areas: activation, adhesion, aggregation, and secretion *(5)*. All these functions occur at a rapid pace, within seconds to minutes after platelets are exposed to biologically relevant stimuli *(6–9)*. They allow platelets to form a hemostatic plug at sites of vascular injury, fulfilling their cardinal function in acute hemostasis *(10)*. Understanding the basic biology of acute platelet function has led to effective clinical approaches for platelet-related diseases, including disorders of platelet number and function *(11)*. They have also markedly expanded our knowledge of how platelets regulate pathophysiological processes including atherosclerosis, diabetes mellitus, and tumor growth and metastasis *(12–15)*.

Platelets Have Roles Beyond Acute Hemostasis

Platelets were initially overlooked in hematology because they are so small and were often missed by microscopy *(16)*. The realization of their role as inflammatory cells was likewise delayed because researchers and pathologists held on to the idea that platelets are merely "critical effectors of clotting" *(17–19)*. Numerous studies over the last decade have now demonstrated that platelets play an active role in antimicrobial host defense, tumor growth and metastasis, the development and progression of coronary artery disease, sepsis, rheumatoid arthritis, and acute respiratory distress syndrome *(13,14,20–25)*. Their involvement in these clinical disorders indicates that platelets subserve inflammatory functions in addition to being acute effectors of hemostasis.

How do platelets participate in vascular inflammation? Two mechanisms are widely accepted. The first is that platelets are a repository of spasmogens, chemotactic factors, chemokines, angiogenic factors, and proteolytic enzymes that participate in the inflammatory process *(5,26)*. These physiologically active substances are derived from granular storage pools or synthesized from membrane phospholipids *(5,26,27)*. The second is that platelets bind target cells and regulate their phenotype during inflammation *(28,29)*. Here we highlight key points and recent discoveries demonstrating that platelets regulate prolonged biological responses through these two mechanisms.

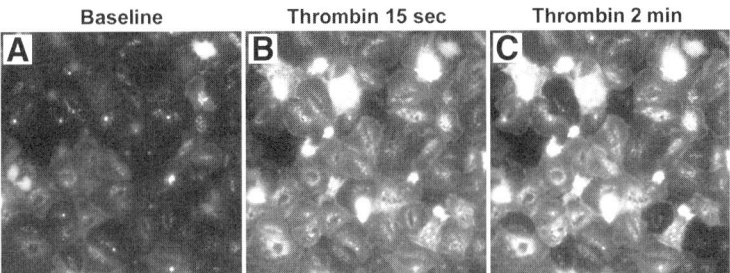

Fig. 1. Adherent platelets respond to delayed agonist administration. Freshly isolated human platelets were incubated with immobilized fibrinogen as previously described *(75)*. After 7 h, the adherent cells were loaded with the fluorescent calcium indicator dye Fura 2 for 1 h. The cells were subsequently stimulated with thrombin (0.1 U/mL) and observed continuously for 2 min. Fluorescence output owing to intracellular calcium fluxes is shown at baseline (**A**) and after thrombin treatment (15 s, **B**; 2 min, **C**). This figure is representative of three experiments and demonstrates that ex vivo, platelets remain viable for prolonged periods after they adhere to extracellular matrices.

SIGNAL-DEPENDENT DEGRANULATION AND LIPID SYNTHESIS

Platelet releasates are derived from intracellular storage pools or generated in phospholipid-rich membranes *(5,26)*. During vessel repair, platelets regulate inflammation by secreting their constituents into the local milieu *(5,27)*. This allows platelets to localize signals spatially and coordinate a temporal sequence of events that, in addition to stabilizing the clot, attracts other leukocytes and initiates vessel growth and repair. It is not clear whether platelets secrete all their constituents at once or whether there is a sustained, submaximal release that occurs over hours. In vitro, thrombin induces robust intracellular calcium fluxes when it is administered 8 h after platelets adhere to immobilized extracellular matrices (Fig. 1), and cultured platelets maintain a constant response to α-thrombin for 24 h with secretory kinetics identical to those of freshly isolated platelets *(30)*. This suggests that under appropriate conditions, platelets can remain functional for extended periods. Although the duration of their functions in vivo is incompletely understood, recent evidence indicates that platelets embedded in maturing arterial thrombi maintain cellular integrity and organelle content for at least 4 h and secrete ATP during this time period *(30)*.

It is likely that the severity of vascular injury, the patterns and levels of platelet agonists in the local milieu, and the half-life of secreted products govern the length of platelet involvement. Nevertheless, it is commonly thought that once platelets are activated at an injured site they rapidly secrete an array of growth and angiogenic factors that include vascular endothelial growth factor family members, platelet-derived growth factor, insulin-like growth factors, epidermal and fibroblast growth factors, hepatocyte growth factor, and transforming growth factor-β_1 *(5,26,27)*. Recent discoveries have demonstrated that activated platelets also release metalloproteinases (MMPs) 1 and 2 *(31,32)*. In addition to remodeling extracellular matrix, MMP-1 amplifies cellular activation responses and directly induces intracellular signaling events *(31)*. Another important platelet releasate is RANTES *(33)*, a chemokine that binds endothelium and attracts leukocytes to the inflamed area *(29,34–38)*. RANTES and P-selectin, an adhesive glycoprotein expressed on the surface of activated platelets and endothelial cells, synergistically induce cytokine synthesis in peripheral blood monocytes *(28,29,39–42)*. CD40 ligand, shed from activated platelets, is another influential factor that directly initiates inflammation of the vessel wall *(39,42)*.

In addition to releasing preformed signaling molecules from storage granules, platelets also generate lipid-based inflammatory products. Among these are products of arachidonic acid that are liberated during platelet activation, including thromboxane A_2 (TXA$_2$) and prostaglandin metabolites *(5,43–45)*. TXA$_2$ amplifies platelet functional responses and vasoconstricts the vessel wall *(5,44–47)*. Suppression of platelet-derived TXA$_2$ in low-density lipoprotein receptor knockout mice markedly retards the development of atherogenesis *(48,49)*. Another lipid-derived mediator, platelet-activating factor (PAF), is synthesized by adherent, activated platelets *(50)*. PAF transmits outside-in signals to intracellular transduction systems in a variety of cell types involved in innate immune and hemostatic processes *(51,52)*. An important signaling pathway elicited by PAF is enhanced gene expression. Monocyte chemotactic protein-1 (MCP-1), interleukin-8 (IL-8), and tumor necrosis factor-α (TNF-α) are synthesized by PAF-stimulated monocytes *(53)*.

ACTIVATED PLATELETS INTERACT WITH TARGET CELLS

Platelet-leukocyte aggregates are readily visible in circulating blood exposed to cigarette smoke *(54)*, during sepsis *(22)*, following transfusion of platelet concentrates *(55)*, and prior to acute myocardial infarction *(56)*. Platelet-leukocyte aggregates are also visible in ruptured atherosclerotic plaques *(57)*, and β_3-integrin-deficient platelets form a monolayer on damaged endothelium that attracts leukocytes and induces neointimal formation *(58)*. The vascular endothelium is a depository for platelets in *ApoE*$^{-/-}$ mice before they development significant atherosclerotic lesions *(59)*, and platelets rosette around tumor cells, enhancing tumor growth and metastasis *(60–64)*.

Do these associations modulate inflammatory outcomes or are they residual side effects of the inflammatory insult? Most studies tip the balance in favor of platelets as triggers and amplifiers of inflammation when they adhere to target cells. Perhaps the most convincing evidence comes from studies demonstrating that activated platelets markedly alter gene expression profiles in endothelial cells and monocytes. In *ApoE*-deficient mice, platelets adhere to the endothelium, preceding the development of atherosclerosis *(59)*. Adhesion coincides with a marked increase in inflammatory gene products in the inflamed area, and blockade of platelet adhesion markedly suppresses atherosclerotic lesion formation *(59)*. Based on in vitro and correlative in vivo evidence, invading leukocytes probably enhance inflammation by multiplying the number and intensity of gene products in the platelet-rich regions *(29,35,36,38,65)*. Platelets adherent to collagen bind and induce MMP-9 synthesis in monocytes, a potent mediator of tissue injury, inflammation, and wound repair *(57)*. Other inflammatory gene products, including IL-8, IL-1β, MCP-1, and macrophage inflammatory protein-1α (MIP-1α), are synthesized by monocytes that are stimulated by activated platelets *(29,57,65)*.

Under most circumstances, expression of these inflammatory proteins requires adhesive interactions that are controlled by platelet-derived P-selectin, and its leukocyte ligand, P-selectin glycoprotein-1 *(28)*. Platelet-derived P-selectin also binds mucin-type glycoproteins on tumor cells, promoting tumor growth and metastasis *(60,61)*. Activated platelets bind dendritic cells and regulate their maturation, a finding that has implications for the roles of platelets during wound healing *(66)*. Platelets also modulate cell survival markers in monocytes as they adhere and are ingested by these phagocytes *(67)*. This process, which occurs over days, demonstrates that the phagocytosis of platelets by monocytes is not an inert response and suggests that platelets regulate inflammatory events even as they are sequestered and removed from the bloodstream *(67)*.

There is Evidence That Platelets Have Prolonged and Sustained Effects in Thrombosis and Inflammation

Can we expect such a specialized cell to do more? Dogma suggests that platelets are "spent" after the initial hemostatic response, merely programmed for rapid function and short survival. This prevailing belief has limited the number of studies that examine long-term functions of platelets (i.e., studies that extend functional analyses beyond 15–30 min post activation). However, the platelet release reaction does not always lead to an irreversible state of platelet dysfunction *(68)*. Activated platelets, reinjected into the circulation, have normal survival curves and retain their capacity to aggregate *(69–71)*. Cultured platelets respond to delayed administration of agonists, hours after initial adhesion, and translational control proteins are continuously phosphorylated in activated platelets (Fig. 1) *(30,72)*. Platelets also retract fibrin-rich clots, an event that can take up to 24 h as platelets exert force on fibrin strands to recanalize vessels obstructed by thrombi *(73)*.

SIGNAL-DEPENDENT PROTEIN SYNTHESIS IN HUMAN PLATELETS: A NEW PARADIGM

We have recently discovered that platelets synthesize inflammatory proteins in response to activating signals as they form fibrin-rich clots *(72,74–76)*. *De novo* synthesis of proteins in platelets occurs via translation of mRNAs that are retained from parent megakaryocytes *(72,74–76)*. Synthesis of some of these proteins requires cellular activation, a process that we term *signal-dependent protein synthesis*. Signal-dependent translation of proteins from constitutive mRNAs occurs in other cell types and may be a critical mechanism for alteration of cellular phenotype *(77)*. In platelets, however, this process suggests new paradigms for their roles in thrombosis, inflammation, and disease.

Protein Synthetic Machinery: Platelets Have Components to Do the Job

Although signal-dependent protein synthesis is a relatively new concept, it has been known for many years that platelets have synthetic potential. In 1967, Francois M. Booyse and Max E. Rafelson demonstrated that resting human platelets constitutively synthesize one-third of their contractile protein pool *(78–83)*. We and others have since confirmed that quiescent platelets synthesize protein *(71,72,74–76,81,82,84–86)*. Synthesis of most proteins involves translation of stable messenger RNAs derived from megakaryocytes *(71,72,74–76,81,82,84)*, although RNA transcription occurs in platelet mitochondria *(87–89)*.

It is generally believed that younger platelets have a higher synthetic potential *(83,84,90–92)*. In this regard, Kieffer et al. *(84)* demonstrated that virtually all proteins revealed by Coomassie blue stain are radiolabeled with amino acids in newly released platelets isolated from patients with idiopathic thrombocytopenic purpura (ITP), suggesting that protein synthesis in newly formed cells is an important determinant of the total protein pool. Although synthesis may decrease with aging, mature platelets also synthesize protein. Belloc et al. *(93)* found that mature platelets isolated from human peripheral blood contain polysomes and synthesize proteins. Booyse and Rafelson *(82,83)* demonstrated that all platelet populations incorporate radiolabeled amino acids into protein, although protein synthesis varied depending on size and density of the cells. Consistent with these findings, immunocytochemistry studies from our laboratory demonstrate that newly synthesized proteins are present in virtually all platelets and are not restricted to a platelet subpopulation (Fig. 2) *(74–76)*. Even though the levels and patterns of synthesis may vary, these data indicate that, independent of their age, platelets can translate mRNA.

Since platelets circulate as anucleate cytoplasts, protein synthetic events primarily occur at the translational level *(75,76,78–83,93)*. Stable messenger RNAs, ribosomes, and translational control proteins are retained as platelets evolve from parent megakaryocytes *(72,75,76,80,85,94)*. RNA-binding fluorochromes stain the entire platelet population isolated from normal donors (our unpublished observations), indicating that RNAs remain with platelets during their entire lifespan in vivo, although transcripts undergo degradation ex vivo (*see* Section "When and Where...," pp.161, 162). cDNA libraries have been developed from platelet mRNA extracts *(95,96)*. Further studies have examined the expression of specific transcripts in platelets *(97–101)*, and more recent cDNA array analyses demonstrate that freshly isolated platelets contain thousands of mRNAs *(72,76,94)*. These data indicate that messenger RNAs with physiologic significance are present and stable in circulating platelets. Platelet RNA can be used as a template for protein synthesis when it is inserted in rabbit reticulocytes in vitro translation systems, indicating that it is functional *(75,96)*. In addition, 5% of total RNA is polyadenylated in platelets isolated from patients with essential thrombocythemia *(96)*, suggesting that the ratio of messenger RNA to total RNA may be higher in platelets compared with other primary human cells and cell lines *(102)*. This may be very important since the relative abundance of platelet RNA is much less than in other cells (*see* Section "What to Expect...," p.163).

Using a cell-free translation system, Booyse and Rafelson *(80)* demonstrated that platelets contain ribosomes and requisite machinery to translate mRNA. In these studies, incorporation of radiolabeled amino acids into protein occurred in platelet lysates, mirroring in vitro translation systems that use rabbit reticulocyte lysates *(80)*. Other investigators have observed ribosomes in circulating platelets *(84,103)*, and we found that all platelet populations stain positive for ribosomal protein S6 and

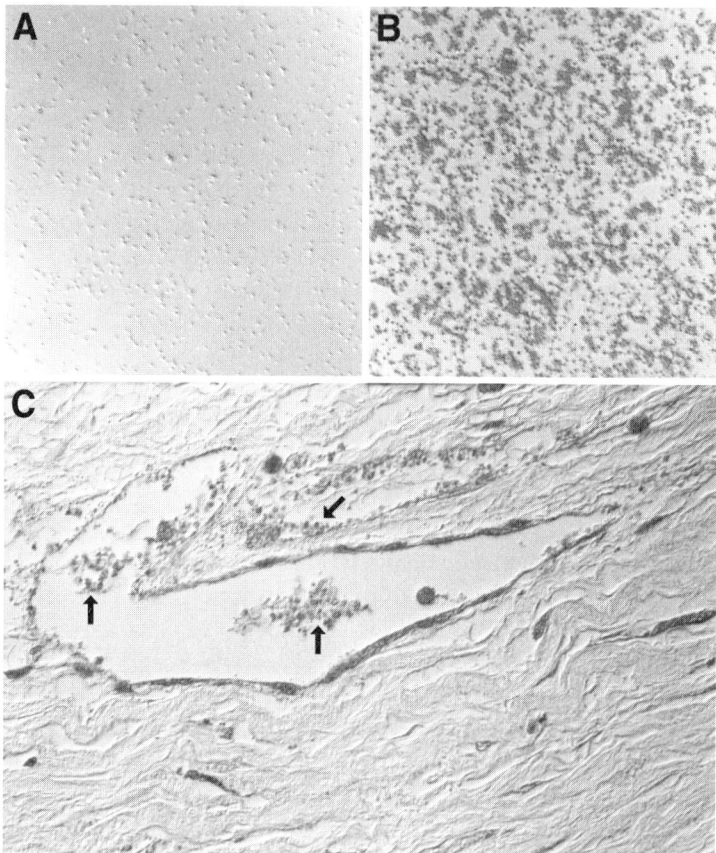

Fig. 2. Bcl-3 is expressed in aggregated platelets in vitro and in vivo. **(A,B)** Immunocytochemical detection of Bcl-3 in platelets ex vivo. Bcl-3 expression was examined in quiescent (A) and thrombin-activated platelets that were freshly isolated from human whole blood (B; 0.1 U/mL for 2 h). B depicts aggregated cells that are positive for Bcl-3. **(C)** Immunohistochemical detection of Bcl-3 in aggregated platelets *in situ*. Tissue sections from vessels resected at the time of surgical intervention in patients with abdominal aortic aneurysms were stained for Bcl-3. Bcl-3 is present in intravascular aggregates and platelets adherent to walls of adventitial microvessels (arrows). Bcl-3 is also present in endothelial cells and leukocytes in this section, consistent with in vitro observations *(153,154)*. (A and B, from ref. *75*, with permission; C, from ref. *74*, with permission. By copyright permission of The Rockefeller University Press.)

the ribosomal P antigen (our unpublished observations), two proteins that bind 40S and 60S ribosomal subunits, respectively *(104,105)*. S6 is the major substrate for protein kinases in eukaryotic ribosomes, including p70, p85, and p90 ribosomal S6 kinases. Platelets express all three

S6 kinase subunits *(106)*. Platelets also express mammalian target of rapamycin (mTOR), the kinase that controls the activity of p70S6 kinase and 4E-BP1 eukaryotic initiation factor-4E (eIF4E)-binding protein-1 (4E-BP1), a protein that represses translation by binding and inhibiting the activity the rate-limiting initiation factor, eIF4E *(107,108)*. Our group *(72,75)* as well as Rosenwald et al. *(85)*, has demonstrated that platelets express 4E-BP1, eIF4E, and eIF-2α. eIF-2α is a critical protein that aids in the transfer of initiator methionyl-tRNA to the 40S ribosomal subunit *(85,109)*.

Signal-Dependent Translation in Platelets: Identifying Products That Regulate Thrombosis and Inflammation

Most studies characterizing platelet protein synthesis have been conducted in quiescent, unstimulated cells. Thrombosthenin, an actomyosin-like contractile protein, was the first synthetic product identified in unstimulated platelets *(79,80)*. More recent products include the major membrane glycoproteins (GPIb, IIb, and IIIa), fibrinogen, thrombospondin, albumin, and von Willebrand factor *(84)*. mRNAs for these proteins are abundantly expressed in platelets (unpublished observations and refs. *94, 96, 99–101,* and *110*), suggesting that constitutive, low-level synthesis may be a mechanism that allows platelets to maintain threshold concentrations of these critical regulatory factors *(84)*.

Although it was clear from earlier reports that platelets have the capacity for basal synthesis of proteins, it was unknown whether they can translate mRNAs in a signal-dependent fashion. As part of ongoing studies of gene regulation in platelet-leukocyte interactions, we made the unexpected discovery that activated platelets expressed B-cell lymphoma 3 (Bcl-3) *(75)*. Bcl-3 protein was expressed within minutes after stimulation of human platelets with thrombin and accumulated for at least 8 h post activation. We found that low levels of Bcl-3 mRNA were expressed in resting platelets and translated into protein in a signal-dependent fashion. Low-abundance transcripts, like Bcl-3, often have features in their untranslated regions (UTRs) that restrict translation until appropriate signals are initiated *(111)*. These include pyrimidine-tracts or extensive secondary structure in their 5'-UTRs or AU-rich elements (AREs) in their 3'-UTRs. In contrast, high-abundant, housekeeping messages, such as actin, have features that predict constitutive translation *(111)*.

We subsequently demonstrated that Bcl-3 protein is expressed in platelets in inflamed vessels, suggesting it may influence vascular repair and remodeling (Fig. 2) *(74)*. Additional experiments in transfected cells demonstrated that Bcl-3 binds the SH3 domain of Fyn *(75)*, a tyrosine kinase that regulates cytoskeletal function in platelets *(112,113)*. Bcl-3 also interacts with Fyn in platelets, suggesting that it scaffolds proteins in the cytoskeletal network. In this regard, Bcl-3-deficient mouse platelets have impaired ability to retract fibrin-rich clots, suggesting that regulated synthesis of this protein modulates platelet functional responses *(114)*. This indicates that Bcl-3, originally described as a nuclear factor-κb (NF-κB) family member *(115)*, has alternative cellular functions. A recent study has identified an activation-dependent NF-κB/IκB-α complex in platelets, a finding that further supports the idea that NF-κB family members have functions beyond transcription *(116)*.

Multiple Proteins Are Synthesized in a Signal-Dependent Fashion in Stimulated Human Platelets

To identify other mRNAs translated in a signal-dependent fashion, we profiled the distribution of mRNAs attached to ribosomes in quiescent and activated platelets by cDNA array analysis and found that IL-1β transcripts are associated with polysomes *(76)*. This finding was intriguing because other investigators had previously reported IL-1β activity in activated platelets, but experiments demonstrating that resting platelets constitutively store the cytokine were lacking *(117–121)*. We found no evidence of constitutive IL-1β protein expression in platelets. However, thrombin or PAF induced the synthesis of pro-IL-1β, a response that was rapid and peaked between 8 and 18 h *(76)*. Immunocytochemical analysis confirmed that platelets synthesize IL-1β *(76)*. We also found that platelets process pro-IL-1β into its biologically active product *(76)*. Mature IL-1β is expressed in platelets that retract the fibrin network of clots, and a portion of IL-1β is released into the extracellular milieu in microparticles and soluble form, where it increases adhesiveness of endothelial cells for polymorphonuclear leukocytes *(76)*. We are currently characterizing mechanisms that control IL-1β translation in stimulated human platelets. Preliminary evidence suggests that IL-1β synthesis is controlled by a pathway dependent on p38-mitogen-activated protein kinase (MAPK), a regulatory feature in other cell types (data not shown and refs. *122* and *123*). Ribosomal profiling experiments also reveal that IL-1β mRNA is associated with polysomes of quiescent cells and is repressed until signals delivered by thrombin or PAF initiate translation and protein synthesis (*see* above and ref. *76*). This demonstrates that translation of IL-1β mRNA occurs at postinitiation checkpoint in platelets, a unique mode of regulation that has also been identified in *Drosophila (124)*.

Other proteins besides Bcl-3 and IL-1β are synthesized by stimulated platelets (*see* next section for specific proteins and refs. *72* and *75*). This

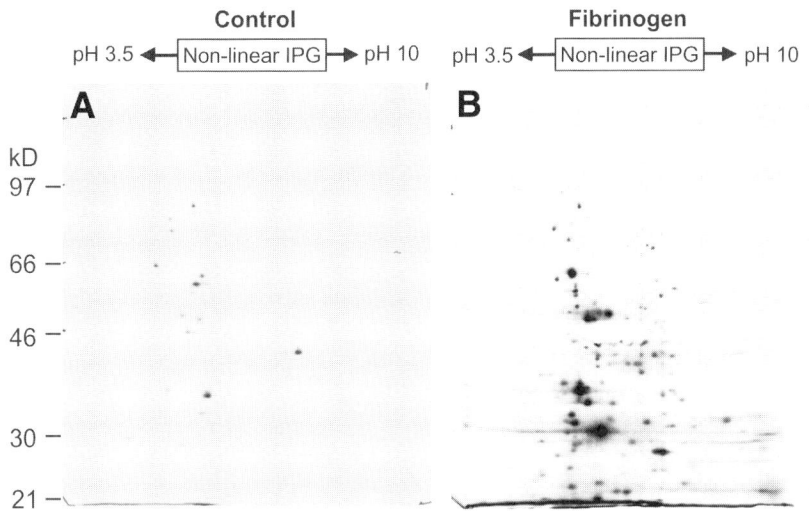

Fig. 3. Adherent platelets synthesize multiple proteins. Freshly isolated human platelets were incubated with [^{35}S]methionine and left in suspension (Control, **A**) or made to adhere to immobilized fibrinogen for 8 h (Fibrinogen, **B**). After the 8-h incubation period, [^{35}S]methionine-labeled proteins were separated by 2D gel electrophoresis. This figure is representative of at least 10 experiments that were conducted in a similar fashion. IPG, immobilized pH gradient.

is most evident by studies from our group demonstrating increased incorporation of [^{35}S]methionine into proteins extracted from adherent platelets compared with quiescent, nonadherent cells (Fig. 3) *(75)*. Protein synthesis is also increased when platelets are stimulated with specific extracellular plasma factors *(86)* or when they phagocytize latex particles *(125)*. These data indicate that additional translated mRNAs important for platelet regulatory responses will be discovered in the future. Intriguing targets include apoptotic gene products that exhibit increased expression as platelets age in vitro *(126,127)* and inducible nitric oxide synthase, a protein whose expression is increased in stimulated platelets *(128,129)*.

ASSESSING THE CLINICAL SIGNIFICANCE OF SIGNAL-DEPENDENT PROTEIN SYNTHESIS BY PLATELETS

Therapeutic Interventions That Modulate Signal-Dependent Protein Synthesis

Patterns and levels of protein synthesis are tightly controlled in platelets through signal-dependent mechanisms. Although characterization of translational control in platelets is far from complete and probably involves multiple levels of regulation, we have identified two pathways that mediate this response: signaling through integrin receptors and regulation by mTOR *(72,74–76)*. Blocking these pathways significantly reduces signal-dependent protein synthesis by platelets *(72,74–76)*.

$\alpha_{IIb}\beta_3$ INHIBITORS: INTEGRIN SIGNALING TO TRANSLATIONAL CHECKPOINTS

$\alpha_{IIb}\beta_3$ inhibitors are indicated as an adjunct to percutaneous coronary intervention to reduce complications attributed to excessive platelet accumulation at the dilated site *(130–132)*. $\alpha_{IIb}\beta_3$ inhibitors currently in use include abciximab (ReoPro®), tirofiban (Aggrastat®), and eptifibatide (Integrilin®) *(132)*. Their primary mode of action is to antagonize fibrinogen binding to $\alpha_{IIb}\beta_3$ integrins, a process that blocks platelet aggregation *(131)*. They have significant beneficial attributes in short-term infusion trials, but long-term studies of oral $\alpha_{IIb}\beta_3$ receptor antagonists have been less effective *(132)*. We found that $\alpha_{IIb}\beta_3$ inhibitors block signal-dependent protein synthesis by platelets *(72,74,76)*. Ligation of $\alpha_{IIb}\beta_3$ integrins during platelet aggregation or adherence to immobilized fibrinogen markedly increases the overall synthetic rate of platelets *(72,75)*. Interruption of this process with abciximab or eptifibatide decreases synthesis, including the generation of Bcl-3 *(74)*. Abciximab, more so than other $\alpha_{IIb}\beta_3$ inhibitors, also abrogates synthesis of IL-1β *(76)*. Dual inhibition of $\alpha_v\beta_3$ and $\alpha_{IIb}\beta_3$ may be involved *(131)* since clot retraction, which markedly increases IL-1β synthesis *(76)*, is modulated by both integrin subfamilies *(133)*.

One mechanism that integrins utilize to increase protein synthesis is spatial targeting of translational factors to mRNA-rich areas *(72,134)*. In quiescent platelets, most mRNAs reside in cytoskeletal networks, dissociated from essential translation factors *(72)*. Engagement of β_3-integrins redistributes translational factors to the transcript-rich cytoskeleton inducing mRNA translation *(72)*. Since most platelets lack a defined endoplasmic reticulum, the cytoskeleton is probably the primary apparatus that supports mRNA translation in platelets *(72)*.

These in vitro results suggest that by curtailing platelet accumulation post angioplasty, $\alpha_{IIb}\beta_3$ inhibitors also prevent secondary accumulation of inflammatory proteins resulting from signal-dependent protein synthesis. The effect of other inhibitors that regulate platelet function (such as aspirin, Aggrenox, and ticlodipine) on signal-dependent protein synthesis is not yet known but will be important as their full inhibitory potential is unveiled.

Inhibition of mTOR: A Novel Platelet Signal Transduction Pathway

Sirolimus (Rapamune®), formerly known as rapamycin, is an immunosuppressive agent indicated for the prophylaxis of organ rejection in renal transplant patients *(135)*. In cells, sirolimus binds to the immunophilin FK binding protein-12 (FKBP-12) to generate an immunosuppressive complex that binds and inactivates mTOR, a key regulatory kinase *(136)*. Inhibition of mTOR suppresses cytokine-driven cell proliferation *(137)*.

Sirolimus-releasing stents represent one of the most promising therapeutic targets for treatment of restenosis *(138–140)*. Intramural delivery of rapamycin during balloon angioplasty also reduces restenosis after balloon dilation, suggesting that acute administration of this immunosuppressant has lasting effects (Buerke et al., ms. submitted). This latter finding also suggests that sirolimus modulates functions of nonproliferating cells such as platelets. Platelet activation and/or adherence increases phosphorylation of targets downstream of mTOR that include p70S6 kinase and 4E-BP1 (our unpublished observations and ref. *72*). Low concentrations of sirolimus block p70S6 kinase and 4E-BP1 phosphorylation without altering the phosphorylation of other signaling proteins or inhibiting acute platelet function (i.e., adherence, aggregation, or secretion; our unpublished observations and ref. *72*). Sirolimus also reduces, but does not eliminate, signal-dependent protein synthesis in platelets, as is expected for an inhibitor of mTOR *(75)*. Signal-dependent translation of Bcl-3 mRNA, which has extensive secondary structure, is blocked by sirolimus *(75)*.

When and Where Does Signal-Dependent Protein Synthesis by Platelets Come Into Play?

Platelets have a variety of different mechanisms to regulate thrombosis and inflammation during vascular injury and repair *(12,141)*. Signal-dependent protein synthesis may enhance, maintain, and in some cases resolve inflammation. Translation of mRNA is tightly controlled by platelets: proteins are differentially synthesized by platelets depending on the adhesive environment and the presence or absence of specific soluble agonists (our unpublished observations and refs. *75* and *76*). In some cases, the amount of synthesized product also increases with the level of soluble agonist in the milieu *(75)*. Thus, the type and severity of vascular injury may elicit synthetic responses in platelets that push an inflammatory reaction in a specific direction. During atherogenesis or tumor cell growth, recurrent adhesive and signaling episodes may also induce sustained synthesis of specific platelet products, such as IL-1β, that maintain thrombosis and inflammation for prolonged periods.

It is clear that platelets isolated from healthy donors are capable of synthesizing proteins that regulate inflammatory outcomes *(76)*. However, it is intriguing to speculate that certain environmental factors or genetic predispositions may increase or decrease the synthetic potential of platelets. In cases of accelerated platelet turnover, newly formed platelets express cyclooxgenase-2 (COX-2), a key synthase that catalyzes the formation of various prostaglandins, and TXA_2, which regulates inflammatory events *(142)*. This indicates that platelet subpopulations differentially express proteins that regulate inflammation. Platelet subpopulations may likewise possess differential synthetic potential. It is known that newly formed platelets from ITP patients have more synthetic potential than platelets from normal subjects *(84)*. Whether ITP platelets correspond to normal young platelets or are generated by a population of megakaryocytes releasing stress platelets of larger size is unclear *(84,143)*. If the latter is true, messenger RNAs derived from megakaryocytes, and their corresponding biosynthetic products may be quite different in ITP platelets vs normal platelets. Environmental stresses, such as hypercholesterolemia or diabetes, or genetic factors may similarly influence the mRNA pool or the function of regulatory translational factors in circulating platelets. It is known that platelets from Glanzmann's thrombasthenic patients have decreased synthetic responses because they lack $\alpha_{IIb}\beta_3$ integrins that drive translation *(74)*. Other inherited or acquired deficiencies may likewise inhibit or enhance platelet synthetic responses, similar to congenital disorders that affect platelet secretion and signal transduction *(144)*.

Protein synthetic events may also be very important during platelet storage and transfusion. Several studies have now demonstrated that platelets undergo regulated apoptosis over several hours, and platelets aged in vitro (i.e., up to 24 h) exhibit increased expression of proapoptotic factors that parallel constitutive diminution of cell function *(126,127,145,146)*. Cycloheximide, a translational inhibitor, prolongs platelet survival *(147)*, suggesting that proapoptotic factors may be synthesized during the initial phases of platelet storage. Another possibility is that over extended periods, stored platelets lose their synthetic potential. We have observed that after approx 24 h of storage, ribosomal RNA begins to degrade, and we are unable to obtain any RNA from platelet concentrates that have been stored for 5 d (our unpublished observations). This suggests the possibility that abnormal platelet function associated with storage may, in part, be owing to loss of key transcripts and a consequent dysfunctional biosynthetic system.

METHODS USED TO ASSESS mRNA TRANSLATION BY PLATELETS

Our group has used a variety of experimental approaches to examine signal-dependent protein synthesis by platelets *(72,74–76)*. Most of the difficulties we have encountered center on the detection and isolation of low-abundant mRNAs and synthesized proteins. Here we highlight strategies and technical approaches routinely used by our laboratory to assess RNA and synthetic pathways in platelets.

What to Expect From Platelet RNA

A primary advantage of working with platelets is that megakaryocytes transfer stable RNA to circulating platelets, and the functionality of the RNA can be examined in the absence of nuclear influences. An inherent difficulty when working with platelet RNA is its relative low abundance compared with other cells *(99)*. For instance, we typically extract 0.01 µg of total RNA from 1×10^7 human platelets using TRIzol isolation procedures. Using the same procedure, approx 10-fold and 100-fold greater amounts are obtained from similar numbers of primary human neutrophils and mononuclear cells, respectively (our unpublished observations and ref. 99). Platelet-specific mRNAs have been confirmed by cDNA cloning, Northern blot analysis, and RNase protection assays *(95,96,110,145,148)*. Owing to the relative low abundance of most messages, however, reverse transcriptase polymerase chain reaction (RT-PCR) is the most common technique used to study platelet mRNAs *(75,76,95,99,100)*, and with the advent of quantitative real-time RT-PCR, accurate copy numbers can be obtained for most transcripts *(94)*. An additional technical hurdle is that it is often difficult to eliminate completely all the proteinacious material that associates with purified RNA when it is isolated from large numbers of platelets. Excessive protein contamination becomes apparent if RNA extracts are exceptionally "sticky," reducing the integrity of purified RNA. Adding proteinase K prior to the isolation procedure markedly reduces this problem.

Measuring the Product

A primary objective is to identify mRNAs that are translated into functional protein, a goal that is not trivial in platelets or other cells. In platelet systems, we initially delineate conditions that induce protein synthesis using standard [^{35}S]methionine protein incorporation studies *(72,75,95,96)*. In these studies, we routinely examine cellular lysates and supernatants *(72,75)* and often separate the proteins by 2-D gel electrophoresis (Fig. 3). We have found that low concentrations of thrombin or PAF induce protein synthesis in washed platelets incubated in suspension with exogenous fibrinogen *(72,76,149)*. Adherence to extra-cellular matrices such as collagen, fibrinogen, and laminin also enhances protein synthetic events, a response that is typically increased when the platelets are costimulated with thrombin or other soluble agonists (Lindemann et al., ms. in preparation). In some cases, we have been able to sequence synthesized proteins directly if they are abundant enough to be detected by colloidal Coomassie- or silver-stained gels run in parallel. We have detected constitutive or regulated synthesis of Rho-GDIα and -β, tropomyosin, actin, and the fibrinogen β-chain by platelets using this method (Lindemann et al., ms. in preparation).

More often than not, however, these staining procedures are not sensitive enough to detect newly synthesized proteins. Therefore, we also employ alternative strategies centered on cDNA array analysis to identify candidate mRNAs under translational control *(72,76,94)*. cDNA array profiling experiments provide patterns of mRNA expression in platelets, and candidate messages under translational control can be predicted based on their relative abundance and unique 5'- and 3'-UTRs (*see* Signal-Dependent Translation in Platelets section above and ref. *77*). A more targeted approach involves cDNA arrays of mRNAs that are associated with polysomes or with specific RNA binding proteins *(76)*. The assumption in the first case is that when mRNAs associate with multiple ribosomes (i.e., polysomes) either they are in a state of active translation *(150)* or the ribosomes are temporarily "stalled" on the message *(151)*, waiting for appropriate signals to be delivered to trigger active translation. We used ribosomal expression profiling to identify IL-1β as a candidate gene under signal-dependent translational control in platelets (*see* ref. *76*).

In addition, we have recently begun profiling mRNAs attached to RNA-binding proteins that regulate translation (Lindemann et al., ms. in preparation). Here, RNA-binding proteins such as eIF4E are immuno-precipitated with specific antibodies, and coprecipitating RNAs are used as templates in cDNA arrays *(152)*. The prediction from other cellular systems is that if mRNAs are actively translated, their association with RNA-binding proteins will be altered. The utility of these functional genomic approaches includes a highly sensitive method of detection, simultaneous interrogation of numerous genes, and a modus operandi to identify genes that are in or near an active translation state.

Once candidate mRNAs have been identified, confirmation that they are synthesized into functional protein is required. One approach is to immunoprecipitate [^{35}S]methionine-labeled products with appropriate antibodies directed against the antigen of interest *(75,76)*. Western analysis and/or enzyme-linked immunosorbent assay can also be used to determine relative amounts of the product *(75,76)*. All these experiments should be done in the presence or absence of translational inhibitors such as puromycin to confirm that regulated expression is owing to protein synthesis *(75,76)*. In select studies, transcriptional inhibitors can be used in parallel *(75)*, although care should be taken when interpreting these experiments since actinomycin D also has nonspecific effects on platelets that may indirectly affect protein synthesis (our unpublished observations). Nevertheless, an advantage of using transcriptional inhibitors is that, depending on the results, contributions of leukocyte contaminants can be eliminated. White blood cell contamination can also be minimized by careful isolation procedures and can be decreased if leukocyte reduction filters or magnetic bead purification steps are installed. However, these latter procedures are expensive, they can prematurely activate the cells, and they extend the duration of the isolation period.

A parallel approach is to localize the antigen in platelets by immunocytochemistry. In most cases, this documents that the candidate protein is synthesized in stimulated platelets (Fig. 2) *(74–76)*. In addition, indirect labeling procedures can be used to increase sensitivity for the detection of low-abundance proteins, and intracellular localization patterns often give clues regarding mechanisms that control the synthesis and/or function of the targeted protein. For instance, we initially observed that Bcl-3 expression was prominent in platelet aggregates compared with single activated platelets (Fig. 2) *(75)*, a finding that led to experiments demonstrating that $\alpha_{IIb}\beta_3$ integrins regulate translational events in platelets *(74)*. Demonstrating function for the synthesized protein is also imperative. For IL-1β, we were able to predict its functional consequences based on its known biology *(76)*. Proline-rich sequences in Bcl-3 strongly suggested it interacted with specific proteins that contain SH3 binding domains *(75)*.

SUMMARY: NEW BIOLOGICAL POTENTIALS FOR ACTIVATED HUMAN PLATELETS

In this review we have made a case that platelets use a variety of functional responses to mediate inflammatory events. A number of the highlighted studies demonstrate that platelets continue to function after their initial hemostatic repertoire is completed. This implies that we previously underestimated the biologic potential of platelets by assuming that these anucleate cytoplasts are always finished with their work immediately after activation. We have focused on one previously unrecognized function of platelets, signal-dependent protein synthesis, which can be rapidly initiated but also proceeds for many hours depending on the protein product (Fig. 4). Ongoing studies in our laboratory and others

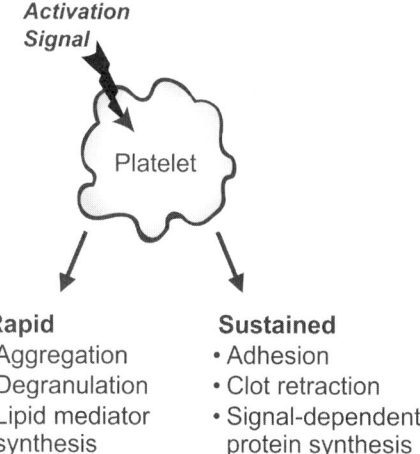

Fig. 4. Pictorial depicting rapid and sustained functions of platelets. See text for details regarding signal-dependent protein synthesis.

will determine how protein synthetic events modulate functional responses in platelets. Our prediction is that other important features of platelets, both immediate and prolonged, will be revealed in the near future as the functional roles of this small, anuclear cell continue to exceed original expectations.

REFERENCES

1. Wintrobe MM. Blood Platelets and coagulation. In: Wintrobe MM, ed. Clinical Hematology. Lea & Febiger, Philadelphia, 1946, pp. 187–238.
2. Bizzozero G. Su di un nuovo elemento morfologico del sangue dei mammiferi e della sua importanza nella trombosi e nella coagulazione. Osservatore 1881;17:785–787.
3. Bizzozero G. Ueber einen neuen Formbestandtheil des Blutes und dessen Rolle bei der Thrombose und der Blutgerinnung. Virchows Arch Pathol Anat Physiol 1882;90:261–332.
4. Coller BS. A brief and highly selective history of ideas about platelets in health and disease. In: Michelson AD, ed. Platelets. Academic Press, San Diego, 2002, pp. xxix–xliii.
5. Zucker MB, Nachmias VT. Platelet activation. Arteriosclerosis 1985;5:2–18.
6. McNicol A. Platelet preparation and estimation of functional responses. In: Watson SP, ed. Platelets: A Practical Approach. IRL Press at Oxford University Press, Oxford, 1996, pp. 1–26.
7. Clemetson KJ. Platelet activation: signal transduction via membrane receptors. Thromb Haemost 1995;74:111–116.
8. Levy-Toledano S. Platelet signal transduction pathways: could we organize them into a 'hierarchy'? Haemostasis 1999;29:4–15.
9. Parise LV. Integrin alpha(IIb)beta(3) signaling in platelet adhesion and aggregation. Curr Opin Cell Biol 1999;11:597–601.

10. Bouchard BA, Butenas S, Mann KG, Tracy PB. Interactions between platelets and the coagulation system. In: Michelson AD, ed. Platelets. Elsevier Science, San Diego, 2002, pp. 229–253.

11. Michelson AD. The clinical approach to disorders of platelet number and function. In: Michelson AD, ed. Platelets. Elsevier Science, San Diego, 2002, pp. 541–545.

12. Ruggeri ZM. Platelets in atherothrombosis. Nat Med 2002;8:1227–1234.

13. Goldschmidt PJ, Lopes N, Crawford LE. Atherosclerosis and coronary heart disease. In: Michelson AD, ed. Platelets. Elsevier Science, San Diego, 2002, pp. 375–398.

14. Karpatkin S. Tumor growth and metastasis. In: Michelson AD, ed. Platelets. Elsevier Science, San Diego, 2002, pp. 491–502.

15. Tschoepe D, Menart-Houtermans, B. Diabetes mellitus. In: Michelson AD, ed. Platelets. Elsevier Science, San Diego, 2002, pp. 435–445.

16. Gordon JLM. Blood platelets as multifunctional cells. In: Gordon JL, ed. Platelets in Biology and Pathology: Elsevier/North-Holland Biomedical, Amsterdam, 1976, pp. 3–22.

17. Herd CM, Page CP. Pulmonary immune cells in health and disease: platelets. Eur Respir J 1994;7:1145–1160.

18. Klinger MH. Platelets and inflammation. Anat Embryol (Berl) 1997;196:1–11.

19. Mannaioni PF, Di Bello MG, Masini E. Platelets and inflammation: role of platelet-derived growth factor, adhesion molecules and histamine. Inflamm Res 1997;46:4–18.

20. Yeaman M, Bayer, AS. Antimicrobial host defense. In: Michelson AD, ed. Platelets. Elsevier Science, San Diego, 2002, pp. 469–490.

21. Nash GF, Turner LF, Scully MF, Kakkar AK. Platelets and cancer. Lancet Oncol 2002;3:425–430.

22. Russwurm S, Vickers J, Meier-Hellmann A, et al. Platelet and leukocyte activation correlate with the severity of septic organ dysfunction. Shock 2002;17:263–268.

23. Vincent JL, Yagushi A, Pradier O. Platelet function in sepsis. Crit Care Med 2002;30:S313–S317.

24. Endresen GK, Forre O. Human platelets in synovial fluid. A focus on the effects of growth factors on the inflammatory responses in rheumatoid arthritis. Clin Exp Rheumatol 1992;10:181–187.

25. Hasleton PS, Roberts TE. Adult respiratory distress syndrome—an update. Histopathology 1999;34:285–294.

26. Reed GL. Platelet secretion. In: Michelson AD, ed. Platelets. Elsevier Science, San Diego, 2002, pp. 181–195.

27. Rendu F, Brohard-Bohn B. The platelet release reaction: granules' constituents, secretion and functions. Platelets 2001;12:261–273.

28. McEver RP. Adhesive interactions of leukocytes, platelets, and the vessel wall during hemostasis and inflammation. Thromb Haemost 2001;86:746–756.

29. Weyrich AS, Elstad MR, McEver RP, et al. Activated platelets signal chemokine synthesis by human monocytes. J Clin Invest 1996;97:1525–1534.

30. McBane RD 2nd, Ford MA, Karnicki K, Stewart M, Owen WG. Fibrinogen, fibrin and crosslinking in aging arterial thrombi. Thromb Haemost 2000;84:83–87.

31. Galt SW, Lindemann S, Allen L, et al. Outside-in signals delivered by matrix metalloproteinase-1 regulate platelet function. Circ Res 2002;90:1093–1099.

32. Sawicki G, Salas E, Murat J, Miszta-Lane H, Radomski MW. Release of gelatinase A during platelet activation mediates aggregation. Nature 1997;386:616–619.

33. Kameyoshi Y, Dorschner A, Mallet AI, Christophers E, Schroder JM. Cytokine RANTES released by thrombin-stimulated platelets is a potent attractant for human eosinophils. J Exp Med 1992;176:587–592.

34. Schall TJ, Bacon K, Toy KJ, Goeddel DV. Selective attraction of monocytes and T lymphocytes of the memory phenotype by cytokine RANTES. Nature 1990;347:669–671.

35. Schober A, Manka D, von Hundelshausen P, et al. Deposition of platelet RANTES triggering monocyte recruitment requires P-selectin and is involved in neointima formation after arterial injury. Circulation 2002;106:1523–1529.

36. von Hundelshausen P, Weber KS, Huo Y, et al. RANTES deposition by platelets triggers monocyte arrest on inflamed and atherosclerotic endothelium. Circulation 2001;103:1772–1777.

37. Bacon KB, Premack BA, Gardner P, Schall TJ. Activation of dual T cell signaling pathways by the chemokine RANTES. Science 1995;269:1727–1730.

38. Weyrich AS, Prescott SM, Zimmerman GA. Platelets, endothelial cells, inflammatory chemokines, and restenosis: complex signaling in the vascular play book. Circulation 2002;106:1433–1435.

39. Henn V, Slupsky JR, Grafe M, et al. CD40 ligand on activated platelets triggers an inflammatory reaction of endothelial cells. Nature 1998;391:591–594.

40. McEver RP. Properties of GMP-140, an inducible granule membrane protein of platelets and endothelium. Blood Cells 1990;16:73–80.

41. McEver RP. Selectins. Curr Opin Immunol 1994;6:75–84.

42. Topol EJ. Aspirin with bypass surgery—from taboo to new standard of care. N Engl J Med 2002;347:1359–1360.

43. FitzGerald GA, Fitzgerald DJ, Lawson JA, Murray R. Thromboxane biosynthesis and antagonism in humans. Adv Prostaglandin Thromboxane Leukot Res 1987; 17A:199–203.

44. Fitzgerald DJ, Wright F, FitzGerald GA. Increased thromboxane biosynthesis during coronary thrombolysis. Evidence that platelet activation and thromboxane A2 modulate the response to tissue-type plasminogen activator in vivo. Circ Res 1989;65:83–94.

45. FitzGerald GA, Murray R, Moran N, et al. Mechanisms of eicosanoid action. Adv Prostaglandin Thromboxane Leukot Res 1991;21B:577–581.

46. Fitzgerald GA, Catella F, Oates JA. Eicosanoid biosynthesis in human cardiovascular disease. Hum Pathol 1987;18:248–252.

47. Patrono C. Aspirin and human platelets: from clinical trials to acetylation of cyclooxygenase and back. Trends Pharmacol Sci 1989;10:453–458.

48. Pratico D, Tillmann C, Zhang ZB, Li H, FitzGerald GA. Acceleration of atherogenesis by COX-1-dependent prostanoid formation in low density lipoprotein receptor knockout mice. Proc Natl Acad Sci USA 2001;98:3358–3363.

49. Cyrus T, Sung S, Zhao L, Funk CD, Tang S, Pratico D. Effect of low-dose aspirin on vascular inflammation, plaque stability, and atherogenesis in low-density lipoprotein receptor-deficient mice. Circulation 2002;106:1282–1287.

50. Ostrovsky L, King AJ, Bond S, et al. A juxtacrine mechanism for neutrophil adhesion on platelets involves platelet-activating factor and a selectin-dependent activation process. Blood 1998;91:3028–3036.

51. Zimmerman GA, Elstad MR, Lorant DE, et al. Platelet-activating factor (PAF): signalling and adhesion in cell-cell interactions. Adv Exp Med Biol 1996;416:297–304.

52. Zimmerman GA, McIntyre TM, Prescott SM, Stafforini DM. The platelet-activating factor signaling system and its regulators in syndromes of inflammation and thrombosis. Crit Care Med 2002;30:S294–S301.

53. Weyrich AS, McIntyre TM, McEver RP, Prescott SM, Zimmerman GA. Monocyte tethering by P-selectin regulates monocyte chemotactic protein-1 and tumor necrosis factor-alpha secretion. Signal integration and NF-kappa B translocation [see comments]. J Clin Invest 1995;95:2297–2303.

54. Lehr HA, Weyrich AS, Saetzler RK, et al. Vitamin C blocks inflammatory platelet-activating factor mimetics created by cigarette smoking [see comments]. J Clin Invest 1997;99:2358–2364.
55. Gutensohn K, Geidel K, Brockmann M, et al. Binding of activated platelets to WBCs in vivo after transfusion. Transfusion 2002;42:1373–1380.
56. Furman MI, Barnard MR, Krueger LA, et al. Circulating monocyte-platelet aggregates are an early marker of acute myocardial infarction. J Am Coll Cardiol 2001;38:1002–1006.
57. Galt SW, Lindemann S, Medd D, et al. Differential regulation of matrix metalloproteinase-9 by monocytes adherent to collagen and platelets. Circ Res 2001;89:509–516.
58. Smyth SS, Reis ED, Zhang W, Fallon JT, Gordon RE, Coller BS. Beta(3)-integrin-deficient mice but not P-selectin-deficient mice develop intimal hyperplasia after vascular injury: correlation with leukocyte recruitment to adherent platelets 1 hour after injury. Circulation 2001;103:2501–2507.
59. Massberg S, Brand K, Gruner S, et al. A critical role of platelet adhesion in the initiation of atherosclerotic lesion formation. J Exp Med 2002;196:887–896.
60. Kim YJ, Borsig L, Han HL, Varki NM, Varki A. Distinct selectin ligands on colon carcinoma mucins can mediate pathological interactions among platelets, leukocytes, and endothelium. Am J Pathol 1999;155:461–472.
61. Kim YJ, Borsig L, Varki NM, Varki A. P-selectin deficiency attenuates tumor growth and metastasis. Proc Natl Acad Sci USA 1998;95:9325–9330.
62. Borsig L, Wong R, Hynes RO, Varki NM, Varki A. Synergistic effects of L- and P-selectin in facilitating tumor metastasis can involve non-mucin ligands and implicate leukocytes as enhancers of metastasis. Proc Natl Acad Sci USA 2002;99:2193–2198.
63. Borsig L, Wong R, Feramisco J, Nadeau DR, Varki NM, Varki A. Heparin and cancer revisited: mechanistic connections involving platelets, P-selectin, carcinoma mucins, and tumor metastasis. Proc Natl Acad Sci USA 2001;98:3352–3357.
64. Hallahan DE, Staba-Hogan MJ, Virudachalam S, Kolchinsky A. X-ray-induced P-selectin localization to the lumen of tumor blood vessels. Cancer Res 1998;58:5216–5220.
65. Neumann FJ, Marx N, Gawaz M, et al. Induction of cytokine expression in leukocytes by binding of thrombin-stimulated platelets. Circulation 1997;95:2387–2394.
66. Hilf N, Singh-Jasuja H, Schwarzmaier P, Gouttefangeas C, Rammensee HG, Schild H. Human platelets express heat shock protein receptors and regulate dendritic cell maturation. Blood 2002;99:3676–3682.
67. Lang D, Dohle F, Terstesse M, et al. Down-regulation of monocyte apoptosis by phagocytosis of platelets: involvement of a caspase-9, caspase-3, and heat shock protein 70-dependent pathway. J Immunol 2002;168:6152–6158.
68. Morgenstern E. Ultracytochemistry of blood platelets. In: Graumann W, Lojda, A, Pearse, AGE, Schiebler, TH, eds. Progress in Histochemistry and Cytochemistry, vol. 12. Gustav Fischer, New York, 1980, pp. 1–86.
69. Packham MA, Guccione MA, Kinlough-Rathbone RL, Mustard JF. Platelet sialic acid and platelet survival after aggregation by ADP. Blood 1980;56:876–880.
70. Kinlough-Rathbone RL, Packham MA, Guccione MA, Richardson M, Harfenist EJ, Mustard JF. Characteristics of thrombin-degranulated human platelets: development of a method that does not use proteolytic enzymes for deaggregation. Thromb Haemost 1991;65:403–410.
71. Born GV. Observations on the change in shape of blood platelets brought about by adenosine diphosphate. J Physiol 1970;209:487–511.

72. Lindemann S, Tolley ND, Eyre JR, Kraiss LW, Mahoney TM, Weyrich AS. Integrins regulate the intracellular distribution of eukaryotic initiation factor 4E in platelets. A checkpoint for translational control. J Biol Chem 2001;276:33947–33951.

73. Seabold JE, Schroder E, Conrad GR, et al. Indium-111 platelet scintigraphy and two-dimensional echocardiography for detection of left ventricular thrombus: influence of clot size and age. J Am Coll Cardiol 1987;9:1057–1066.

74. Pabla R, Weyrich AS, Dixon DA, et al. Integrin-dependent control of translation: engagement of integrin alphaIIbbeta3 regulates synthesis of proteins in activated human platelets. J Cell Biol 1999;144:175–184.

75. Weyrich AS, Dixon DA, Pabla R, et al. Signal-dependent translation of a regulatory protein, Bcl-3, in activated human platelets. Proc Natl Acad Sci USA 1998;95:5556–5561.

76. Lindemann S, Tolley ND, Dixon DA, et al. Activated platelets mediate inflammatory signaling by regulated interleukin 1 beta synthesis. J Cell Biol 2001;154:485–490.

77. Mahoney TS, Weyrich AS, Dixon DA, McIntyre T, Prescott SM, Zimmerman GA. Cell adhesion regulates gene expression at translational checkpoints in human myeloid leukocytes. Proc Natl Acad Sci USA 2001;98:10284–10289.

78. Booyse FM, Rafelson ME Jr. Stable messenger RNA in the synthesis of contractile protein in human platelets. Biochim Biophys Acta 1967;145:188–190.

79. Booyse F, Rafelson ME, Jr. In vitro incorporation of amino-acids into the contractile protein of human blood platelets. Nature 1967;215:283–284.

80. Booyse FM, Rafelson ME Jr. Studies on human platelets. I. Synthesis of platelet protein in a cell-free system. Biochim Biophys Acta 1968;166:689–697.

81. Booyse FM, Hoveke TP, Rafelson ME. Studies on human platelets. II. Protein synthetic activity of various platelet populations. Biochim Biophys Acta 1968;157:660–663.

82. Booyse FM, Rafelson ME. Protein synthesis and platelet function. In: Johnson SA, ed. Dynamics of Thrombus Formation and Dissolution. JB Lippincott, Philadelphia, 1969, p. 149.

83. Booyse FM, Zschocke D, Hoveke TP, Rafelson ME. Studies on human platelets. IV. Protein synthesis in maturing human platelets. Thromb Diath Haemorrh 1971;26:167–176.

84. Kieffer N, Guichard J, Farcet JP, Vainchenker W, Breton-Gorius J. Biosynthesis of major platelet proteins in human blood platelets. Eur J Biochem 1987;164:189–195.

85. Rosenwald IB, Pechet L, Han A, et al. Expression of translation initiation factors elF-4E and elF-2alpha and a potential physiologic role of continuous protein synthesis in human platelets. Thromb Haemost 2001;85:142–151.

86. Plow EF. Extracellular factors influencing the in vitro protein synthesis of platelets. Thromb Haemost 1979;42:666–678.

87. Schneider W, Dries R, Scheurlen PG. [New findings on nucleic acid synthesis in human blood platelets]. Verh Dtsch Ges Inn Med 1972;78:696–698.

88. Schneider W, Dries R, Kulenkampff G. Studies on the protein and nucleic acid synthesis of normal human blood platelets. Acta Univ Carol Med Monogr 1972;53:113–137.

89. Soslau G. De novo synthesis of DNA in human platelets. Arch Biochem Biophys 1983;226:252–256.

90. Karpatkin S. Heterogeneity of human platelets. I. Metabolic and kinetic evidence suggestive of young and old platelets. J Clin Invest 1969;48:1073–1082.

91. Kienast J, Schmitz G. Flow cytometric analysis of thiazole orange uptake by platelets: a diagnostic aid in the evaluation of thrombocytopenic disorders. Blood 1990;75:116–121.

92. Steiner M, Baldini M. Protein synthesis in aging blood platelets. Blood 1969;33:628–633.
93. Belloc F, Hourdille P, Boisseau MR, Bernard P. Protein synthesis in human platelets correlation with platelet size. Nouv Rev Fr Hematol 1982;24:369–373.
94. Gnatenko DV, Dunn JJ, McCorkle SR, Weissmann D, Perrotta PL, Bahou WF. Transcript profiling of human platelets using microarray and serial analysis of gene expression. Blood 2002;14:14.
95. Power CA, Clemetson JM, Clemetson KJ, Wells TN. Chemokine and chemokine receptor mRNA expression in human platelets. Cytokine 1995;7:479–482.
96. Roth GJ, Hickey MJ, Chung DW, Hickstein DD. Circulating human blood platelets retain appreciable amounts of poly (A)+ RNA. Biochem Biophys Res Commun 1989;160:705–710.
97. Soslau G, Morgan DA, Jaffe JS, Brodsky I, Wang Y. Cytokine mRNA expression in human platelets and a megakaryocytic cell line and cytokine modulation of platelet function. Cytokine 1997;9:405–411.
98. Santoso S, Kalb R, Kiefel V, Mueller-Eckhardt C. The presence of messenger RNA for HLA class I in human platelets and its capability for protein biosynthesis. Br J Haematol 1993;84:451–456.
99. Sottile J, Mosher DF, Fullenweider J, George JN. Human platelets contain mRNA transcripts for platelet factor 4 and actin. Thromb Haemost 1989;62:1100–1102.
100. Newman PJ, Gorski J, White GC 2nd, Gidwitz S, Cretney CJ, Aster RH. Enzymatic amplification of platelet-specific messenger RNA using the polymerase chain reaction. J Clin Invest 1988;82:739–743.
101. Konkle BA, Schick PK, He X, Liu RJ, Mazur EM. Plasminogen activator inhibitor-1 mRNA is expressed in platelets and megakaryocytes and the megakaryoblastic cell line CHRF-288. Arterioscler Thromb 1993;13:669–674.
102. Ausubel F, Brent R, Kingston RE, et al. Preparation and analysis of RNA. In: Chanda V, ed. Current Protocols in Molecular Biology, vol. 1: John Wiley, New York, 1987–1998, pp. 4.5.1–4.5.2.
103. Ts'ao CH. Rough endoplasmic reticulum and ribosomes in blood platelets. Scand J Haematol 1971;8:134–140.
104. Jeno P, Ballou LM, Novak-Hofer I, Thomas G. Identification and characterization of a mitogen-activated S6 kinase. Proc Natl Acad Sci USA 1988;85:406–410.
105. Nguyen YH, Mills AA, Stanbridge EJ. Assembly of the QM protein onto the 60S ribosomal subunit occurs in the cytoplasm. J Cell Biochem 1998;68:281–285.
106. Papkoff J, Chen RH, Blenis J, Forsman J. p42 mitogen-activated protein kinase and p90 ribosomal S6 kinase are selectively phosphorylated and activated during thrombin-induced platelet activation and aggregation. Mol Cell Biol 1994;14:463–472.
107. Gingras AC, Gygi SP, Raught B, et al. Regulation of 4E-BP1 phosphorylation: a novel two-step mechanism. Genes Dev 1999;13:1422–1437.
108. Gingras A-C, Raught B, Sonenberg N. eIF4 initiation factors: effectors of mRNA recruitment to ribosomes and regulators of translation. Annu Rev Biochem 1999;68:913–963.
109. Hinnebusch A. Initiator methionyl-tRNA binding to ribosomes. In: Sonenberg N, Hershey JWB, Mathews MB, eds. Translational Control of Gene Expression. Cold Spring Harbor Laboratory Press, Cold Spring Harbor, 2000, pp. 185–243.
110. Djaffar I, Vilette D, Bray PF, Rosa JP. Quantitative isolation of RNA from human platelets. Thromb Res 1991;62:127–135.
111. Kochetov AV, Ischenko IV, Vorobiev DG, et al. Eukaryotic mRNAs encoding abundant and scarce proteins are statistically dissimilar in many structural features. FEBS Lett 1998;440:351–355.

112. Bertagnolli ME, Hudson LA, Stetsenko GY. Selective association of the tyrosine kinases Src, Fyn, and Lyn with integrin-rich actin cytoskeletons of activated, nonaggregated platelets. Biochem Biophys Res Commun 1999;260:790–798.

113. Kralisz U, Cierniewski CS. Activity of pp60c-src and association of pp60c-src, pp54/58lyn, pp60fyn, and pp72syk with the cytoskeleton in platelets activated by collagen. IUBMB Life 2000;49:33–42.

114. Weyrich AS, Lindemann S, Tolley ND, et al. Translational control in platelets: signaling through mTOR regulates clot retraction. In: First Conference on Arteriosclerosis, Thrombosis, and Vascular Biology, Denver, Colorado, May 20–22, 2000.

115. Lenardo M, Siebenlist U. Bcl-3-mediated nuclear regulation of the NF-kappa B trans-activating factor. Immunol Today 1994;15:145–147.

116. Liu F, Morris S, Epps J, Carroll R. Demonstration of an activation regulated NF-kappaB/I-kappaBalpha complex in human platelets. Thromb Res 2002;106:199.

117. Gawaz M, Brand K, Dickfeld T, et al. Platelets induce alterations of chemotactic and adhesive properties of endothelial cells mediated through an interleukin-1-dependent mechanism. Implications for atherogenesis. Atherosclerosis 2000;148:75–85.

118. Hawrylowicz CM, Santoro SA, Platt FM, Unanue ER. Activated platelets express IL-1 activity. J Immunol 1989;143:4015–4018.

119. Hawrylowicz CM, Howells GL, Feldmann M. Platelet-derived interleukin 1 induces human endothelial adhesion molecule expression and cytokine production. J Exp Med 1991;174:785–790.

120. Kaplanski G, Porat R, Aiura K, Erban JK, Gelfand JA, Dinarello CA. Activated platelets induce endothelial secretion of interleukin-8 in vitro via an interleukin-1-mediated event. Blood 1993;81:2492–2495.

121. Loppnow H, Bil R, Hirt S, et al. Platelet-derived interleukin-1 induces cytokine production, but not proliferation of human vascular smooth muscle cells. Blood 1998;91:134–141.

122. Kaspar RL, Gehrke L. Peripheral blood mononuclear cells stimulated with C5a or lipopolysaccharide to synthesize equivalent levels of IL-1 beta mRNA show unequal IL-1 beta protein accumulation but similar polyribosome profiles. J Immunol 1994;153:277–286.

123. Lee JC, Laydon JT, McDonnell PC, et al. A protein kinase involved in the regulation of inflammatory cytokine biosynthesis. Nature 1994;372:739–746.

124. Clark IE, Wyckoff D, Gavis ER. Synthesis of the posterior determinant Nanos is spatially restricted by a novel cotranslational regulatory mechanism. Curr Biol 2000;10:1311–1314.

125. Bessler H, Agam G, Djaldetti M. Increased protein synthesis by human platelets during phagocytosis of latex particles in vitro. Thromb Haemost 1976;35:350–357.

126. Plenchette S, Moutet M, Benguella M, et al. Early increase in DcR2 expression and late activation of caspases in the platelet storage lesion. Leukemia 2001;15:1572–1581.

127. Brown SB, Clarke MC, Magowan L, Sanderson H, Savill J. Constitutive death of platelets leading to scavenger receptor-mediated phagocytosis. A caspase-independent cell clearance program. J Biol Chem 2000;275:5987–5996.

128. Chen LY, Mehta JL. Further evidence of the presence of constitutive and inducible nitric oxide synthase isoforms in human platelets. J Cardiovasc Pharmacol 1996;27:154–158.

129. Mehta JL, Chen LY, Kone BC, Mehta P, Turner P. Identification of constitutive and inducible forms of nitric oxide synthase in human platelets. J Lab Clin Med 1995;125:370–377.

130. Coller BS. Platelet GPIIb/IIIa antagonists: the first anti-integrin receptor therapeutics. J Clin Invest 1997;100:S57–S60.
131. Coller BS. Platelet GPIIb/IIIa antagonists: the first anti-integrin receptor therapeutics. J Clin Invest 1997;99:1467–1471.
132. Fitzgerald DJ. Vascular biology of thrombosis: the role of platelet-vessel wall adhesion. Neurology 2001;57:S1–S4.
133. Chen YP, O'Toole TE, Leong L, Liu BQ, Diaz-Gonzalez F, Ginsberg MH. Beta 3 integrin-mediated fibrin clot retraction by nucleated cells: differing behavior of alpha IIb beta 3 and alpha v beta 3. Blood 1995;86:2606–2615.
134. Chicurel ME, Singer RH, Meyer CJ, Ingber DE. Integrin binding and mechanical tension induce movement of mRNA and ribosomes to focal adhesions. Nature 1998;392:730–733.
135. Saunders RN, Metcalfe MS, Nicholson ML. Rapamycin in transplantation: a review of the evidence. Kidney Int 2001;59:3–16.
136. Abraham RT, Wiederrecht GJ. Immunopharmacology of rapamycin. Annu Rev Immunol 1996;14:483–510.
137. Brown EJ, Schreiber SL. A signaling pathway to translational control. Cell 1996;86:517–520.
138. Curfman GD. Sirolimus-eluting coronary stents. N Engl J Med 2002;346:1770–1771.
139. Suzuki T, Kopia G, Hayashi S, et al. Stent-based delivery of sirolimus reduces neointimal formation in a porcine coronary model. Circulation 2001;104:1188–1193.
140. Morice MC, Serruys PW, Sousa JE, et al. A randomized comparison of a sirolimus-eluting stent with a standard stent for coronary revascularization. N Engl J Med 2002;346:1773–1780.
141. Pinedo HM, Verheul HM, D'Amato RJ, Folkman J. Involvement of platelets in tumour angiogenesis? Lancet 1998;352:1775–1777.
142. Rocca B, Secchiero P, Ciabattoni G, et al. Cyclooxygenase-2 expression is induced during human megakaryopoiesis and characterizes newly formed platelets. Proc Natl Acad Sci USA 2002;99:7634–7639.
143. Corash L, Shafer B. Use of asplenic rabbits to demonstrate that platelet age and density are related. Blood 1982;60:166–1671.
144. Rao AK, Gabbeta J. Congenital disorders of platelet signal transduction. Arterioscler Thromb Vasc Biol 2000;20:285–289.
145. Li J, Xia Y, Bertino AM, Coburn JP, Kuter DJ. The mechanism of apoptosis in human platelets during storage. Transfusion 2000;40:1320–1329.
146. Pereira J, Soto M, Palomo I, et al. Platelet aging in vivo is associated with activation of apoptotic pathways: studies in a model of suppressed thrombopoiesis in dogs. Thromb Haemost 2002;87:905–909.
147. Seghatchian J, Krailadsiri P. Platelet storage lesion and apoptosis: are they related? Transfus Apheresis Sci 2001;24:103–105.
148. Dixon DA, Tolley ND, Zimmerman GA. Convenient and rapid ribonuclease protection assay for use with primary cell cultures. Biotechniques 2001;31:992–993.
149. Wintrobe MM. Blood platelets and coagulation. In: Wintrobe MM, ed. Clinical Hematology. Lea & Febiger, Philadelphia, 1946, pp. 187–216.
150. Miyamoto S, Qin J, Safer B. Detection of early gene expression changes during activation of human primary lymphocytes by in vitro synthesis of proteins from polysome-associated mRNAs. Protein Sci 2001;10:423–433.
151. Wolin SL, Walter P. Ribosome pausing and stacking during translation of a eukaryotic mRNA. EMBO J 1988;7:3559–3569.

152. Tenenbaum SA, Carson CC, Lager PJ, Keene JD. Identifying mRNA subsets in messenger ribonucleoprotein complexes by using cDNA arrays. Proc Natl Acad Sci USA 2000;97:14085–14090.
153. Pan J, McEver RP. Regulation of the human P-selectin promoter by Bcl-3 and specific homodimeric members of the NF-kappa B/Rel family. J Biol Chem 1995;270:23077–23083.
154. Ohno H, Takimoto G, McKeithan TW. The candidate proto-oncogene bcl-3 is related to genes implicated in cell lineage determination and cell cycle control. Cell 1990;60:991–997.

7 Phosphoproteomics of Human Platelets

Katrin Marcus, PhD, and Helmut E. Meyer, PhD

CONTENTS

INTRODUCTION
PROTEIN SEPARATION
MASS SPECTROMETRY
POSTTRANSLATIONALLY MODIFIED PROTEINS
IDENTIFICATION OF PHOSPHORYLATED PLATELET PROTEINS
CONCLUDING REMARKS
NOTES
REFERENCES

INTRODUCTION

Platelets circulate freely in the blood, playing a critical role in wound healing by forming plugs and initiating repair processes and in underlying thrombotic diseases such as myocardial infarction or stroke *(1)*. Normally platelets are found in the blood in a nonadhesive, resting state. Interactions with structures in the subendothelial matrix initiate a rapid platelet activation, resulting in the formation of vascular plugs and release of intracellular substances that initiate repair processes. Genetic defects may result in bleeding disorders such as Glanzmann's thrombasthenia and Bernard-Soulier syndrome *(2)*. The high clinical relevance of arterial thrombosis, the limited knowledge about the underlying mechanisms at the molecular level, and the small number of available antiplatelet drugs *(3)* show the necessity for gaining more profound insights into this system. One important event in regulating the platelet

From: *Contemporary Cardiology:*
Platelet Function: Assessment, Diagnosis, and Treatment
Edited by: M. Quinn and D. Fitzgerald © Humana Press Inc., Totowa, NJ

function is the phosphorylation/dephosphorylation of multiple proteins on various tyrosine, serine, and threonine residues within intracellular signaling cascades. To understand the exact mechanisms, it is essential to identify proteins involved in the signaling pathways and to localize their phosphorylation sites.

PROTEIN SEPARATION

As platelets arise through membrane budding of megakaryocytes, they are anucleated cells, and protein synthesis proceeds only partially by residual mRNA in mitochondria and megakaryocytes. Thus, genome and transcriptome analysis of platelets will be largely unsuccessful, and significant analysis is preferentially performed on the protein level. In 1996, Wilkins and Williams *(4)* created the term *proteome*, denoting the protein complement of a genome. Modern, large-scale proteome analysis consists of three major steps—2D polyacrylamide gel electrophoresis (2D-PAGE), image analysis, and mass spectrometry (MS) (*see* detailed descriptions in refs. *5* and *6*). Such analysis offers a huge potential for an almost complete overview of the proteins present in a given sample *(7)*. It is well known that one gene will result in a variety of protein products in consequence of alternative splicing of the prae-mRNA or the introduction of posttranslational modifications, e.g., sugars and phosphates, or controlled proteolysis, contributing to a complex protein pattern. Consequently, proteome analysis must incorporate analysis of protein expression patterns, posttranslational modifications, and protein quantitation. Presently, 2D-PAGE is the method of choice for separation of an extensive protein population and subsequent comparative proteome analysis of different functional states (e.g., treated/ untreated cells, healthy/diseased tissue). This technique comprises two different separation steps. In the first step, isoelectric focusing (IEF), the proteins are separated by charge; in the second, commonly SDS-PAGE, they are separated by their molecular weight.

Two different methods for separation in the first dimension exist so far—the method of Klose *(8)* and O'Farrell *(9)*, whereby the pH gradient is created via carrier ampholytes during IEF, and the method of Görg et al. *(10)*, using immobilized pH gradients in the first dimension. The detection of phosphorylated proteins after separation by gel electrophoresis can be performed using different techniques, e.g., staining with phospho-specific dyes like "Stains all" *(11)* or phospho-staining kits (e.g., Pierce, Perbio Science, Bonn, Germany). Unfortunately, these detection methods are not applicable to in vivo analysis of phosphorylated proteins owing to their lack of sensitivity. In another approach, phosphorylated proteins can be visualized on gels or on membranes using anti-phosphoamino acid-specific antibodies. Alternatively, protein populations can be separated by 2D-PAGE before and after enzymatic removal of the phospho group (12). "Disappearing" spots in the subsequent differential analysis indicate the modified proteins. Finally, phosphoproteins can be visualized by radioactive labeling with ^{32}P-orthophosphate, as we describe here. To date, this labeling procedure has been the method of choice for specific and highly sensitive detection of phosphorylation in a global proteomics study, as all phosphorylated proteins with a sufficient basic turnover can be detected easily and rapidly.

MASS SPECTROMETRY

Further protein analysis is performed by MS, which provides characteristic and reliable protein data. In the protein and peptide analysis, two different techniques are of particular importance: matrix-assisted laser desorption/ionization mass spectrometry (MALDI-MS) (13,14) and electrospray ionization mass spectrometry (ESI-MS) (15). Advantages of MS compared with other techniques for protein identification are its short analysis time, its high sensitivity (down to attomole amounts), and its feasibility for automation.

MALDI-MS is a very fast method and is therefore suitable for high-throughput proteome analysis. Thus MALDI-MS is generally used for the analysis of relatively simple protein mixtures and for identification via peptide mass fingerprinting (PMF) (16,17) after in gel digestion of the electrophoretically separated proteins and extraction of the generated peptides. Evaluation of PMF data is done automatically by screening a database via specific database search algorithms like ProFound (http://prowl.rockefeller.edu/cgi-bin/ProFound) (18) or Mascot (www.matrixscience.com) (19). These database searches compare theoretical data generated from protein or DNA databases with experimentally obtained data and may result in an unambiguous identification of the protein.

The significance of a database search result increases with increasing sequence coverage of the identified protein and increasing mass accuracy between experimental and theoretical data. When the sample contains more than one protein, an unequivocal identification of all protein components in parallel causes problems using MALDI-MS. Therefore, it would be essential to analyze single peptides by fragmentation experiments via MALDI-postsource decay (PSD) (20,21). Hence, fragmentation of peptides generally occurs at the peptide bond, and the fragmention analysis facilitates the determination of the primary peptide structure/ sequence. Depending on the destination of the charge after the ionization process and decay, various ion types can be differentiated (22). C-terminally charged ions are indicated as *x*-, *y*-, and *z*-ions and N-terminally charged ions as *a*-, *b*-, and *c*-ions. Analysis of these fragmentation data is also done via special database search programs like SEQUEST™ *(23,24)* or Mascot *(19)*, comparing theoretically produced MS/MS fragmentation patterns with the experimentally obtained data.

ESI-MS is well suited for coupling with liquid chromatography (LC) *(25)* since the analyte molecules are available in solution. Integrated LC-ESI-MS systems are preferred for the analysis of complex samples. By using miniaturized high-performance liquid chromatography (HPLC) systems, femtomole amounts of proteins/peptides can be detected *(26)*. One major advantage of online LC-ESI-MS/MS (fragmentation) analyses lies in the generation of a high quantity of fragment ion spectra, providing a great deal of information about the peptide sequence. The MS/MS spectra are available for identification of the protein by searching databases with the aforementioned database search tools. With this technique, simultaneous detection of several proteins in a mixture is possible.

POSTTRANSLATIONALLY MODIFIED PROTEINS

One of the biggest challenges in proteomics today is the detection and analysis of posttranslationally modified proteins (i.e., glycoproteins and phosphoproteins), including the classification of the particular modification as well as its localization. Modified proteins often appear as "pearl-necklet" spots in the 2D gel owing to their changed migration behavior caused by the modified charge state and molecular weight. The complexity of an MS analysis depends on the character of the modification: modifications such as N-terminal acetylation and oxidations may be detected even by PMF analyses. Glycosylations or phosphorylations lead to signal suppression of the modified peptide owing to their low ionization rate in the concomitant presence of the unmodified species. Often one protein spot in the gel contains various protein species merging because of the same modification at different positions in the polypeptide chain. After proteolysis of the protein, a complex peptide pattern arises whereby the modified peptides are found only with a very low abundance compared with the unmodified ones, additionally complicating the analysis of modified peptides.

For minimization of such suppression effects and quantity problems, isolation and/or enrichment of the modified peptides is essential prior to the MS analysis *(27)*. To date a variety of methods for the analysis of phosphoproteins and phosphopeptides have been described *(28)*, such as enzymatic dephosphorylation *(29,30)*, parent ion scanning *(31,32)*, or neutral loss scanning *(33,34)*. In most of these methods enrichment of the phosphoproteins, or phosphopeptides by specific antibodies *(35,36)*

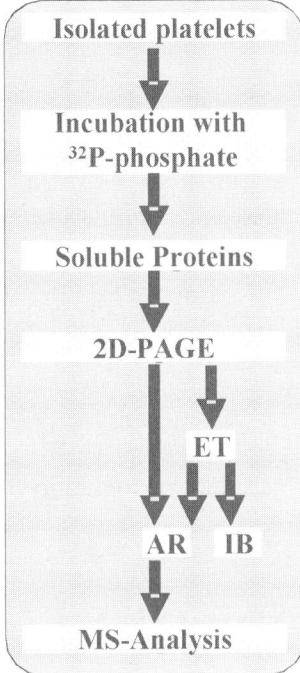

Fig. 1. Strategy for the analysis of phosphorylated platelet proteins. Following incubation of the platelets with ^{32}P-orthophosphate, the protein separation was done by 2D-PAGE. For further analysis, two gels of the same sample were run in parallel. One of the gels was used for autoradiography (AR), and the phosphorylated spots detected were analyzed by mass spectrometry (MS). Proteins separated in parallel were transferred to a nitrocellulose membrane by electrotransfer (ET), and the phosphorylated proteins were also detected by AR. For discrimination of serine-/threonine-phosphorylated and tyrosine-phosphorylated proteins, immunostaining was performed using an antiphosphotyrosine antibody. IB, immunoblot.

or immobilized metal ion affinity chromatography (IMAC) *(37,38)* prior to the analysis is required to localize the phosphorylation site unequivocally.

IDENTIFICATION OF PHOSPHORYLATED PLATELET PROTEINS

We describe below a strategy for the successful detection and identification of phosphorylated platelet proteins as well as the localization of their phosphorylation sites using proteomic techniques (Fig. 1). The phosphoproteins are first labeled with radioactive ^{32}P orthophosphate. After protein separation by 2D-PAGE, the phosphoproteins are directly assigned by detection of ^{32}P radioactivity via autoradiography. Further characterization is performed via immunodetection of tyrosine-phos-phorylated proteins. The steps involved are discussed in detail on the following pages.

Sample Preparation and 2D-PAGE

The description of a biological system requires the characterization of a complex mixture of thousands of proteins. To get a wide and preferably complete overview of the proteins present in the respective cell systems, an analysis strategy must be established. All parameters involved in the separation procedure—sample preparation, IEF, and SDS-PAGE—are to be optimized and standardized.

Every additional manipulation during the sample preparation process holds the risk of protein loss or protein modification, resulting in artificial differences in the protein pattern and causing incorrect results. As no universally applicable sample preparation method exists for proteome analyses, an individual sample preparation method must be adapted to every particular project. Generally, an efficient and reproducible separation of the proteins is required for differential proteome analysis. For a detailed description of sample preparation and 2D-PAGE, *see* Marcus et al. *(6,39)* and therefore will be mentioned here briefly (*see* Notes 1, 2).

Human platelets should be prepared from volunteers free from medication. After the platelets are resuspended in Tyrode's buffer (10 mM HEPES, 137 mM NaCl, 2.7 mM KCl, 1 mM EDTA, 5 mM glucose, pH 7.4), they are incubated in 1 mL of labeling solution (1 mCi ^{32}P-phosphate in 2 mL of 2X Tyrode's buffer) for 1 h at 37°C and afterwards topped up to 10 mL with 1X Tyrode's buffer. Sedimentation of the cells is performed by centrifugation (10 min at 420g). For further analysis, one half of the cells is activated with thrombin, and the other half is used as control (*see* Note 3). After cell lysis, 2D separation of the platelet proteins using immobilized pH gradient (IPG) strips is optimized under pH 3–10, 6–11, and 4–7. The optimal parameters for the different pH gradients are summarized in Table 1 (*see* Notes 4–6).

Autoradiography and Immunoblotting

Radioactive labeling with ^{32}P-phosphate is the method of choice for specific and highly sensitive detection of phosphorylation. Since platelets are anucleated cells, cell culture trials are not possible, and the radioactive labeling has to be done after isolation of the platelets. Optimal detection of the phosphorylated proteins is either by film and consecutive autoradiography or by phosphoimagers. When phosphoimagers are used, a quantitative differential analysis is possible via specific image analysis tools, whereas with direct autoradiography a quantitative analy-

Table 1
Summary of the Conditions for 2D-PAGE for Different pH Gradients

pH	Rehydration solution	IEF	SDS-PAGE
3.0–10.0	8 M urea 2 M thiourea 2% CHAPS 100 mM DTT 0.8% Servalyte (3–10)	Anodic sample application Cover with oil 80 kVh	Equilibration time: 15 min Gel: 11% T; 2.5% C 240 min at 350 mA
4.0–7.0	8 M urea 2 M thiourea 2% CHAPS 100 mM DTT 0.8% Servalyte (4–7)	Anodic sample application Cover with oil 80 kVh	Equilibration time: 15 min Gel: 11% T; 2.5% C 240 min, 350 mA
6.0–11.0	8 M urea 2 M thiourea 2% CHAPS 100 mM DTT 0.4% Servalyte (6–9, 9–11)	Anodic sample application Cover with oil 30 kVh	Equilibration time: 20 min Gel: 11% T; 2.5% C 240 min, 350 mA

Abbreviations : CHAPS, 3[3-cholaminopropyl diethylammonio]-1-propane sulfonate; DTT, dithiothreitol.

sis is hardly possible, owing to the low dynamic range of the films. The gels should be dried after fixing without staining to avoid extensive washing of the gel pieces, which could cause sample loss (*see* Note 7). To ensure high reproducibility of the method, a sufficient quantity of gels should be produced (at least three gels of both states). The autoradiograms provide a general presentation of all kinds of phosphorylated protein species (Fig. 2). Thus, no distinction among O-phosphates (serine, threonine, and tyrosine phosphates), N-phosphates (arginine, lysine, and histidine phosphates), S-phosphates (cysteine phosphates), or acyl-phosphates (aspartic acid and glutamic acid phosphates) is possible. Because identification of N-, S-, and acyl-phosphates after gel electrophoresis is not feasible *(40)*, supplementary attention should be paid to the analysis of O-phosphates. Further discrimination of tyrosine-phosphorylated proteins on the one hand and serine- and threonine-phosphorylated proteins on the other hand can be performed by subsequent immunoblotting using a group-specific antiphosphotyrosine antibody (e.g., clone 4G10, Upstate Biotechnology, Lake Placid, NY). Indeed, using antiphosphothreonine and antiphosphoserine antibodies

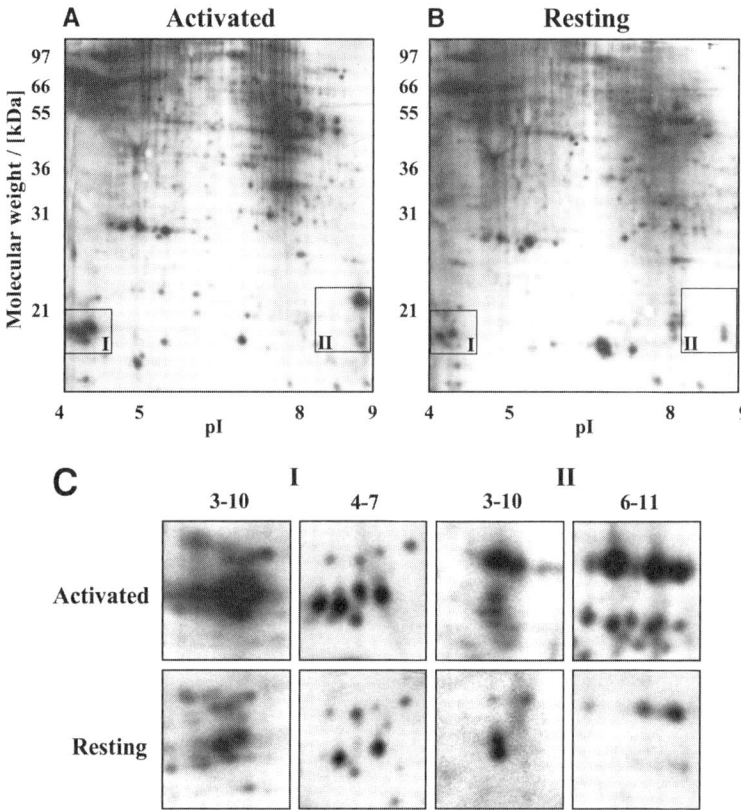

Fig. 2. Autoradiography following 2D-PAGE of human platelet proteins after ^{32}P-orthophosphate labeling in pH area 3–10 compared with areas 4–7 and 6–11. **(A)** Autoradiography of the 2D gel in pH area 3–10 after application of 400 µg protein of thrombin-stimulated platelets. **(B)** Autoradiography of the 2D gel in pH area 3–10 after application of 400 µg protein of resting platelets. **(C)** Upscaled parts I + II in pH area 3–10 and the corresponding regions in pH areas 4–7 and 6–11. pH areas 4–7 and 6–11 showed far better protein separations, particularly in the acidic and basic border regions.

for immunoblotting is not indicated, owing to their sequence specificity. Thus, phosphoserine and phosphothreonine can only be identified specifically in the context of a larger epitope (sequence specificity), precluding whole phosphoproteome analysis.

In our hands the electroblotting procedure described by Dunn *(41)* using the semidry-technique with a discontinuous buffer system *(42)* is very effective.

1. Proteins are transferred from the 2D-PAGE to nitrocellulose (pore size 0.2 µm, Hybond ECL, Amersham Biosciences) and kept for 1 h at a constant current of 0.8 mA/cm^2 and a maximum voltage of 25 V using

the 2117-250 Novablot Electrophoretic Transfer Kit (Amersham Biosciences).

2. The blocked membrane (blocking solution: 10% [w/v] nonfat milk powder in TBS [10 mM Tris-HCl, 150 mM NaCl, pH 7.6]) is incubated with the primary antiphosphotyrosine antibody (clone 4G10, Upstate Biotechnology) at a dilution of 1:2000 in TBS-T (TBS + 0.05% Tween-20, pH 7.6, 3% [w/v] nonfat milk powder) for 1.5 h at room temperature (RT).

3. The antimouse horseradish peroxidase (HRP)-conjugated secondary antibody (Sigma Aldrich, Deisenhofen, Germany) is used at a dilution of 1:5000 (in TBS-T, 1% [w/v] nonfat milk powder) for 1 h at RT.

4. Chemiluminescence detection of peroxidase activity is carried out with the SuperSignal® West Dura Substrate (Pierce, Rockford, IL) according to the manufacturer's instructions.

Several different signals are detected in the pH areas 4–7 and 6–11 (Fig. 3), and all 134 proteins can be identified in the subsequent MS analyses (*see* next heading).

Mass Spectrometry and Localization of Phosphorylation Sites

MS approaches via PMF or fragmentation analyses require proteolytic digestion prior to acquisition of the MS data. The reason for analyzing peptides rather than proteins is that gel-separated proteins are difficult to elute and analyze by MS, and also the molecular weight of proteins is not usually sufficient for database identification. For this purpose the protein spots of interest have to be excised from the gel, and interfering substances such as sodium dodecyl sulfate (SDS) and/or dye have to be removed. Furthermore, the optimal pH range for the protease used has to be adjusted. In most studies trypsin is used for the in-gel digest, as it generates peptides of ideal size (10–15 amino acids) for MS analyses. In the present study, the washing and digestion procedure described below seemed to be most effective.

Analysis of the samples by MS requires specialized equipment and a great deal of experience in order to achieve high sensitivity. The detection and characterization of posttranslational modifications such as phosphorylation is one of the most challenging and fruitful areas of proteomics today. As phosphorylation is an important mechanism in a number of signal transduction events, it is important to apply the appropriate tools and techniques for the phosphoproteins and phosphopeptide analysis. As already described, the reversible in vivo phosphorylation occurs in the cell just substoichometrically. That means the ratio of the phosphorylated compared with the nonphosphorylated species is only about 1–5% *(43)* and localization of phosphorylation sites in vivo via MS approaches is only possible after enrichment of the phosphorylated spe-

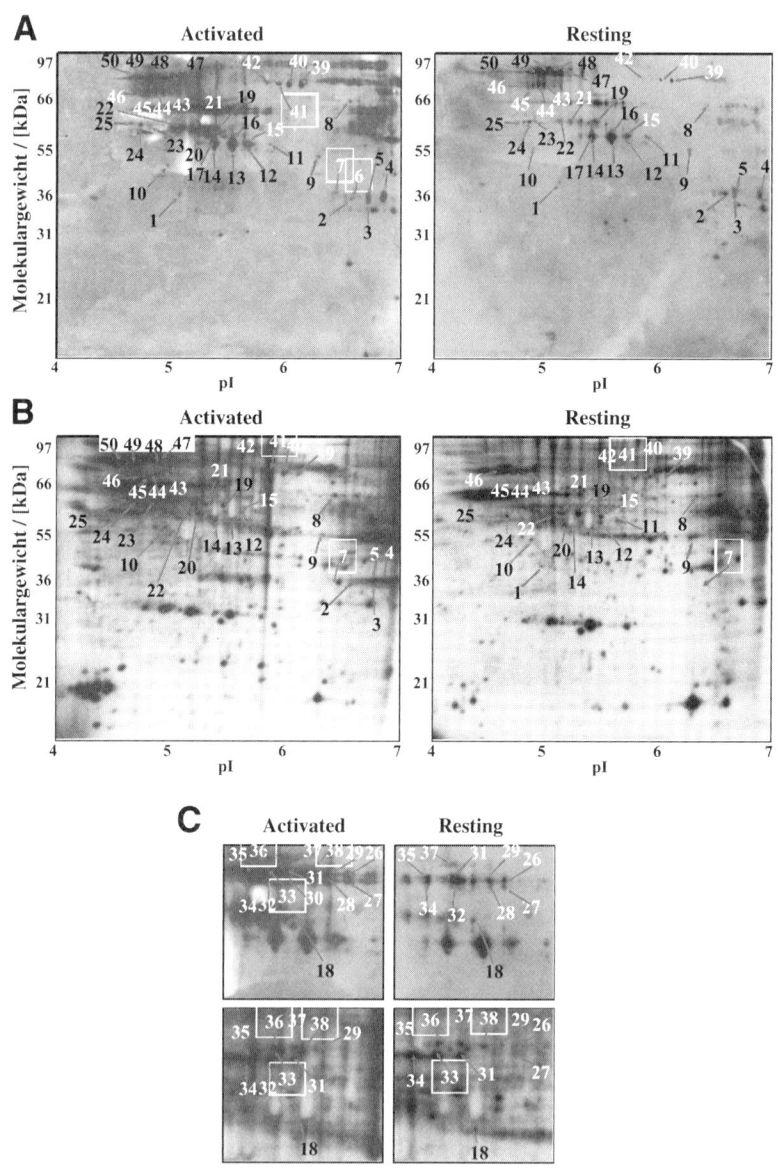

Fig. 3. Autoradiography and antiphosphotyrosine immunoblot after 2D separation of resting and activated platelets in pH area 4–7. (**A**) Antiphosphotyrosine immunoblot of the 2D gels in pH area 4–7 after application of 400 µg protein (left: activated platelets; right: resting platelets). (**B**) To the in A demonstrated immunoblots corresponding autoradiograms (left: activated; right: resting). (**C**) Up-scaled sections (MW 40–55 kDa, pI 5.4–5.9) from the immunoblots and autoradiograms shown in A and B to get a better overview. Corresponding spots in the immunoblot and the autoradiograms are numbered.

cies or prior separation of the phosphopeptides and the nonphosphorylated peptides *(27,44)*. The application of specific antibodies for the enrichment of phosphoproteins and phosphopeptides is restricted to phosphotyrosine residues, owing to the antibodies' particular specificity (*see* Sample Preparation and 2D-PAGE section above).

Another identification strategy combines in vivo and in vitro experiments involving radiolabeling of cell extracts and the protein of interest with the kinase of interest followed by blotting, autoradiography, and MS identification of the phosphorylated spots *(45,46)*. An inference of the in vivo phosphorylation site might not be possible with this method because the ^{32}P-orthophosphate is not introduced under native conditions. Therefore biochemical examination of the in vivo function of the localized phosphorylation sites using mutation analysis, for example, is always required for verification of its biological relevance and functionality. Separation of phosphorylated from nonphosphorylated peptides is another possibility to overcome the problems arising when analyzing phosphopeptides (*see* Sample Preparation and 2D-PAGE section above).

With regard to these problems, we chose the nano-LC-ESI-MS method for this work (*see* Note 8). This technique facilitates online coupling of the MS analysis directly after peptide separation by nano-HPLC without any additional manual manipulation, which carries the risk of sample loss. During the measurements, a huge number of ion spectra fragments and thus highly specific data are created, resulting in unambiguous identification of the proteins. The sensitivity of this technique is increased by miniaturizing the HPLC columns and ion sources applied. With this assembly, 25 fmol of phosphorylated casein peptides can be detected, demonstrating higher sensitivity than, i.e., the IMAC method, which is described for handling amounts of phosphopeptides on the picomole and subpicomole level *(47)* (*see* Note 9).

1. The gel spots are washed twice with 10 μL digestion buffer (10 m*M* NH$_4$HCO$_3$) and 10 μL modified digestion buffer (10 m*M* NH$_4$HCO$_3$/ acetonitrile 1:1).
2. The gel pieces are shrunk in the vacuum and reswollen with 2 μL protease solution (0.05 μg/μL trypsin, Promega, Madison, WI; *see* Note 10).
3. Digestion is performed for 10–12 h at 37°C.
4. Then 8 μL of 5% formic acid is added to the gel piece twice (successively), and the peptides are extracted for 15 min in the sonication bath.
5. The supernatants are pooled in a sample vessel for automatic sample application and either directly used for further MS analysis or stored at –80°C.
6. Analysis of the peptides is carried out using an ESI-ion trap mass spectrometer (LCQ^{TM} Classic, Thermo Finnigan, San Jose, CA) directly coupled to a nano-HPLC system (LC-Packings, Dionex, Idstein, Germany).

7. The peptides are automatically transferred from the autosampler (Famos™, LC-Packings, Dionex) to the preconcentration column (nano-precolumn™, 0.3 mm I.D. × 1 mm, C18 PepMap™).

8. After preconcentration and washing for 10 min (40 μL/min, 0.1% trifluoro acetic acid [TFA]), the peptides are injected automatically on a nano-HPLC column (75 μm I.D. × 250 mm, C_{18} PepMap™, 300-Å pore size, 5-μm particle size, LC-Packings, Dionex) using the Switchos™ system (LC-Packings, Dionex).

9. The inert HPLC pump (Ultimate™, LC-Packings, Dionex) is driven with a flow rate of 160 nL/min.

10. The gradient (solution A: 0.1% formic acid [FA] vs solution B: 0.1% FA, 84% acetonitrile) starts at 5% solution B and rises to 50% solution B in 90 min. A dual-channel UV detector (LC-Packings, Dionex) with a 3-nL flow cell (LC Packings, Dionex) at 215 nm (peptide bond) and 295 nm (tryptophan side chains) wavelength is used.

11. Separated peptides are transferred to the mass spectrometer via a heated capillary and a metal back-coated glass needle (PicoTip™, cat. no. S360-20-10, New Objective Incorporated, Cambridge, MA).

12. The following ESI parameters are used: spray voltage 1.8–2.15 kV, capillary temperature 200°C, capillary voltage 42 V, and tube lens offset 30 V, with the electron multiplier set to –950 V. The collision time is set automatically depending on the mass of the parent ion. Trapping time is set to 200 ms and the automatic gain control to 10^7.

13. The data are collected in centroid mode with one full-MS experiment followed by three MS/MS spectra of the three most intensive ions (intensity at least 3×10^5). Dynamic exclusion is used for the data collection with exclusion duration of 5 min and an exclusion mass of ± 1.5 Da.

14. For automatic interpretation of fragment ion spectra, the SEQUEST algorithm (23,24), version 27, is used to screen the NCBI protein database (weekly updated version). The parameters used are: average masses, a mass tolerance of ±1.5 Dalton for the parent ions and ±1.5 Dalton for the fragment ions, no restriction for the protease used, carbamidomethylation of cysteine residues as fixed modification, oxidation of methionine, and phosphorylation of serine, threonine, and tyrosine as differential modifications. The number of maximal missed cleavages is set to 1. Weighting factors for the b-, y-, and a-ions are set to 1.

Using this technique, 134 different proteins were identified, 21 of which were already described to be phosphorylated on Ser, Thr, or Tyr residues. Some of the proteins identified are given in Table 2. The pro-

Table 2
A Sample of Proteins Identified in This Study
by Nano-LC-ESI-MS/MS Analysis[a]

Protein	Molecular weight (kDa)	NCBI accession no	pI
Aldolase A	39.3	gil229674	8.4
Annexin XI	54.4	gil4557317	6.5
ARP2/3, subunit 21	20.5	gil5031597	8.8
ARP 3	47.4	gil5031573	5.6
ATP synthase	59.8	gil15030240	9.1
β-Integrin-coupled serine/threonine kinase	51.4	gil4758606	8.3
Breast cancer-associated protein (BRAP1)	61.7	gil7705296	5.1
Calretikulin	48	gil4757900	4.3
CAP1	51.7	gil5453595	8.1
Cofilin 1	18.5	gil5031635	8.2
Coronin	53.3	gil11346452	6.7
Cortactin	61.6	gil4885205	5.2
Cystein-rich protein 1	20.6	gil4758086	8.9
Destrin	17	gil5802966	9.1
Enolase 2	47.3	gil5803011	4.9
Fibrinogen, α	69.8	gil11761629	8.2
Fibrinogen, β	55.9	gil11761631	8.5
Fibrinogen, γ	49.5	gil71827	5.7
Gelsolin	85.7	gil4504165	5.9
HS71	70.1	gil462325	5.5
Hypothetical protein FLJ22570	53.3	gil13376308	7.9
LASP-1	29.8	gil2135552	6.1
Myosin, regulatory light chain	19.8	gil5453740	4.7
Pleckstrin p47	36.5	gil13637534	8.5
Profilin	36.5	gil4826898	8.4
RSP-1 protein (ras supressor)	36.7	gil6912638	6.9
Talin	36.7	gil4235275	5.8
Tyrosin-phosphatase 1C	36.9	gil557900	7.3
VASP	36.9	gil11414808	9.1
WD repeat protein 1	36.9	gil12652891	6.2

[a]Proteins in italics are known to be phosphorylated.

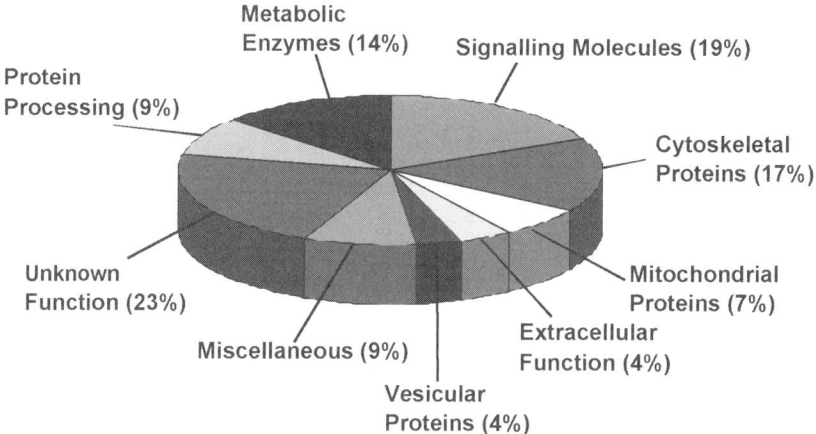

Fig. 4. Classification of phosphorylated proteins after differential proteome analysis of resting and thrombin-stimulated human platelets. One hundred and thirty seven protein samples were analysed, and 134 different proteins were identified.

teins could be classified into different categories based on their particular function (Fig. 4): cytoskeletal proteins (17%), mitochondrial proteins (7%), extracellular proteins (4%), vesicular proteins (4%), metabolic enzymes (14%), signaling molecules (19%), proteins involved in protein processing (9%), proteins with unknown function (23%), and miscellaneous (9%). For further information and identifications *see* ref. *39.* It is noteworthy that the molecular weight and/or pI detected for a variety of proteins diverged from the theoretical measured values. This could be attributed to point mutations, posttranslational modifications, and protein degradation. For some of the proteins, a functional proteolysis has already been described in the literature *(48,49).*

Additionally, platelets have an average lifetime of about 7 d, and therefore a particular percentage of in vivo protein degradation is possible. In some cases more than one protein was detected in a single spot. In these cases no prediction was possible as to which of the identified proteins changed its phosphorylation state after thrombin stimulation.

Besides the successful identification of potentially phosphorylated proteins, localization of several phosphorylation sites was successfully performed for some of the proteins by using nano-LC-ESI-MS/MS. Several characteristics of phosphorylated peptides are very helpful for the detection and localization of phosphorylation sites. Thus, in most of the analyses the phosphopeptide as well as the nonphosphorylated peptide appear, and in most cases the phosphopeptide elutes later in the HPLC separations. The occurrence of both forms (phosphorylated and nonphosphorylated) allows a direct comparison of both spectra, facilitating the localization of a given phosphorylation site. Another important attribute is the specific loss of –98 Dalton arising from a facile loss of H_3PO_4 from the phosphopeptide in singly charged ions or –49 Dalton in doubly charged ions. Under the conditions for MS, serine and threonine phosphates are not stable and show very intensive signals at m/z –98 Dalton, corresponding to the creation of dehydroalanine from phosphoserine or dehydro-α-aminobutyric acid from phosphothreonine, respectively. An additional, less intense signal infrequently occurs at m/z –80 Dalton caused by the loss of HPO_3^- *(45,50)*. These secessions are likewise echoed in the *b*- and *y*-ion series of the spectra, and with this information an unambiguous assignment of the phosphorylated residue is usually possible (Figs. 5–7).

In the present study nine phosphorylation sites in five different proteins were localized (Table 3; *see* Note 11).

Cortactin

In several spots the actin-binding protein cortactin was identified. The human form of cortactin—EMS1—was identified as an oncogene often amplified in human colon carcinomas and tumor cells *(51)* and seems to be involved in the signal transduction caused by extracellular stimuli such as thrombin, integrins, or epidermal growth factor (EGF) *(52)*. With regard to cortactin, overall three different phosphorylation sites were localized in this study. On the basis of the MS/MS spectra of the nonphosphorylated and the phosphorylated peptide, a phosphorylation of Ser-418 was detected (results not shown). Additionally, two further phosphorylations were localized at Thr-401 and Ser-405 (Fig. 5). These sites were already described to be phosphorylated by extracellular signal-regulated kinase (ERK) in vivo and in vitro *(53)*. Although the exact role of this phosphorylation is not clear, it probably has an important function in regulation of the subcellular localization of cortactin *(54)*. Additionally, a tyrosine phosphorylation of cortactin by the tyrosine kinase pp60c-src at different tyrosine residues (Tyr-421, Tyr-466, and Tyr-482) is known to be responsible for its reduced actin-crosslink activity *(55)*. In the present study cortactin was unambiguously detected in the antiphosphotyrosine immunoblots in different spots, and hence a tyrosine phosphorylation was confirmed. Localization of one of these tyrosine phosphorylation sites was not possible owing to the low protein quantity.

Myosin Regulatory Light Chain

The phosphorylation site of myosin regulatory light chain (RLC) was localized in this study (Fig. 6). The MS/MS spectra of the

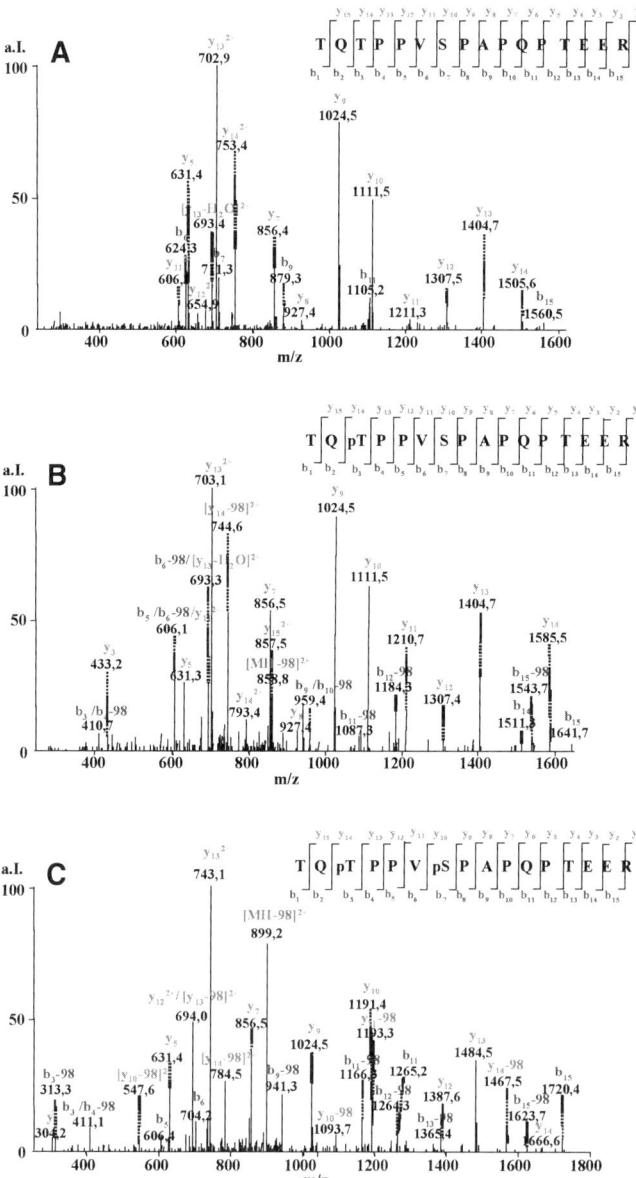

Fig. 5. Localization of the cortactin phosphorylation sites. **(A)** Fragment ion spectrum of the nonphosphorylated peptide TQTPPVSPAPQPTEER of cortactin. **(B)** Fragment spectrum of the phosphopeptide TQpTPPVSPA PQPTEER. **(C)** Fragment ion spectrum of the bis-phosphorylated peptide TQpTPPVpSPAPQPTEER. Owing to the secessions of –98 Dalton, Thr-401 (Thr-3 in the spectrum) and Ser-405 (Ser-7 in the spectrum) were seen to be phosphorylated.

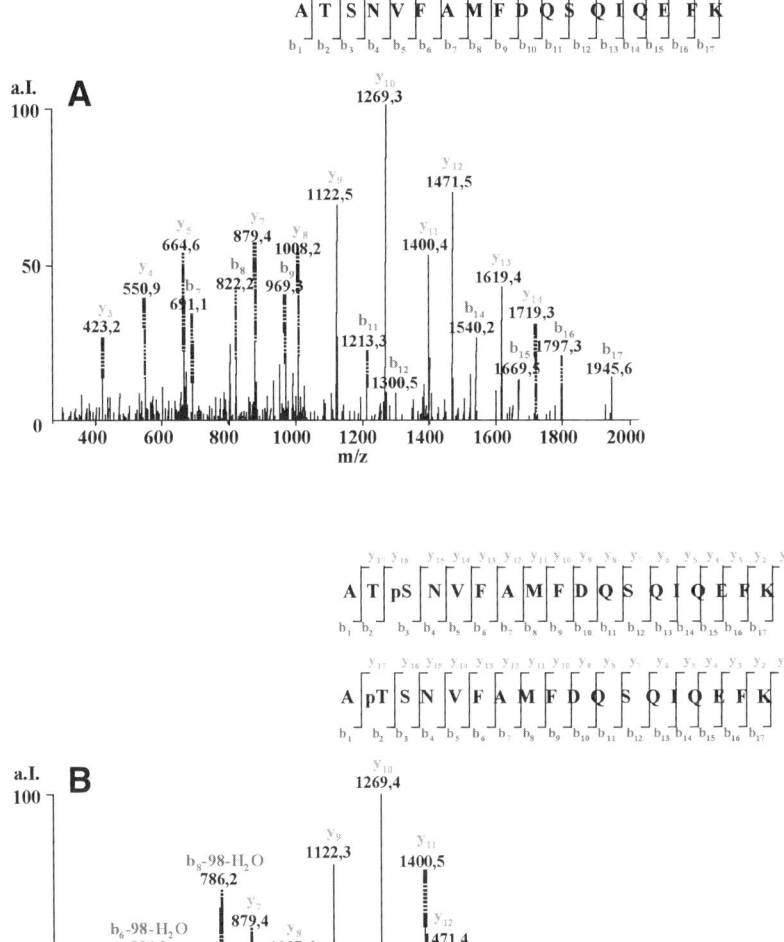

Fig. 6. Localization of the phosphorylation sites of the myosin regulatory light chain (RLC). **(A)** Fragment ion spectrum of the nonphosphorylated peptide ATSNVFAMFDQSQIQEFK of the RLC. **(B)** Fragment spectrum of the phosphorylated peptides ApTSNVFAMFDQSQIQEFK or ATpSN VFAMFDQSQIQEFK. As no secession of –98 Dalton was observed until y_{13}, a phosphorylation of Ser-13 was excluded. On the basis of the MS/MS spectrum, the exact site of phosphorylation could not be determined.

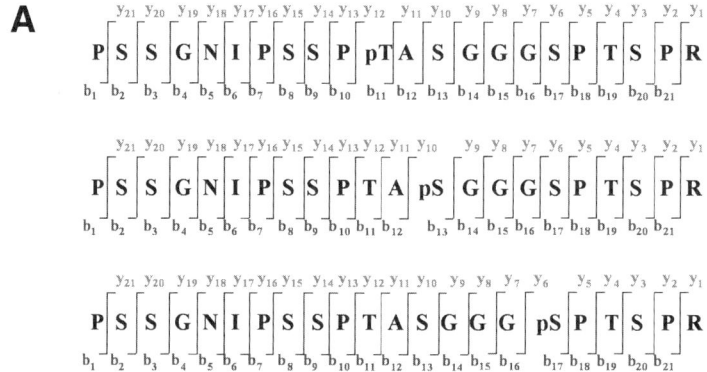

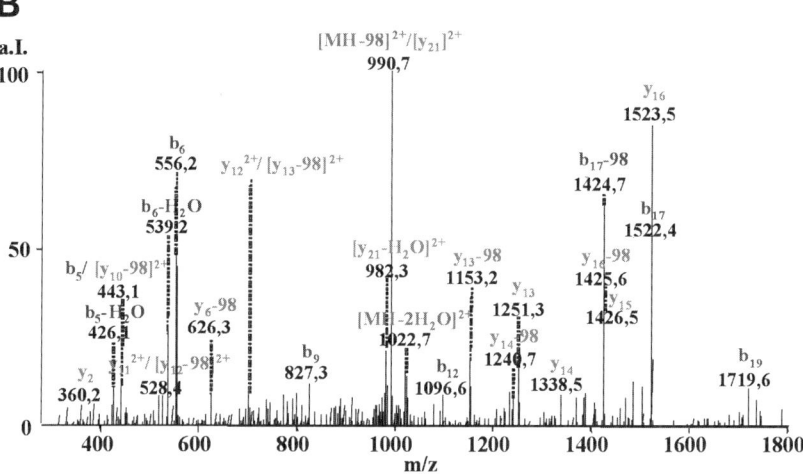

Fig. 7. (A) Fragment spectrum of a phosphopeptide of breast cancer-associated protein (BRAP). As a secession of –98 Dalton was observed until y_{13} and a b_{17}-98 was detected, phosphorylation of Ser-428 (Ser-2), Ser-429 (Ser-3), Ser-434 (Ser-8), Ser-435 (Ser-9), Thr-445 (Thr-19), and Ser-446 (Ser-20) could be excluded. **(B)** Localization of the phosphorylation sites of BRAP. On the basis of the MS/MS spectrum, an unequivocal localization of the site of phosphorylation was not possible, and therefore Thr-437 (Thr-11), Ser-439 (Ser-13), or Ser-443 (Ser-17) might be phosphorylated.

nonphosphorylated peptide ATSNVFAMFDQSQIQEFK and the corresponding phosphopeptides A**p**TSNVFAMFDQSQIQEFK or AT**pS**NVFAMFDQSQIQEFK are demonstrated in Fig. 6A and B, respectively. This peptide contained three possible phosphorylation sites (Thr-2, Ser-3, and Ser-12). The comparison of the two spectra revealed Thr-2 or Ser-3 as phosphorylated residues. As no secession of –98 Dalton

Table 3
Summary of All Detected Phosphopeptides and
Their Corresponding Phosphorylation Sites

Protein	Amino acid sequence of the identified phosphopeptides	m/z (Dalton)	Phosphorylated amino acid residue
Fibrinogen, α chain	ADpSGEGDFLAEGGGVR	1617.6	Ser-3
Myosin, regulatory light chain	ApTSNVFAMFDQSQIQEFK/ ATpSNVFAMFDQSQIQEFK	2172.3 2172.3	Thr-18 or Ser-19
Cortactin	LPSpSPVYEDAASFK	1591.0	Ser-418
	TQpTPPVSPAPQPTEER	1816.3	Thr-401
	TQpTPPVpSPAPQPTEER	1881.8	Thr-401/Ser-405
Hypothetical protein FJ22570	ATpSLPSLDTPGELR	1537.6	Ser-330
Breast cancer-assoiated protein (BRAP1)	PSSGNIPSSPpTASGGGSPTSPR/ PSSGNIPSSPTApSGGGSPTSPR/ PSSGNIPSSPTASGGGpSPTSPR	2079.1	Thr-11 or Ser-13 or Ser-17

was observed until y_{13}, a phosphorylation of Ser-13 could be excluded. On the basis of the fragment ion spectrum, the exact site of phosphorylation could not be determined (*see* Note 12). Potentially, a mixture of both monophosphorylated peptides was detected. Both amino acid residues are known to be phosphorylated by the myosin light chain kinase (MLCK) in resting platelets *(56)*.

Besides the detection of the phosphorylation sites already described, various up to now unknown phosphorylated amino acids were detected, e.g., in the hypothetical protein FLJ22570 (results not shown) and the breast cancer-associated protein (BRAP1) (Fig. 7).

BREAST CANCER-ASSOCIATED PROTEIN

The function of BRAP1 is completely unknown up to now. The detection of this protein in the antiphosphotyrosine immunoblot hinted at a tyrosine phosphorylation site. Actually, a phosphoserine or phosphothreonine was detected at positions 437, 439, or 443. Interpretation of the phosphopeptide fragment spectrum of BRAP1 was complicated owing to strong internal fragmentation because of the existence of many proline and glycine residues. In the *y*-ion series, a splitting of –98 Dalton from y_{13} and in the *b*-ion series from b_{17} occurred, and hence Ser-428, Ser-429, Ser-434, Ser-435, Thr-445, and Ser-446 (in the spectrum Ser-2, Ser-3, Ser-8, Ser-9, Thr-11, and Ser-20) were excluded as possibilities for phosphorylation (Fig. 7B). A decision as to whether Thr-437,

Ser-439, or Ser-443 (in the spectrum Thr-11, Ser-13, and Ser-17, respectively) were phosphorylated was not possible on the basis of the data acquired, and the existence of all three monophosphorylated peptides could not be excluded. Table 3 shows a summary of all localized phosphorylation sites.

CONCLUDING REMARKS

Proteomics provides a powerful set of tools for the characterization of phosphorylated proteins. Despite the importance of developing techniques for phosphoprotein and phosphopeptide analysis, the identification of phosphorylated proteins from such global approaches is only the first step in characterizing these important protein species. It is important to verify the involvement of the proteins identified and to prove the localized phosphorylation sites in regard to their functionality. Such studies may be performed by using antibodies against the protein of interest and/or overexpression of wild-type and mutant forms of epitope-tagged proteins to examine their role in signal transduction pathways.

NOTES

1. For preparation of all solutions and buffers, use chemicals of the highest quality and clean vials to avoid introduction of contamination. In every step clean vials and equipment should be used to prevent contamination of the sample.
2. Gloves should be worn in all preparation steps to reduce the risk of contamination by keratins. However, only unpowdered gloves should be used, as such powders very often contain milk proteins or amino acids, which could falsify the analyses.
3. Do not use glass vials when working with platelets, to ensure that no unintentional activation takes place.
4. Never heat urea solutions above 37°C, to reduce the risk of protein carbamylation.
5. Sample can be applied using sample cups or by in-gel sample rehydration. In the technique described in ref. 6, the sample is introduced in the rehydration solution and directly soaked into the strip during the overnight rehydration step. In our experience much better results are obtained when using sample cups. After in-gel rehydration, a strong horizontal smear is observed caused by actin. Best results were achieved when applying the sample with sample cups near the isoelectric point of the main protein component (actin). Diluting the sample with rehydration solution and covering it with silicone oil minimized protein precipitation at the application point.

6. When one is analyzing phosphoproteins, phosphatase inhibitors have to be added to the samples to avoid loss of phosphate groups owing to phosphatase cleavage.

7. Extended washing (destaining) of the gel piece may result in protein loss, especially of proteins with molecular weights less than 30 kDa.

8. Nano-LC columns with low flow rates should be used for the analysis of small protein/peptide amounts to avoid sample dilution.

9. Further limitations concerning the IMAC technique include the possible loss of phosphopeptides owing to their inability to bind to the IMAC column, difficulty in the elution of some multiply phosphorylated peptides, and background from unphosphorylated peptides (typically acidic peptides) that have affinity for immobilized metal ions.

10. The liquid volume should correspond to approximately three times the volume of the dried gel piece.

11. In addition to the low abundance of phosphorylated protein species, MS analysis of a digest of a given protein rarely results in 100% sequence coverage, and the regions of interest are easily missed. Moreover, negatively charged modifications in general can hinder proteolytic digestion by trypsin (28).

12. Serine and threonine residues occur quite commonly in proteins. The chance that a given tryptic peptide has multiple serine and threonine residues is thus quite high. Even if a peptide is determined to be phosphorylated, it may not be possible to localize the phosphogroup unequivocally.

REFERENCES

1. Brown AS, Erusalimsky JD, Martin JF. In: von Bruchhausen F, Walter U, eds. Platelets and Their Factors. Springer-Verlag, Berlin, 1997, pp. 3–19.

2. Nurden AT. Inherited abnormalities of platelets. Thromb Haemost 1999;82:468–480.

3. Fitzgerald DJ. Vascular biology of thrombosis: the role of platelet-vessel wall adhesion. Neurology 2001;57:S1–S4.

4. Wilkins M, Sanchez JC, Gooley AA, et al. Progress with proteome projects: why all proteins expressed by a genome should be identified and how to do it. Biotechnol Genet Eng Rev 1996;13:19–50.

5. Blackstock W, Weir MP. Proteomics: quantitative and physical mapping of cellular proteins. Tibtech 1999;17:121–127.

6. Marcus K, Meyer HE. (2003) Two-dimensional polyacrylamide gel electrophoresis for platelet proteomics. In: Gibbins J, Mahaut-Smith MP, eds. Platelets and Megacaryocytes, *Vol. 2, Perspectives and Techniques*. Methods in Biology Series. Humana, Totowa, NJ.

7. Lottspeich F. Proteome analysis: a pathway to the functional analysis of proteins. Angew Chem Int Ed Eng 1999;38:2476–2492.

8. Klose J. Protein mapping by combined isoelectric focusing and electrophoresis of mouse tissues. A novel approach to testing for induced point mutation in mammals. Humangenetik 1975;26:231–243.

9. O'Farrell PH. High resolution two-dimensional electrophoresis of proteins. J Biol Chem 1975;250:4007–4021.

10. Görg A, Postel W, Günther S. Two-dimensional electrophoresis with immobilized pH gradients of leaf proteins from barley (*Hordeum vulgare*): method, reproducibility and genetic aspects. Electrophoresis 1988;9:531–546.

11. Campell KP, MacLennan DH, Jorgensen AO. Staining of Ca^{2+} binding proteins, calsequestrin, calmodulin, torponin C and S-100 with the cationic carbocyanine dye 'Stains-all'. J Biol Chem 1983;258:11267–11273.

12. Karas M, Hillenkamp F. Laser desorption ionization of proteins with molecular mass exceeding 10,000 daltons. Anal Chem 1988;60:2299–2301.

13. Yamagata A, Kristensen DB, Takeda Y, et al. Mapping of phosphorylated proteins on two-dimensional polyacrylamide gels using protein phosphatase. Proteomics 2002;2:1267–1276.

14. Karas M, Gluckmann M, Schafer J. Ionization in matrix-assisted laser desorption/ ionization: singly charged molecular ions are the lucky survivors. J Mass Spectrom 2000;35:1–12.

15. Fenn JB. Electrospray ionization for mass spectrometry of large biomolecules. Science 1989;246:64–71.

16. Shevchenko A, Jensen ON, Podtelejnikov AV, et al. Linking genome and proteome by mass spectrometry: large-scale identification of yeast proteins from two dimensional gels. Proc Natl Acad Sci USA 1996;93:14440–14445.

17. Jensen ON, Larsen MR, Roepstorff P. Mass spectrometric identification and microcharacterization of proteins from electrophoretic gels: strategies and applications. Proteins 1998;2:74–89.

18. Zhang W, Chait BT. ProFound: an expert system for protein identification using mass spectrometric peptide mapping information. Anal Chem 2000;72:2482–2489.

19. Creasy DM, Cottrell JS. Error tolerant searching of uninterpreted tandem mass spectrometry data. Proteomics 2002;10:1426–1434.

20. Spengler B, Kirsch D. Peptides sequencing by matrix assisted laser desorption mass spectrometry. Rapid Commun Mass Spectrom 1992;6:105–108.

21. Kaufmann R, Kirsch D, Spengler B. Sequencing of peptides in a time of flight mass spectrometer: evaluation of postsource decay following matrix assisted laser desorption/ionization (MALDI). Int J Mass Spectrom Ion Proc 1994;131:355–385.

22. Biemann K. Mass spectrometry of peptides and proteins. Annu Rev Biochem 1992;61:977–1010.

23. Eng J, McCormack AL, Yates JR III. An approach to correlate tandem mass spectral data of peptides with amino acid sequences in a protein database. J Am Soc Mass Spectrom 1994;5:976–989.

24. Yates JR III, Eng JK, McCormack AL, Schieltz D. Method to correlate tandem mass spectra of modified peptides to amino acid sequences in the protein database. Anal Chem 1995;67:1426–1436.

25. Linscheid M. Die Kopplung von Flüssigkeitschromatographie mit Massenspektrometrie. CLB Chemie Labor Biotechnik 1990;41:125–133.

26. Wilm M, Shevchenko A, Houthaeve T, et al. Femtomole sequencing of proteins from polyacrylamide gels by nano-electrospray mass spectrometry. Nature 1996;379:466–469.

27. Mortz E, Sareneva T, Haebel S, Julkunen I, Roepstorff P. Mass spectrometric characterization of glycosylated interferon-gamma variants separated by gel electrophoresis. Electrophoresis 1996;17:925–931.

28. McLachlin DT, Chait BT. Analysis of phosphorylated proteins and peptides by mass spectrometry. Curr Opin Chem Biol 2001;5:591–602.

29. Jensen ON, Larsen MR, Roepstorff P. Mass spectrometric identification and microcharacterization of proteins from electrophoretic gels: strategies and applications. Proteins 1998;2:74–89.
30. Kussmann M, Hauser K, Kissmehl R, Breed J, Plattner H, Roepstorff P. Comparison of in vivo and in vitro phosphorylation of the exocytosis-sensitive protein PP63/ parafusin by differential MALDI mass spectrometric peptide mapping. Biochemistry 1999;38:7780–7790.
31. Wilm M, Neubauer G, Mann M. Parent ion scans of unseparated peptide mixtures. Anal Chem 1996;68:527–533
32. Steen H, Küster B, Fernandez M, Pandey A, Mann M. Quadrupole time-of-flight versus triple-quadrupole mass spectrometry for the determination of phosphopeptides by precursor ion scanning. Anal Chem 2001;73:1440–1448.
33. Hunter AP, Games DE. Chromatographic and mass spectrometric methods for the identification of phosphorylation sites in phosphoproteins. Rapid Commun Mass Spectrom 1994;8:559–570.
34. Schlosser A, Pipkorn R, Bossemeyer D, Lehmann WD. Analysis of protein phosphorylation by a combination of elastase digestion and neutral loss tandem mass spectrometry. Anal Chem 2001;73:170–176.
35. Larsen MR, Roepstorff P. Mass spectrometric identification of proteins and characterization of their post-translational modifications in proteome analysis Fresenius. J Anal Chem 2000;366:677–690.
36. Pandey A, Andersen JS, Mann M. Use of mass spectrometry to study signaling pathways. STKE 2001;37:PL1.
37. Figeys D, Gygi SP, Zhang Y, Watts J, Gu M, Aebersold R. Electrophoresis combined with novel mass spectrometry techniques: powerful tools for the analysis of proteins and . Electrophoresis 1998;19:1811–1818.
38. Posewitz MC, Tempst P. Immobilized gallium(III) affinity chromatography of phosphopeptides. Anal Chem 1999;71:2883–2892.
39. Marcus K, Moebius J, Meyer HE. Differential analysis of phosphorylated proteins in resting and thrombin-stimulated human platelets. Anal Bioanal Chem 2003;376:973–993.
40. Sickmann A, Meyer HE. Phosphoamino acid analysis. Proteomics 2001;2:200–206.
41. Dunn MJ. Electroblotting of proteins from 2-D polyacrylamide gels. Methods Mol Biol 1999;112:313–318.
42. Kyhse-Andersen J. Electroblotting of multiple gels: a simple apparatus without buffer tank for rapid transfer of proteins from polyacrylamide to nitrocellulose. J Biochem Biophys Methods 1984;3–4:203–209.
43. Marcus K, Immler D, Sternberger J, Meyer HE. Identification of platelet proteins separated by two-dimensional gel electrophoresis and analyzed by matrix assisted laser desorption/ionization-time of flight-mass spectrometry and detection of tyrosine-phosphorylated proteins. Electrophoresis 2000;21:2622–2636.
44. Yan JX, Packer NH, Gooley AA, Williams KL. Protein phosphorylation: technologies for the identification of phosphoamino acids. J Chromatogr A 1998;808:23–41.
45. Butt E, Bernhardt M, Smolenski A, et al. Endothelial nitric-oxide synthase (type III) is activated and becomes calcium independent upon phosphorylation by cyclic nucleotide-dependent protein kinases. J Biol Chem 2000;275:5179–5187.
46. Lehr S, Kotzka J, Herkner A, et al. Identification of major tyrosine phosphorylation sites in the human insulin receptor substrate Gab-1 by insulin receptor kinase in vitro. Biochemistry 2000;39:10898–10907.
47. Butt E, Gambaryan S, Gottfert N, Galler A, Marcus K, Meyer HE. Actin binding of human LIM and SH3 protein is regulated by cGMP- and cAMP-dependent protein kinase phosphorylation on serine 146. J Biol Chem 2003;278:15601–15607.

48. Fujitani K, Kambayashi J, Sakon M, et al. Identification of mu-, m-calpains and calpastatin and capture of mu-calpain activation in endothelial cells. J Cell Biochem 1997;66:197–209.

49. Hayashi M, Suzuki H, Kawashima S, Saido TC, Inomata M. The behaviour of calpain-generated N- and C-terminal fragments of talin in integrin-mediated signaling pathways. Arch Biochem Biophys 1999;15:133–142.

50. Annan RS, Carr SA. Phosphopeptide analysis by matrix-assisted laser desorption time-of-flight mass spectrometry. Anal Chem 1996;68:3413–3421.

51. Schuuring E, Verhoeven E, Litvinov S, Michalides RJ. The product of the EMS1 gene, amplified and overexpressed in human carcinomas, is homologous to a v-src substrate and is located in cell-substratum contact sites. Mol Cell Biol 1993;13:2891–2898.

52. Huang C, Liu J, Haudenschild CC, Zhan X. The role of tyrosine phosphorylation of cortactin in the locomotion of endothelial cells. J Biol Chem 1998;273:25770–25776.

53. Campbell DH, Sutherland RL, Daly RJ. Signaling pathways and structural domains required for phosphorylation of EMS1/cortactin. Cancer Res 1999;59:5376–5385.

54. van Damme H, Brok H, Schuuring-Scholtes E, Schuuring E. The redistribution of cortactin into cell-matrix contact sites in human carcinoma cells with 11q13 amplification is associated with both overexpression and post-translational modification. J Biol Chem 1997;272:7374–7380.

55. Huang C, Ni Y, Wang T, Gao Y, Haudenschild CC, Zhan X. Down-regulation of the filamentous actin cross-linking activity of cortactin by Src-mediated tyrosine phosphorylation. J Biol Chem 1997;272:13911–13915.

56. Naka M, Saitoh M, Hidaka H. Two phosphorylated forms of myosin in thrombin-stimulated platelet. Arch Biochem Biophys 1988;261:235–240.

II ASSESSING PLATELET FUNCTION

8   Platelet Function Studies

Dermot Cox, PhD

INTRODUCTION

Platelets play an essential role in hemostasis and thrombosis *(1)*. A defect in platelet function can result in platelets that are unresponsive or hypersensitive. Characterization of a defect is an important first step in the treatment of the disorder. Although defects usually present as bleeding or bruising, the existence of a defect is not always obvious. This is particularly a problem with thrombocytopenia, owing to heparin or a glycoprotein (GP)IIb-IIIa antagonist. In these cases the bleeding may be mistaken for the pharmacological effects of the drug.

Abnormal Platelet Function

Abnormal platelet function can present as a bleeding disorder or as a thrombotic disorder. A bleeding disorder is usually attributable to a reduced platelet count (thrombocytopenia), nonfunctioning platelets, or

From: *Contemporary Cardiology:*
Platelet Function: Assessment, Diagnosis, and Treatment
Edited by: M. Quinn and D. Fitzgerald © Humana Press Inc., Totowa, NJ

the presence of platelet inhibitors. A thrombotic disorder is attributable to platelets with increased activity.

THROMBOCYTOPENIA

A low platelet count can be caused by excessive consumption of platelets or failure to produce platelets. Excessive consumption is usually owing to ongoing thrombosis, e.g., disseminated intravascular coagulation, or the presence of antiplatelet antibodies that lead to removal of antibody-bound platelets from the circulation. A decrease in platelet production can be owing to a hereditary defect or can be drug-induced.

NONRESPONSIVE PLATELETS

Platelets can be defective because of hereditary disorders (2). The most common defect is Glanzmann's thrombasthenia, which is caused by a deficiency of GPIIb-IIIa (3). As GPIIb-IIIa is the platelet fibrinogen receptor, the result is that platelets fail to aggregate, producing a bleeding disorder. Another, much less common, bleeding disorder is Bernard-Soulier syndrome, which is caused by a defect in GPIb, the von Willebrand factor (vWF) receptor (4). It is characterized by thrombocytopenia and giant platelets. Although the platelets aggregate normally, the severe thrombocytopenia and the inability to bind to immobilized vWF are responsible for the bleeding problems associated with this disease. A number of other functional defects in platelets are rare and difficult to diagnose.

PLATELET INHIBITORS

The presence of antiplatelet agents will also lead to bleeding problems. The most used antiplatelet agent is aspirin, which irreversibly inhibits cyclooxygenase (COX) (5). This results in inhibition of thromboxane production, which is an essential mediator of platelet activation. Another inhibitor is clopidogrel (6), which irreversibly inhibits the ADP receptor on platelets. ADP is released upon platelet activation and is essential for amplification of the aggregation response. The third class of antiplatelet agents is GPIIb-IIIa antagonists (7). These inhibit platelet aggregation by inhibiting fibrinogen binding to GPIIb-IIIa.

PLATELET HYPERACTIVITY

Increased platelet activity is usually owing to an increase in local levels of prothrombotic stimuli. These include soluble mediators released from other platelets or damaged tissue as well as exposed subendothelial matrix. One of the most serious sources of thrombogenic material is ruptured atherosclerotic plaque (8).

Characterization of Platelet Function

Many devices are available for assessing platelet function; these include laboratory-based systems such as aggregometers and bedside or point-of-care devices. The methods primarily used to determine the platelet count and assess platelet function are flow cytometry and microscopy.

THE PLATELET COUNT

The first step in assessing a patient's platelet function, especially if he or she presents with a bleeding problem, is to perform a platelet count. This can be done with a hemocytometer, but more commonly it is performed with an electronic particle counter. Although thrombocytopenia is defined as a count of less than 150,000 platelets/µL, bleeding problems do not usually appear with counts above 50,000 platelets/µL, unless there is a functional defect as well. It is important to confirm thrombocytopenia by repeating the count using citrated blood and by examining a slide. A normal citrate count or evidence of platelet clumps under the microscope would suggest pseudothrombocytopenia, which is caused by an effect of EDTA on the platelet and appears to have no clinical significance *(9)*.

Investigation of Thrombocytopenia

Once thrombocytopenia is confirmed, it is necessary to determine the cause. Thrombocytopenia can be caused by increased consumption or decreased synthesis of platelets, and it can be associated with a platelet defect. Thrombocytopenia accompanied by giant platelets would suggest Bernard-Soulier syndrome, which is a deficiency of GPIb *(4)*. Thrombocytopenia owing to excessive consumption is characterized by evidence of platelet activation or the presence of antiplatelet antibodies. Increased platelet consumption is also accompanied by increased synthesis of platelets. These new platelets tend to be bigger and contain more nucleic acid than the older platelets. They are analogous to red cell reticulocytes and are known as platelet reticulocytes *(10)*. Increased consumption is characterized by increased levels of platelet reticulocytes. Drugs such as heparin, quinine, and GPIIb-IIIa antagonists can be responsible for thrombocytopenia. In these cases the cause is drug-dependent antibodies. In heparin-induced thrombocytopenia (HIT), antibodies are formed to a complex of platelet factor-4 (PF-4) and heparin *(11)*. When bound to the PF-4-heparin complex, these antibodies can activate platelets through the Fc receptor. The activated platelets are cleared from the system. In the case of GPIIb-IIIa antagonists, an antibody to the drug-receptor complex is formed *(12)*. These antibody-bound platelets are removed from the circulation. A similar scenario occurs with quinine: either GPIb-IX-V or GPIIb-IIIa can be the target for quinine *(13)*. A decreased synthesis of platelets will usually present with normal levels of platelet reticulocytes without evidence of platelet activation.

DETECTION OF ANTIPLATELET ANTIBODIES

The platelet-associated immunoglobin (PAIg) assay measures antibody on the surface of a patient's platelets, usually with an antihuman Ig antibody and flow cytometry *(14)*. This assay is hampered by the low levels of circulating platelets that have bound Ig on their surface owing to the rapid clearance of such platelets from the circulation. Alternatively, plasma from a patient is mixed with platelets from a healthy donor, and antibodies on the platelet surface are detected by flow cytometry. However, foreign donor platelets may contain antigens unrelated to the drug target, or may not contain the same polymorphisms as the patient. Platelet lysates can be used to measure antiplatelet antibodies in serum from patients using enzyme-linked immunosorbent assay (ELISA) *(15)*. This assay is often used to screen positive samples from the PAIg or antiplatelet antibody assays. In this case immobilized antigen such as GPIIb-IIIa or PF-4 can be used to confirm the presence of antibodies.

DETECTION OF PLATELET-ACTIVATING ANTIBODIES

Antiplatelet antibodies that activate platelets can be detected by their ability to induce platelet aggregation or to release serotonin. The serotonin release assay is highly sensitive but has limited use, as it is more difficult to perform but is often used for HIT *(16)*. Platelet aggregation is often used in screening for HIT, in which the addition of patient plasma, heparin, and donor platelets can lead to platelet aggregation *(16,17)*. This assay does not work for GPIIb-IIIa antagonist-dependent antibodies, as these drugs inhibit aggregation, but it is commonly used for HIT.

DETECTION OF PLATELET RETICULOCYTES

Platelet reticulocytes can be detected using flow cytometry by their characteristic size and high nucleic acid content. They are usually detected by staining with thiazole orange. Platelet fluorescence is measured by flow cytometry and compared with a normal sample *(10)*.

PLATELET FUNCTION TESTS

Assays to assess platelet function are all based on the detection of platelet aggregate formation after stimulation with an agonist. These assays all use different technologies to detect this aggregate formation.

Some are laboratory-based technologies, but more recently small, rapid, point-of-care devices have been developed. The appropriate device can make assessment of platelet function more widely available, as the existing laboratory-based assays are only found in larger hospitals.

Platelet Aggregation

Platelet aggregometry is based on a turbidimetric technique devised by Born in 1962 (18) and utilizes the principle that the absorbance of a suspension is dependent on the number of particles rather than on their size. As aggregation occurs, the number of particles decreases, and light transmission increases. Blood is usually collected in sodium citrate, and platelet-rich plasma (PRP) is prepared by centrifugation at a low speed (850g for 3 min or 100g for 10 min). This PRP is added to a cuvet with a stirrer and stirred (900–1200 rpm) while agonist is added. Platelet-poor plasma (PPP) is used as a blank for the aggregometer. Modifications of this assay have also been developed including an impedance-based method and bedside assays.

THROMBOCYTOPENIA

Aggregation may be influenced by the platelet count. Aggregometry requires platelet counts between 200,000 and 400,000 platelets/μL. Some researchers adjust the platelet count to ensure it is within these levels for the sake of uniformity, and there is evidence that the platelet count may affect the degree of inhibition by GPIIb-IIIa antagonists (19). Whereas diluting a sample with a high platelet concentration is relatively simple, concentrating a dilute platelet sample is difficult without activating the sample. However, platelet aggregometers will still give a response with counts as low as 50,000 platelets/μL, although this response will be attenuated. In the case of blood from a patient with Bernard-Soulier syndrome, there are problems in preparing PRP, as the platelets sediment with the white cells. The solution is to allow the blood to settle under gravity. Usually within 2–3 h there is sufficient PRP for an aggregation test.

RELIABILITY

The aggregation response that is obtained depends on a number of factors. Some samples can give 90% aggregation and others only 40%, but it cannot be concluded that a 40% response represents nonfunctional platelets. Variation between samples has been estimated to have a standard deviation ranging from 3.6 to 7.7%, with day-to-day variation accounting for the majority of the variation, followed by operator variability (20). The sources of this variation include sample preparation, dietary factors including high levels of lipids in the sample, smoking, drinking and aging of the sample.

Agonists

The choice of platelet agonist is very important when one is performing a platelet function study. Agonists generate a response through two signaling systems. One is dependent on phospholipase A_2 (PLA_2) and utilizes COX and thromboxane synthase to produce the platelet agonist thromboxane A_2, which leads to further activation of platelets through its receptor. The other system is dependent on phospholipase C (PLC) and results in the production of inositol triphosphate (IP_3) and diacylglycerol (DAG). These in turn activate the IP_3 receptor and protein kinase C, respectively. Agonists can act via one or other pathway, and some agonists act via PLA_2 at low concentration and PLC at high concentration. The term *weak agonist* applies to agonists using PLA_2 only, and *strong agonists* applies to those using PLC with or without PLA_2 activity *(21)*.

Thrombin is a strong platelet agonist and can generate a response when no other agonist can. In gel-filtered platelets, aggregation occurs with concentrations of 0.01–0.05 U/mL thrombin and is inhibited by anti-GPIb antibodies *(22)*. At concentrations above 0.2 U/mL, anti-GPIb antibodies have no effect, and the response is dependent on protease-activated receptors (PARs) 1 and 4 *(23)*. In PRP, higher concentrations of thrombin are needed owing to neutralization of thrombin by antithrombin III. Here 0.2–0.4 U/mL is the lowest concentration that will induce platelet aggregation. As an alternative to thrombin, a thrombin receptor-activating peptide (TRAP) can be used. This is the peptide exposed by thrombin on the amino terminal of the PAR-1 receptor. TRAP is synthesized as the hexapeptide SFLLRN and is used in the range 5–20 μ*M*. This mimics the actions of thrombin on the PAR-1 without the problems of coagulation *(23)*. Either thrombin or TRAP should always be used in platelet function studies, as this is the maximum response possible from the platelets.

Collagen is also a strong agonist and activates platelets through the integrin $\alpha_2\beta_1$ and GPVI. $\alpha_2\beta_1$ signals via PLA_2 and is inhibited by aspirin, whereas GPVI signals through PLC and is unaffected by aspirin *(24)*. There are a number of different collagens with different affinities for the two receptors; thus, the response to collagen depends on the source of collagen and the concentration used. If it is to be used, collagen from different suppliers should be tested for activity.

ADP is the most common platelet agonist used. At 3–5 μ*M*, ADP-induced aggregation is strongly PLA_2 dependent, whereas at 20 μ*M* it is PLC dependent. However, platelets lose their responsiveness to ADP after a few hours *(25)*. Platelet sensitivity can be prolonged by storing PRP at room temperature in a tube with minimum air space.

Arachidonic acid. The action of PLA$_2$ is to cleave arachidonic acid from the cell membrane and make it available as a substrate for COX. Thus, arachidonic acid is a useful agonist for studying the integrity of the COX pathway. Arachidonic acid can be obtained in the acid form soluble in organic solvents or as sodium arachidonate, which is water soluble.

Ristocetin. The interaction between platelet GPIb and vWF occurs under high shear and requires immobilized vWF. Ristocetin is an antibiotic that binds to vWF, allowing it to bind to GPIb without the need for shear. When paraformaldehyde-fixed platelets are used, the response is agglutination rather than aggregation *(26,27)*, is independent of GPIIb-IIIa, and can be used as a measure of GPIb function. Botrocetin is a snake venom and another vWF modulator that can be used in agglutination studies *(27,28)*, but its expense means that it is usually only used as a research tool.

Functional studies should be performed with at least two agonists, usually low-dose ADP and TRAP/thrombin to test both the PLA$_2$ and PLC pathways. Usually it is advisable to include collagen in the analysis as well. A normal response to these agonists and a normal platelet count suggest that there is no major platelet disorder. If necessary, a profile using the full range of agonists can be performed to identify an agonist-specific defect. Arachidonic acid is also a useful agonist, as it does not require functional agonist receptors. If there is a difference between the response to ADP and TRAP, the usual explanation is the presence of aspirin, or clopidogrel. Patients may be unaware of taking aspirin, as it is often present in cold/flu and other remedies. If both ADP and TRAP are very low, this suggests a defect in GPIIb-IIIa, especially if the platelet count is normal. A low platelet count will give a reduced aggregation response. If ADP/TRAP aggregation is present and botrocetin/ristocetin aggregation is absent, then a diagnosis of Bernard-Solier syndrome is likely, especially if thrombocytopenia is present. Further tests will focus on studying the activation process of the platelets and quantification of platelet receptors by flow cytometry.

ANTICOAGULANT

There are a number of anticoagulants available, but the standard anticoagulant for platelet aggregometry is 3.8% sodium citrate. It is, however, possible to perform aggregation studies with blood anticoagulated with antithrombins such as heparin, low-molecular-weight heparin, hirudin, and D-phenylalanyl-L-prolyl-L-arginine-chloromethyl ketone (PPACK) *(29)*, although some agonists do not give as good a response *(30)*. Some GPIIb-IIIa antagonists show different potencies in citrate and heparin anticoagulated blood *(31,32)*. This appears to be owing to chelation of calcium from GPIIb-IIIa; the resulting conformational change increases the affinity for eptifibatide. If an antithrombin is used to maintain physiological calcium levels, it is important to choose the appropriate agonist, ideally high-dose ADP, collagen, or TRAP. The alternative is to recalcify citrated PRP immediately prior to aggregation. This works well, as aggregation occurs more rapidly than coagulation *(30)*.

Whole Blood Aggregometry

One of the difficulties with platelet aggregometry is the need to prepare PRP and the lack of sensitivity of the light transmission method. A recent alternative is whole blood aggregometry, which measures changes in impedance across two wires as platelet aggregates form on them. These devices are manufactured by the Chrono-Log Corporation (Havertown, PA). This technique has the advantage of being rapid, as no sample preparation is required; it is potentially more relevant physiologically as all the components of the blood are present *(33,34)*.

Loss of Single Platelets Method

A platelet aggregometer measures the changes in light transmission when a suspension of platelets aggregate. However, its sensitivity is such that only aggregates of around eight platelets are detected. Using a particle counter to compare the platelet count before and after activation, it is possible to measure the loss of single platelets with a very high sensitivity. This method measures microthrombus formation rather than macrothrombus formation. In some cases platelets will form microthrombi (full aggregation by platelet count) but not macrothrombi (no aggregation by light transmission). The advantages of this method are that there is no need for a platelet aggregometer (although it is necessary to stir the sample after the addition of agonist) and it is very useful for thrombocytopenic samples. It is also more sensitive than light transmission aggregometry. However, it cannot be used for samples from patients with Bernard-Solier syndrome as their platelets are too large and are usually not detected by the particle counter *(32,35)*.

Bedside/Point-of-Care Devices

A number of devices have been developed to allow a rapid assessment of platelet function. These were primarily developed to allow the measurement of inhibition owing to antiplatelet agents. However, these devices can be used to measure platelet function as well.

The loss-of-single platelet method for assessing platelet function has been commercialized as the ICHOR (Plateletworks) point-of-care assay *(36)* by Helena Laboratories, Beaumont, TX.

The Ultegra™ Rapid Platelet Function Analyzer is a bedside device to monitor platelet inhibition by GPIIb-IIIa antagonists *(41)*. This assay is based on TRAP-induced platelet aggregation. It consists of a cartridge containing blue beads coated with fibrinogen, a magnetic stirrer, and TRAP. Whole blood is added to the cartridge, and the resulting activated platelets bind to the coated beads, forming aggregates. Aggregation is detected by monitoring the loss of the blue beads by the turbidimetric method using filters to analyze the blue portion of the spectrum *(38)*. This device is made by the Accumetrics Corporation (San Diego) and received Food and Drug Administration approval in 1999. The advantage of this assay is that it only uses a small volume of whole blood and requires no sample preparation; as it is a bedside device, testing is convenient.

Factors Affecting Platelet Responses

The response of platelets to agonist stimulation is greatly influenced by environmental factors that can either increase or decrease platelet activation. Smoking is one of the most common environmental factors influencing platelet function and has been shown to increase the platelet activation *(39–41)*. Dietary factors are also important modulators of platelet function. Folic acid deficiency *(46)* and low intake of vitamin B_{12}, especially in conjunction with hyperhomocysteinemia *(47)* and oxidant stress *(48)*, all increase platelet activation. Vitamins C *(49)* and E *(50)*, iron deficiency *(51,52)*, alcohol *(53,54)*, garlic *(55,56)*, fish *(57)*, and caffeine consumption *(58)* all decrease platelet activation. Exercise can increase platelet reactivity *(59,60)*. Hypercholesterolemia increases platelet activation and atorvastin reduces it *(61)*.

Factors intrinsic to the patient can also affect platelet function. These include depression *(62)*, which enhances platelet activity, and the menstrual cycle *(63)*. Polymorphisms of platelet receptors also alter the response of platelets to agonists *(64)*. Some studies have shown an increased sensitivity of platelets with the PLA polymorphism in GPIIIa *(65,66)*, a polymorphism in the collagen receptor has been shown to increase responsiveness to collagen by increasing the density of $\alpha_2\beta_1$ collagen receptors on the platelet surface and may be related to resistance to aspirin *(67)*, and the Kozak polymorphism in GPIbα is associated with the levels of GPIb on the surface of platelets and may be implicated in enhanced platelet function *(68)*.

FLOW CYTOMETRY

Evidence of platelet dysfunction requires further studies to determine the cause of the dysfunction. One likely cause is a hereditary deficiency of membrane proteins such as Glanzmann's thrombasthenia (GPIIb-

IIIa) or Bernard-Soulier syndrome (GPIb). The easiest way to detect this is by flow cytometry. A quantitative flow cytometry kit from BioCytex (Marseille, France) allows for accurate determination of the number of GPIIb-IIIa, GPIb, and $\alpha_2\beta_1$ (collagen receptors) *(69,70)*. The kit comes with four antibodies (anti GPIIIa, anti-GPIb, anti-α_2, and isotype control), a fluorescein isothiocyanate-labeled secondary antibody, and calibrator beads. The assay uses whole blood and is a no-wash method. The calibration beads contain four populations of beads with different, known amounts of mouse antibody attached. When stained simultaneously with the sample, these beads allow the mean fluorescence value to be converted into molecules of antibody bound and therefore the number of receptors on the platelet. This assay is rapid and highly sensitive. It requires small volumes of blood (~1 mL) and is therefore very effective for screening young children and is not affected by thrombocytopenia. It can detect reduced levels of receptors as well as absolute deficiency. However, it does not distinguish between functional and nonfunctional receptors, which requires data from aggregation studies. The assay also allows for alterations in platelet size since reduction in all three receptors is likely to be caused by small platelets size, but reduction in only one is likely to be caused by a defect in that particular receptor.

TEMPLATE BLEEDING TIME

The template bleeding time is the only in vivo assay of platelet function *(71)*. Bleeding time is measured using a device that provides a standardized cut to the skin. The two principle methods are the Ivy and Simplate methods *(72)*, and the bleeding time is the time taken for bleeding to stop (normally 8–12 min). The template bleeding time is not a sensitive assay and only detects severe levels of platelet dysfunction. However, it is not popular with patients, as it is painful and can lead to scarring. The template bleeding time is also a poor predictor of bleeding events. In a clinical study with abciximab, it was found that prolongation of the bleeding time was a poor predictor of bleeding events *(73)*, and bleeding time was also shown to be a poor predictor of blood loss during surgery *(74)*. Thus, prolongation of bleeding time can indicate strong inhibition of platelet function but does not predict bleeding events.

PLATELET ACTIVATION AND SECRETION

When platelets are exposed to an agonist they become activated. If a weak agonist is used, this results in conversion of GPIIb-IIIa into an activated form in which it has a higher affinity for soluble fibrinogen. If a strong agonist is used, platelets undergo degranulation, which involves fusion of the granules (α and dense granules and lysosomes) with the membrane followed by release of their contents *(75)*. Platelets also undergo a process that is similar to apoptosis *(76)*. This involves membrane flip-flop, with the exposure of intracellular membrane components including annexin V and phospholipids (these are important in coagulation) *(77,78)*. Also, a form of membrane blebbing occurs, resulting in microparticle formation. There are a number of methods of measuring platelet activation, and most currently used methods involve flow cytometry.

The standard method is to use a marker of granule release. The two markers usually used are P-selectin (CD62p), a marker of α-granule release, or CD63 antigen, a marker of dense granule release *(75)*. Neither of these proteins is expressed on resting platelets, but they become exposed after activation-mediated degranulation. P-selectin is expressed at higher levels than CD63 antigen, but it is prone to shedding. There are two methods of analysis. One is to measure the fluorescence intensity of the platelets after binding a fluorescent-labeled CD62p or CD63 antibody *(79)*. This can be quantified using the platelet calibrator kit from BioCytex. The alternative is to determine the number of platelets that express either protein at any level, i.e., the percent positive cells. Another option is to stain the platelets with the anti-GPIIb-IIIa antibody PAC-1 *(80)*. This antibody recognizes the activated form of GPIIb-IIIa.

Another flow cytometric assay measures the level of VASP phosphorylation in platelets. VASP (vasodilator-stimulated phosphoprotein) is an actin regulatory protein that plays an essential role in platelet aggregation *(81)*. Its phosphorylation is mediated by platelet stimulation with nitric oxide and prostacyclin. Dephosphorylation is mediated by activation with ADP. The phosphorylation status of VASP can be determined using a quantitative flow cytometry kit (PlateletVASP) from BioCytex (Marseille, France).

Alternatives to the flow cytometry assays are the serotonin release assay, the chemiluminescence assay and calcium fluorometry. In the serotonin release assay platelets are incubated in ^{14}C-serotonin, which is then taken up into the α-granules *(16)*. The radioactivity in the supernatant after stimulation of a platelet suspension is a measure of activation of the platelet. It is also possible to get a whole blood aggregometer that incorporates a chemiluminescence detector. Whole blood lumiaggregometry allows for monitoring aggregation by the impedance method and ATP secretion simultaneously *(34)*. Secretion is measured by a chemiluminescent assay using luciferase. Another alternative is to load washed platelets with Fura-2-am, which is a membrane-permeable, calcium-dependent fluorochrome. (Inside the platelet it is converted to Fura, which is membrane impermeable.) When platelets are stimulated, there is a calcium influx that causes an increase in fluorescence intensity from the platelets. However, this method requires a dedicated calcium fluorometer *(82)*.

If a patients' platelets fail to aggregate, it is useful to try one of the above techniques. This will determine whether the problem is a failure to activate the platelets or a failure of the activated platelets to aggregate.

MICROSCOPY STUDIES

Electron microscopy can aid in the diagnosis of defects in the platelet ultrastructure. It allows the shape of the platelet to be determined, which can aid in diagnosis, e.g., many giant platelet syndromes have round platelets, whereas in the gray platelet syndrome, platelets are enlarged and discoid shaped *(74)*. The α-granules can be visualized; their absence suggests gray platelet syndrome. Examination of the white blood cells in a blood smear is also important in the diagnosis of platelet disorders. Neutrophil inclusions are associated with May-Hegglin anomaly *(84)*, and leukocyte inclusions are associated with Fechtner's and Sebastian's syndromes *(76)*.

SHEAR-DEPENDENT ASSAYS

As the circulatory system is not static, platelets continuously experience shear conditions as they circulate through the vasculature. In fact they experience a range of shear conditions from low shear in veins to high shear in stenosed arteries. Some of the functions of platelets are designed to operate under these shear conditions only. In particular, the interaction of GPIb on platelets with immobilized von Willebrand factor only occurs under shear. As a result shear based systems have been developed to assess platelet function. These include the cone and plate viscometer *(86)* and systems that flow blood through flow chambers. However, the cone and plate viscometer is a large expensive machine and, while it is easy to use and only requires small volumes of blood, it would not be found in most hospital laboratories. The flow chamber systems require large volumes of blood and usually use confocal microscopy with real-time video capture to a computer. As a result it is a very expensive system and only used for research. The cone and plate viscometer has been used to measure ex vivo platelet function in healthy volunteers *(87)* and in patients post surgery *(88)* and with unstable angina *(89)*. The flow chamber system has been used in healthy volunteers *(56,90)*.

The Platelet Function Analyzer PFA-100™, from Dade International (Miami, FL) is an automated system for monitoring platelet responsiveness. It consists of a membrane that is coated with collagen-adrenaline or collagen-ADP. Whole blood is aspirated through a hole pierced in the membrane under high shear and the time to closure, which is due to the formation of a platelet plug, is a measure of platelet function *(91,92)*. This device has the advantage of using small volumes of whole blood directly applied to a cartridge.

ANTIPLATELET AGENTS

Monitoring antiplatelet agent activity is very important as it ensures that adequate protection is being provided for the patient, and it prevents bleeding complications owing to high levels of these drugs in the plasma. Three main classes of antiplatelet agents are used today. The most widely used is aspirin, which irreversibly inhibits COX. This inhibits thromboxane production and aggregation by weak agonists. However, aggregation by a strong agonist is not affected *(5)*. Clopidogrel is a recently approved antiplatelet agent and acts by irreversibly inhibiting the platelet ADP receptor *(93)*. Finally, GPIIb-III antagonists (abciximab, eptifibatide, and tirofiban) prevent fibrinogen binding and inhibit aggregation in response to all agonists *(7)*.

Aspirin

Monitoring inhibition by aspirin is important, as it is the most widely used antiplatelet agent. Recently there have been reports that some patients are resistant to the effects of aspirin *(94,95)*, and the prognosis of these patients is worse than that of those sensitive to aspirin *(96)*. The easiest way to monitor sensitivity to aspirin is to compare platelet aggregation with TRAP and arachidonic acid or low-dose ADP. Even 75 mg of aspirin daily should produce 100% inhibition of arachidonic acid-induced aggregation compared with TRAP. The PFA-100 is often used to monitor sensitivity to aspirin with the collagen-adrenaline cartridge *(97,99)*. Many cases of aspirin resistance have been detected using this device, and there are concerns that aspirin resistance may be an artifact of the PFA. More recently the Ultegra system has been modified to produce a device suitable for monitoring aspirin inhibition. The VerifyNow® system uses the Ultegra system with arachidonic acid as an agonist. It has been successfully used to monitor aspirin responsiveness in patients *(100)*. A problem with aspirin resistance is that it is assay dependent and often there is little correlation between assays and the Ultegra and PFA-100 give higher incidences than aggregation *(101)*. However, this may be attributable to a lack of sensitivity with aggregation.

True aspirin resistance only occurs when the drug does not completely inhibit thromboxane formation. Failure to inhibit platelet aggregation can be owing to involvement of the PLC pathway in response to the agonist rather than a failure of aspirin to inhibit COX. Thus, measurement of COX activity by measuring thromboxane B_2 production is the most reliable method to detect aspirin resistance. Thromboxane B_2 production can easily be measured by radioimmunoassay (RIA)/ELISA *(102)*. Measuring serum thromboxane B_2 by ELISA has been used to study the effects of aspirin *(103)*, coated aspirin *(104)*, and aspirin and nimesulide *(105)*, although urinary thromboxane levels were shown not to predict aspirin resistance *(106)*.

Clopidogrel

The recent approval of clopidogrel has provided an alternative for patients intolerant of aspirin. Its effects are easily measured by comparing aggregation in response to high-dose ADP ($20 \mu M$) with the response to TRAP. Clopidogrel should provide complete inhibition. In some cases a combination of aspirin and clopidogrel is used for high-risk patients. The inhibition by the different drugs can be monitored by performing platelet aggregation with three agonists: TRAP, ADP ($20 \mu M$), and arachidonic acid. The ADP-induced aggregation detects inhibition by clopidogrel only, whereas arachidonic acid-induced aggregation detects inhibition owing to aspirin. With the collagen-ADP cartridges, the effects of clopidogrel can be monitored with the PFA-100 *(79)*. The Ultegra system has been modified to produce the VerfiyNow® $P_2 Y_{12}$ assay. This is similar to the aspirin assay except that it uses cationic propyl gallate as the agonist and is currently under clinical development. The VASP phosphorylation assay (BioCytex) has also been used to assess clopidogrel resistance *(107,108)*.

GPIIb-IIIa Antagonists

Recent evidence suggests that monitoring treatment of patients with GPIIb-IIIa antagonists is desirable, as many may be underdosed *(109)*. These drugs have steep dose-response relationships, and overdosing can lead to severe bleeding problems. Platelet aggregation can be used to monitor the effects of GPIIb-IIIa antagonists. Although they will inhibit aggregation induced by any agonist, their inhibitory concentration of 50% (IC_{50}) value is dependent on the agonist used. There can be a significant difference between IC_{50} values obtained with low-dose ADP and TRAP. The Ultegra™ has been successfully used to monitor orbofiban, abciximab, eptifibatide, and tirofiban *(110–113)* levels in blood. It gives results similar to platelet aggregation, but the IC_{50} value tends to be lower.

The receptor occupancy assay (BioCytex) is a flow cytometry-based assay that can be used to monitor treatment with GPIIb-IIIa antagonists.

It was also shown that inhibition of greater than 95% in the Ultegra was associated with a reduction in major adverse cardiac events *(113)*. This assay uses three antibodies: an isotype control and two anti-GPIIb-IIIa antibodies. One of these antibodies, MAb2, recognizes a drug-dependent ligand-induced binding site. The epitope for this antibody disappears when a GPIIb-IIIa antagonist binds to the receptor. Both eptifibatide and tirofiban inhibit binding of MAb2, whereas abciximab has no effect. The third antibody in the kit (MAb1) competes with abciximab and is not inhibited by small-molecule antagonists. The kit also includes calibration beads that allows antibody binding to be converted to number of receptors. Together these three antibodies can determine the number of occupied receptors, the total number of receptors, and the percent receptor occupancy *(114)*. The advantages of this assay are that it requires small amounts of whole blood (50 µL) and does not require a baseline sample to estimate percent inhibition. In addition, it gives the number of free receptors as well, which may be more relevant than percent inhibition. If blood is activated with an agonist such as TRAP prior to use in the assay, it allows comparison of inhibition in resting and activated samples. The receptor occupancy assay has been use to measure GPIIb-IIIa receptor occupancy by xemilofiban *(109)*, orbofiban *(115)*, and abciximab *(116)*.

CONCLUSIONS

A patient presenting with a history of bleeding problems should be screened for platelet abnormalities. The initial test is a full blood count, which will indicate the existence of thrombocytopenia. However, only a very low platelet count (<50,000 platelets/µL) can explain bleeding problems. It is necessary to investigate the cause of thrombocytopenia. Evidence of platelet activation and increased levels of reticulated platelets suggests consumption of platelets, whereas no evidence of platelet activation and normal levels of reticulated platelets suggest decreased production of platelets. Thrombocytopenia owing to excessive platelet consumption is usually caused by antiplatelet antibodies that can be identified by flow cytometry or ELISA. A drug-dependent mechanism should be considered.

If the bleeding cannot be explained by thrombocytopenia, then it is necessary to perform functional studies. Although point-of-care assays such as the PFA-100 can be used, the best assay is platelet aggregation. This is can be traditional turbidimetric aggregation, impedance-based, or the loss-of-single-platelets method. A strong agonist such as TRAP and a weak agonist such as low-dose ADP should be used. Ideally, a full profile including arachidonic acid, adrenaline, collagen, and ristocetin should be obtained. If test results suggest Bernard-Soulier syndrome or

Glanzmann's thrombasthenia, then quantitative flow cytometry will confirm the diagnosis and the extent of the defect. If possible, the gene can then be sequenced to identify the mutation involved. If there is no evidence of Bernard-Soulier syndrome or Glanzmann's thrombasthenia, then electron micrographs should be obtained to look for characteristic ultrastructural defects.

Although in many cases identification of a platelet abnormality is irrelevant to a patient's treatment, which is usually platelet concentrates to prevent bleeding; in some cases it is important to know the precise diagnosis. For example, in the case of Fechtner's and Epstein's syndromes, there is an associated nephritis (117) and loss of hearing (118), making early diagnosis important. In the case of a drug-induced thrombocytopenia such as HIT, early diagnosis allows alternative medicines to be used.

REFERENCES

1. George JN. Platelets. Lancet 2000;355:1531–1539.
2. Clemetson K, Clemetson J. Molecular abnormalities in Glanzmann's thrombasthenia, Bernard-Soulier syndrome, and platelet-type von Willebrand's disease. Curr Opin Hematol 1994;1:388–393.
3. Coller B, Seligsohn U, Peretz H, Newman P. Glanzmann thrombasthenia: new insights from an historical perspective. Semin Hematol 1994;31:301–311.
4. Lopez JA, Andrews RK, Afshar-Kharghan V, Berndt MC. Bernard-Soulier syndrome. Blood 1998;91:4397–4418.
5. Awtry EH, Loscalzo J. Aspirin. Circulation 2000;101:1206–1218.
6. Mehta SR, Yusuf S, Peters RJG, et al. Effects of pretreatment with clopidogrel and aspirin followed by long-term therapy in patients undergoing percutaneous coronary intervention: the PCI-CURE study. Lancet 2001;358:527–533.
7. Topol EJ, Byzova TV, Plow EF. Platelet GPIIb-IIIa blockers. Lancet 1999; 353:227–231.
8. Corti R, Farkouh ME, Badimon JJ. The vulnerable plaque and acute coronary syndromes. Am J Med 2002;113:668–680.
9. Sane DC, Damaraju LV, Topol EJ, et al. Occurrence and clinical significance of pseudothrombocytopenia during abciximab therapy. J Am Coll Cardiol 2000;36:75–83.
10. Ault KA, Rinder HM, Mitchell J, Carmody MB, Vary CP, Hillman RS. The significance of platelets with increased RNA content (reticulated platelets). A measure of the rate of thrombopoiesis. Am J Clin Pathol 1992;98:637–646.
11. Kelton JG. Heparin-induced thrombocytopenia: an overview. Blood Rev 2002;16:77–80.
12. Billheimer JT, Dicker IB, Wynn R, et al. Evidence that thrombocytopenia observed in humans treated with orally bioavailable glycoprotein IIb/IIIa antagonists is immune mediated. Blood 2002;99:3540–3546.
13. Peterson JA, Nyree CE, Newman PJ, Aster RH. A site involving the "hybrid" and PSI homology domains of GPIIIa (beta 3-integrin subunit) is a common target for antibodies associated with quinine-induced immune thrombocytopenia. Blood 2003;101:937–942.
14. Ault K. Flow cytometric analysis of platelets. In: Bauer K, Duque R, Shankey T, eds. Clinical Flow Cytometry—Principles and Application: Williams & Wilkins, Baltimore, 1993, pp. 387–403.

15. Bessos H, Perez S, Armstrong-Fisher S, Urbaniak S, Turner M. The development of a quantitative ELISA for antibodies against human platelet antigen type 1a. Transfusion 2003;43:350–356.

16. Griffiths E, Dzik W. Assays for heparin-induced thrombocytopenia. Transfusion Med 1997;7:1–11.

17. Nguyen P, Lecompte T. Heparin-induced thrombocytopenia: a survey of tests employed and attitudes in haematology laboratories. NR Fr Hematol 1994;36:353–357.

18. Born G. The aggregation of blood platelets by adenosine diphosphate and its reversal. Nature 1962;194:927.

19. Kereiakes D, Broderick T, Roth E, et al. High platelet count in platelet-rich plasma reduces measured platelet inhibition by abciximab but not tirofiban nor eptifibatide glycoprotein IIb/IIIa receptor antagonists. J Thromb Thrombol 2000;9:149–155.

20. Nicholson N, Panzer-Knodle S, Haas N, et al. Assessment of platelet function assays. Am Heart J 1998;135:S170–S178.

21. Siess W. Molecular mechanisms of platelet activation. Physiol Rev 1989;69:58–178.

22. Mazzucato M, Marco L, Masotti A, Pradella P, Bahou W, Ruggeri Z. Characterization of the initial alpha-thrombin interaction with glycoprotein Ib alpha in relation to platelet activation. J Biol Chem 1998;273:1880–1887.

23. Furman M, Liu L, Benoit S, Becker R, Barnard M, Michelson A. The cleaved peptide of the thrombin receptor is a strong platelet agonist. Proc Natl Acad Sci USA 1998;95:3082–3087.

24. Inoue K, Ozaki Y, Satoh K, Wu Y, Yatomi Y, Shin Y, Morita T. Signal transduction pathways mediated by glycoprotein Ia/IIa in human platelets: comparison with those of glycoprotein VI. Biochem Biophys Res Commun 1999;256:114–120.

25. Baurand A, Eckly A, Bari N, et al. Desensitization of the platelet aggregation response to ADP: differential down-regulation of the P2Y1 and P2cyc receptors. Thromb Haemost 2000;84:484–491.

26. Berndt M, Du X, Booth W. Ristocetin-dependent reconstitution of binding of von Willebrand factor to purified human platelet membrane glycoprotein Ib-IX complex. Biochemistry 1988;27:633–640.

27. Thomas K, Tune E, Choong S. Parallel determination of von Willebrand factor—ristocetin and botrocetin cofactors. Thromb Res 1994;75:401–408.

28. Andrews R, Booth W, Gorman J, Castaldi P, Berndt M. Purification of botrocetin from *Bothrops jararaca* venom. Analysis of the botrocetin-mediated interaction between von Willebrand factor and the human platelet membrane glycoprotein Ib-IX complex. Biochemistry 1989;28:8317–8326.

29. Glusa E, Markwardt F. Platelet functions in recombinant hirudin-anticoagulated blood. Haemostasis 1990;20:112-118.

30. Cox D, Douglas C, Preston F. The effects of anticoagulation on platelet aggregation. Thromb Haemost 1997;77:301.

31. Phillips D, Teng W, Arfsten A, et al. Effect of Ca^{2+} on GP IIb-IIIa interactions with integrilin: enhanced GPIIb-IIIa binding and inhibition of platelet aggregation by reductions in the concentration of ionized calcium in plasma anticoagulated with citrate. Circulation 1997;96:1488–1494.

32. Storey R, Wilcox R, Heptinstall S. Differential effects of glycoprotein IIb/IIIa antagonists on platelet microaggregate and macroaggregate formation and effect of anticoagulant on antagonist potency. Circulation 1998;98:1616–1621.

33. Mascelli M, Worley S, Veriabo N, et al. Rapid assessment of platelet function with a modified whole-blood aggregometer in percutaneous transluminal coronary angioplasty patients receiving anti-GP IIb/IIIa therapy. Circulation 1997;96:3860–3866.

34. Podczasy J, Lee J, Vucenik I. Evaluation of whole-blood lumiaggregation. Clin Appl Thromb Hemost 1997;3:190–195.

35. Storey R, May J, Wilcox R, Heptinstall S. A whole blood assay of inhibition of platelet aggregation by glycoprotein IIb/IIIa antagonists: comparison with other aggregation methodologies. Thromb Haemost 1999;82:1307–1311.

36. Carville D, Schleckser P, Guyer K, Corsello M, Walsh M. Whole blood platelet function assay on the ICHOR point-of-care hematology analyzer. J Extra Corporal Technol 1998;30:171–177.

37. White MM, Krishnan R, Kueter TJ, Jacoski MV, Jennings LK. The Use of the Point of Care Helena ICHOR/Plateletworks(R) and the Accumetrics Ultergra(R) RPFA for Assessment of Platelet Function with GPIIb-IIIa Antagonists. J Thromb Thrombolysis 2005;18:163–169.

38. Ostrowsky J. Foes J, Warchol M, Tsarovsky G, Blay J. Plateletworks platelet function test compared to the thromboelastograph for prediction of postoperative outcomes. J Extra Corpor Technol 2004;36:149–152.

39. Ray MJ, Walters DL, Bett N, Cameron J, Wood P, Aroney C. Point-of-care testing shows clinically relevant variation in the degree of inhibition of platelets by standard-dose abciximab therapy during percutaneous coronary intervention. Catheter Cardiovasc Interv 2004;62:150–154.

40. Lennon MJ, Gibbs NM, Weightman WM, McGuire D, Michalopoulos N. A comparison of Plateletworks and platelet aggregometry for the assessment of aspirin-related platelet dysfunction in cardiac surgical patients. J Cardiothorac Vasc Anesth 2004;18:136–140.

41. Steinhubl S, Keriakes D. Ultegra rapid platelet function analyzer. In: Michelson A, ed. Platelets: Academic Press, 2002:317–322.

42. Smith J, Steinhubl S, Lincoff A, et al. Rapid platelet-function assay an automated and quantitative cartridge-based method. Circulation 1999;99:620–625.

43. Putter M, Grotemeyer K, Wurthwein G, Araghi-Niknam M, Watson R, Hosseini SPR. Inhibition of smoking-induced platelet aggregation by aspirin and pycnogenol. Thromb Res 1999;95:155–161.

44. Fusegawa Y, Goto S, Handa S, Kawada T, Ando Y. Platelet spontaneous aggregation in platelet-rich plasma is increased in habitual smokers. Thromb Res 1999;93:271–278.

45. Pernerstorfer T, Stohlawetz P, Stummvoll G, et al. Low-dose aspirin does not lower in vivo platelet activation in healthy smokers. Br J Haematol 1998;102:1229–1231.

46. Durand P, Prost M, Blache D. Folic acid deficiency enhances oral contraceptive-induced platelet hyperactivity. Arterioscler Thromb Vasc Biol 1997;17:1939–1946.

47. Mezzano D, Kosiel K, Martinez C, et al. Cardiovascular risk factors in vegetarians. Normalization of hyperhomocysteinemia with vitamin B(12) and reduction of platelet aggregation with n-3 fatty acids. Thromb Res 2000;100:153–160.

48. Cipollone F, Ciabattoni G, Patrignani P, et al. Oxidant stress and aspirin-insensitive thromboxane biosynthesis in severe unstable angina. Circulation 2000;102:1007–1013.

49. Wilkinson I, Megson I, MacCallum H, Sogo N, Cockcroft J, Webb D. Oral vitamin C reduces arterial stiffness and platelet aggregation in humans. J Cardiovasc Pharmacol 1999;34:690–693.

50. Pignatelli P, Pulcinelli F, Lenti L, Gazzaniga P, Violi F. Vitamin E inhibits collagen-induced platelet activation by blunting hydrogen peroxide. Arterioscler Thromb Vasc Biol 1999;19:2542–2547.

51. Kabakus N, Yilmaz B, Caliskan U. Investigation of platelet aggregation by impedance and optic methods in children with iron deficiency anaemia. Haematologia (Budap) 2000;30:107–115.

52. Kurekci A, Atay A, Sarici S, Zeybek C, Koseoglu V, Ozcan O. Effect of iron therapy on the whole blood platelet aggregation in infants with iron deficiency ancmia. Thromb Res 2000;97:281–285.

53. Nguyen A, Packham M, Rand M. Effects of ethanol on platelet responses associated with adhesion to collagen. Thromb Res 1999;95:303–314.

54. Zhang Q, Das K, Siddiqui S, Myers A. Effects of acute, moderate ethanol consumption on human platelet aggregation in platelet-rich plasma and whole blood. Alcohol Clin Exp Res 2000;24:528–534.

55. Ali M, Bordia T, Mustafa T. Effect of raw versus boiled aqueous extract of garlic and onion on platelet aggregation. Prostaglandins Leukotriene Med 1999;60:43–47.

56. Steiner M, Li W. Aged garlic extract, a modulator of cardiovascular risk factors: a dose-finding study on the effects of AGE on platelet functions. J Nutr 2001; 131:980S–984S.

57. Mori T, Beilin L, Burke V, Morris J, Ritchie J. Interactions between dietary fat, fish, and fish oils and their effects on platelet function in men at risk of cardiovascular disease. Arterioscler Thromb Vasc Biol 1997;17:279–286.

58. Varani K, Portaluppi F, Gessi S, et al. Dose and time effects of caffeine intake on human platelet adenosine A(2A) receptors: functional and biochemical aspects. Circulation 2000;102:285–289.

59. Li N, Wallen N, Hjemdahl P. Evidence for prothrombotic effects of exercise and limited protection by aspirin. Circulation 1999;100:1374–1379.

60. Hurlen M, Seljeflot I, Arnesen H. Increased platelet aggregability during exercise in patients with previous myocardial infarction. Lack of inhibition by aspirin. Thromb Res 2000;99:487–494.

61. Sanguigni V, Pignatelli P, Lenti L, et al. Short-term treatment with atorvastatin reduces platelet CD40 ligand and thrombin generation in hypercholesterolemic patients. Circulation 2005;111:412–419.

62. Musselman D, Tomer A, Manatunga A, et al. Exaggerated platelet reactivity in major depression. Am J Psychiatry 1996;153:1313–1317.

63. Faraday N, Goldschmidt-Clermont P, Bray P. Gender differences in platelet GPIIb-IIIa activation. Thromb Haemost 1997;77:748–754.

64. Bray P. Platelet glycoprotein polymorphisms as risk factors for thrombosis. Curr Opin Hematol 2000;7:284–289.

65. Feng D, Lindpaintner K, Larson M, et al. Increased platelet aggregability associated with platelet GPIIIa PlA2 polymorphism: the Framingham Offspring Study. Arterioscler Thromb Vasc Biol 1999;19:1142–1147.

66. Michelson A, Furman M, Goldschmidt-Clermont P, et al. Platelet GP IIIa Pl(A) polymorphisms display different sensitivities to agonists. Circulation 2000;101:1013–1018.

67. Kritzik M, Savage B, Nugent D, Santoso S, Ruggeri Z, Kunicki T. Nucleotide polymorphisms in the alpha2 gene define multiple alleles that are associated with differences in platelet alpha2 beta1 density. Blood 1998;92:2382–2388.

68. Afshar-Kharghan V, Li C, Khoshnevis-Asl M, Lopez J. Kozak sequence polymorphism of the glycoprotein (GP) Ibalpha gene is a major determinant of the plasma membrane levels of the platelet GPIb-IX-V complex. Blood 1999;94:186–191.

69. Kerrigan SW, Douglas I, Wray A, et al. A role for glycoprotein Ib in *Streptococcus sanguis*-induced platelet aggregation. Blood 2002;100:509–516.

70. Moran N, Morateck PA, Deering A, et al. Surface expression of glycoprotein Ibalpha is dependent on glycoprotein Ibbeta: evidence from a novel mutation causing Bernard-Soulier syndrome. Blood 2000;96:532–539.

71. Lind S. The bleeding time. In: Michelson A, ed. Platelets: Academic Press, San Diego, 2002;pp. 283–287.

72. Sramek R, Sramek A, Koster T, Briet E, Rosendaal F. A randomized and blinded comparison of three bleeding time techniques: the Ivy method, and the Simplate II method in two directions. Thromb Haemost 1992;67:514–518.

73. Bernardi M, Califf R, Kleiman N, Ellis S, Topol E. Lack of usefulness of prolonged bleeding times in predicting hemorrhagic events in patients receiving the 7E3 glycoprotein IIb/IIIa platelet antibody. The TAMI Study Group. Am J Cardiol 1993;72:1121–1125.

74. De Caterina R, Lanza M, Manca G, Strata G, Maffei S, Salvatore L. Bleeding time and bleeding: an analysis of the relationship of the bleeding time test with parameters of surgical bleeding. Blood 1994;84:3363–3370.

75. Rendu F. The platelet release reaction: granules' constituents, secretion and functions. Platelets 2001;12:261–273.

76. Pereira J, Soto M, Palomo I, et al. Platelet aging in vivo is associated with activation of apoptotic pathways: studies in a model of suppressed thrombopoiesis in dogs. Thromb Haemost 2002;87:905–909.

77. Trotter P, Orchard M, Walker J. Thrombin stimulates the intracellular relocation of annexin V in human platelets. Biochim Biophys Acta 1994;1222:135–140.

78. Hemker H, van Rijn J, Rosing J, van Dieijen G, Bevers E, Zwaal R. Platelet membrane involvement in blood coagulation. Blood Cells 1983;9:303–317.

79. Grau AJ, Reiners S, Lichy C, Buggle F, Ruf A, Jilma B. Platelet function under aspirin, clopidogrel, and both after ischemic stroke: a case-crossover study—synergistic antiplatelet effects of clopidogrel and aspirin detected with the PFA-100 in stroke patients. Stroke 2003;34:849–854.

80. Holthe MR, Staff AC, Berge LN, Lyberg T. Different levels of platelet activation in preeclamptic, normotensive pregnant, and nonpregnant women. Am J Obstet Gynecol 2004;190:1128–1134.

81. Obergfell A, Judd BA, del Pozo MA, et al. The molecular adapter SLP-76 relays signals from platelet integrin $\alpha_{IIb}\beta_3$ to the actin cytoskeleton. J Biol Chem 2001;276:5916–5923.

82. Gende O. Capacitative calcium influx and intracellular pH cross-talk in human platelets. Platelets 2003;14:9–14.

83. Drouin A, Favier R, Masse J-M, et al. Newly recognized cellular abnormalities in the gray platelet syndrome. Blood 2001;98:1382–1391.

84. So C, Wong K. May-Hegglin anomaly. Br J Haematol 2003;120:373.

85. White J, Mattson J, Nichols W, Luban N, Greinacher A. A variant of the Sebastian platelet syndrome with unique neutrophil inclusions. Platelets 2002;13:121–127.

86. Shankaran H, Alexandridis P, Neelamegham S. Aspects of hydrodynamic shear regulating shear-induced platelet activation and self-association of von Willebrand factor in suspension. Blood 2003;101:2637–2645.

87. Goto S, Tamura N, Eto K, Ikeda Y, Handa S. Functional significance of adenosine 5'-diphosphate receptor (P2Y(12)) in platelet activation initiated by binding of von Willebrand factor to platelet GP Ibα induced by conditions of high shear rate. Circulation 2002;105:2531–2536.

88. Ikeda M, Iwamoto S, Imamura H, Furukawa H, Kawasaki T. Increased platelet aggregation and production of platelet-derived microparticles after surgery for upper gastrointestinal malignancy. J. Surg Res 2003;115:174–183.

89. Eto K, Ochiai M. Isshiki T, et al. Platelet aggregability under shear is enhanced in patients with unstable angina pectoris who developed acute myocardial infarction. Jpn Circ J 2001;65:279–282.

90. Sakakibara M, Goto S, Eto K, et al. Application of ex vivo flow chamber system for assessment of stent thrombosis. Arterioscler Thromb Vasc Biol 2002; 22:1360–1364.

91. Kundu S, Heilmann E, Sio R, Garcia C, Ostegaard R. Characterization of an in vitro platelet function analyzer, PFA-100™. Clin App Thromb/Hemost 1996;2:241–249.

92. Francis J. Platelet function analyzer (PFA)-100. In: Michelson A, ed. Platelets, Academic Press, San Diego, 2002; pp. 325–332.
93. Quinn M, Fitzgerald D. Ticlopidine and Clopidogrel. Circulation 1999; 100:1667–1672.
94. Hankey GJ, Eikelboom JW. Aspirin resistance. BMJ 2004;328:477–479.
95. Campbell CL, Steinhubl SR. Variability in response to aspirin: do we understand the clinical relevance? J Throm Haemost 2005;3:665–669.
96. Eikelboom JW, Hirsh J, Weitz JI, et al. Aspirin-resistant thromboxane biosynthesis and the risk of myocardial infarction, stroke, or cardiovascular death in patients at high risk for cardiovascular events. Circulation 2002;105:1650–1655.
97. Marshall P, Williams A, Dixon R, et al. A comparison of the effects of aspirin on bleeding time measured using the Simplate method and closure time measured using the PFA-100, in healthy volunteers. Br J Clin Pharmacol 1997;44:151–155.
98. Homoncik M, Jilma B, Hergovich N, Stohlawetz P, Panzer S, Speiser W. Monitoring of aspirin (ASA) pharmacodynamics with the platelet function analyzer PFA-100. Thromb Haemost 2000;83:316–321.
99. Sambola A, Heras M, Escolar G, et al. The PFA-100 detects sub-optimal antiplatelet responses in patients on aspirin. Platelets 2004;15:439–446.
100. Malinin A, Spergling M, Muhlestein B, Steinhubl S, Serebruany V. Assessing aspirin responsiveness in subjects with multiple risk factors for vascular disease with a rapid platelet function analyzer. Blood Coagul Fibrinolysis 2004;15:295–301.
101. Harrison P, Segal H, Blasbery, et al. Screening for aspirin responsiveness after transient ischemic attack and stroke. Comparison of 2 point-of-care platelet function tests with optical aggregometry. Stroke 2005, in press.
102. Ciabattoni G, Maclouf J, Catella F, FitzGerald G, Patrono C. Radioimmunoassay of 11-dehydrothromboxane B2 in human plasma and urine. Biochimica Biophysic Acta 1987;918:293–297.
103. Feldman M, Cryer B. Aspirin absorption rates and platelet inhibition times with 325-mg buffered aspirin tablets (chewed or swallowed intact) and with buffered aspirin solution. Am J Cardiol 1999;84:404–409.
104. Brown N, May J, Wilcox R, Allan L, Wilson A, Kiff P, Heptinstall S. Comparison of antiplatelet activity of microencapsulated aspirin 162.5 Mg (Caspac XL), with enteric coated aspirin 75 mg and 150 mg in patients with atherosclerosis. Br J Clin Pharmacol 1999;48:57–62.
105. Belton O, Byrne D, Kearney D, Leahy A, Fitzgerald D. Cyclooxygenase-1 and -2-dependent prostacyclin formation in patients with atherosclerosis. Circulation 2000;102:840–845.
106. Bruno A, McConnell JP, Cohen SN, et al. Serial urinary 11-dehydrothromboxane B2, aspirin dose, and vascular events in blacks after recent cerebral infarction. Stroke 2004;35:727–730.
107. Aleil B, Ravanat C, Cazenave JP, et al. Flow cytometric analysis of intraplatelet VASP phosphorylation for the detection of clopidogrel resistance in patients with ischemic cardiovascular diseases. J Thromb Haemost 2005;3:85–92.
108. Geiger J, Teichmann L, Grossmann R, et al. Monitoring of clopidogrel action: comparison of methods. Clin Chem 2005, in press.
109. Quinn M, Cox D, Foley J, Fitzgerald D. Glycoprotein IIb/IIIa receptor number and occupancy during chronic administration of an oral antagonist. J Pharmacol Exp Ther 2000;295:670–676.
110. Theroux P, Gosselin G, Nasmith J, et al. The Accumetrics Rapid Platelet Function Analyzer (RPFA®) to monitor platelet aggregation during oral administration of a GPIIb/IIIa antagonist. J Am Coll Cardiol 1999;33:330A.
111. Kereiakes D, Mueller M, Howard W, et al. Efficacy of abciximab induced platelet blockade using a rapid point of care assay. J Thromb Thrombol 1999;7:265–275.

112. Steinhubl S, Kottke-Marchant K, Molitterno D, et al. Attainment and maintenance of platelet inhibition through standard dosing of abciximab in diabetic and non-diabetic patients undergoing percutaneous coronary intervention. Circulation 1999;100:1977–1982.

113. Steinhubl SR, Talley JD, Braden GA, Tcheng JE, Casterella PJ, Moliterno DJ, Navetta FI, Berger PB, Popma JJ, Dangas G, Gallo R, Sane DC, Saucedo JF, Jia G, Lincoff AM, Theroux P, Holmes DR, Teirstein PS, Kereiakes DJ. Point-of-care measured platelet inhibition correlates with a reduced risk of an adverse cardiac event after percutaneous coronary intervention: results of the GOLD (AU-Assessing Ultegra) multicenter study. Circulation 2001;103:2372–2578.

114. Quinn M, Deering A, Stewart M, Cox D, Foley B, Fitzgerald D. Quantifying GPIIb/IIIa receptor binding using 2 monoclonal antibodies: discriminating abciximab and small molecular weight antagonists. Circulation 1999;99:2231–2238.

115. Cox D, Smith R, Quinn M, Theroux P, Crean P, Fitzgerald D. Evidence of platelet activation during treatment with a GPIIb/IIIa antagonist in patients presenting with acute coronary syndromes. J Am Coll Cardiol 2000;36:1514–1519.

116. Hezard N, Metz D, Nazeyrollas P, et al. Free and total platelet glycoprotein IIb/IIIa measurement in whole blood by quantitative flow cytometry during and after infusion of c7E3 Fab in patients undergoing PTCA. Thromb Haemost 1999;81:869–873.

117. Ghiggeri G, Caridi G, Magrini U, et al. Genetics, clinical and pathological features of glomerulonephritis associated with mutations of nonmuscle myosin IIA (Fechtner syndrome). Am J Kidney Dis 2003;41:95–104.

118. Deutsch S, Rideau A, Bochaton-Piallat M, et al. D1424N MYH9 mutation results in an unstable protein responsible for the phenotypes in May-Hegglin anomaly/Fechtner syndrome. Blood 2003;102:529–534.

9 Platelet Function Under Flow

José A. López, MD, Ian del Conde, MD, and Jing-Fei Dong, MD, PhD

CONTENTS

INTRODUCTION

As vertebrates have evolved high-pressure, high-flow circulatory systems, an extraordinarily effective hemostatic system has developed alongside to protect these organisms from hemorrhage. More than a century's worth of evidence indicates that platelets are the blood cells chiefly responsible for maintaining hemostasis and causing thrombosis. Platelets are geared to monitor vascular integrity and effect hemostasis in the arterial circulation, as injuries to arteries (rather than veins) are much more likely to result in circulatory collapse and death. Furthermore, deployment of the hemostatic mechanism in the setting of vascular disease—particularly that caused by atherosclerosis—is largely responsible for the tremendous disease burden associated with vascular disease, being the culminating event in myocardial infarction and stroke. In this chapter, we review the characteristics of blood flow that influence

From: *Contemporary Cardiology:*
Platelet Function: Assessment, Diagnosis, and Treatment
Edited by: M. Quinn and D. Fitzgerald © Humana Press Inc., Totowa, NJ

Velocity Profile   **Shear Rate (Stress) Profile**

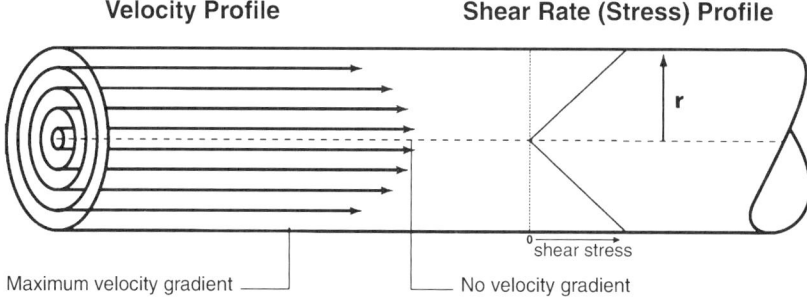

Fig. 1. Flow of an idealized fluid. The series of adjacent laminae have a parabolic velocity profile, with the fluid velocity greatest at the center of the tube and approaching zero at the vessel wall. Note the linear inverse relationship between the velocity and shear rate profiles.

platelet function and the cellular and molecular determinants that allow the platelets to carry out their hemostatic functions under flow.

HYDRODYNAMICS OF BLOOD FLOW

Sir Isaac Newton proposed that the flow of idealized fluids can be modeled by considering the fluid as being composed of an infinite number of adjacent layers (laminae) of infinitesimal thickness. In a tubular structure like a blood vessel, these laminae would constitute a series of concentric tubes, each of uniform velocity (Fig. 1). The velocity profile of these laminae in a plane transecting the center of the tube is parabolic, with the fluid velocity greatest at the center of the tube and diminishing to zero at the wall (Fig. 1). The force per unit area that tends to impede the flow of the laminae past each other, the *shear stress*, is proportional to the relative velocity between two adjacent layers, the *shear rate*. Thus, because the difference in flow between adjacent layers is greatest at the wall, that is also the site of greatest shear stress. The shear rate is a velocity gradient, representing the distance moved in the direction of flow divided by the distance between laminae. Conventionally, this is represented as cm per s per cm. Because the distance units (cm) cancel, the units of shear stress are inverse seconds (s^{-1}). The ratio of shear rate to shear stress is the viscosity of the fluid, representing the friction between layers.

In an idealized, *newtonian* fluid, the relationship between shear rate and shear stress remains constant regardless of shear rate, that is, the shear rate does not influence the viscosity (*see* just below). However, in non-newtonian fluids, such as blood, viscosity decreases with increasing

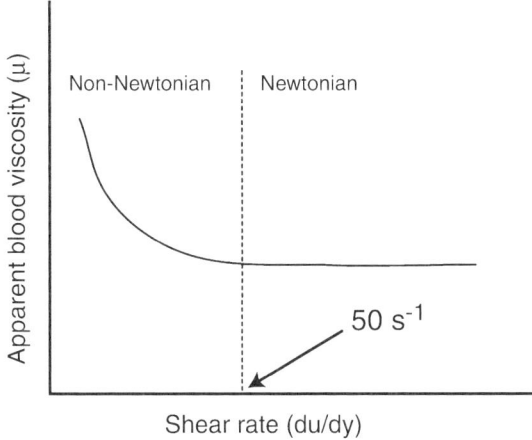

Fig. 2. Relationship between apparent viscosity and shear rate in blood. At low shear rates, the viscosity of blood, a non-newtonian fluid, increases with decreasing shear rates. At higher shear rates, however, it adopts more newtonian characteristics.

shear stress. This shear thinning phenomenon is most significant in the low shear range, resulting from a high content of erythrocytes (Fig. 2). The first derivative of the velocity profile is the shear rate, du/dt (note the linear inverse relationship between shear rate and velocity profile shown in Fig. 1). The shear stress at any point in the fluid stream is thus related to the velocity profile and to the shear rate by the equation.

$$\tau = \mu(du/dy)$$

where du/dy is the shear rate, μ is the viscosity, and u represents the axial velocity at a radial position y in the flood stream. The shear stress thus varies from 0 at the centerline to a maximum at the vessel wall.

Discussions of the effect of shear stress on platelet function often involve the terms *wall shear rate* and *wall shear stress*. These are useful because they can be expressed in terms of the volumetric flow rate and thus can be calculated for all vessels in which the flow rate and diameter can be measured. This relationship is represented by the equation:

$$\tau_w = 4\mu Q/\pi r^3$$

where τ_w is the wall shear stress, Q is the volumetric flow rate, and r is the vessel radius. Table 1 depicts the ranges in mean wall shear rates and shear stresses throughout the human vasculature.

Although these values are calculated based on volumetric flow rates and vessel diameters, in smaller blood vessels the values may overesti-

Table 1
Estimated Ranges of Wall Shear Rates and Stresses
at Different Sites of the Vasculature[a]

Blood vessel	Wall shear rate per second	Wall shear stress (dynes/cm^2)
Large arteries	300–800	11.4–30.4
Arterioles	500–1,600	19.0–60.8
Veins	20–200	0.76–7.6
Stenotic vessels	800–10,000	30.4–380

[a]The viscosity of blood is assumed to be 0.038 Poise (4).

mate actual shear rates, owing to alterations in viscosity related to the cellular content of the blood.

Blood circulates in a cardiovascular system consisting of vessels of various inner diameters and branching patterns. The patterns of flow are thus quite complex. Because of the periodic pumping action of the heart, blood flow in large arteries is pulsatile but becomes almost constant in small arterioles (diameter of 10–50 μm), in which it adopts more newtonian characteristics (1–3).

In addition to wall shear stress, the vascular endothelial cells, especially in arteries, are also subjected to tensile stress produced by the expansion and contraction of the vessel wall (4). This stretching force regulates the functions of the endothelial cells and the genes they express (5–7). Finally, at the areas of curves and branch points, regions of secondary flow are found, characterized by low wall shear stress and directional oscillation (3). Examples of these sites are the site of bifurcation of the carotids and iliacs and in the coronary tree. It is in these areas that atherosclerotic lesions commonly develop (3).

Blood cells of different sizes travel at different speeds depending on their axial location in the blood stream. Cells near the vessel wall move significantly more slowly than those traveling at the center of the fluid stream (2). In this cellular gradient, platelets, the smallest cellular component of blood, travel near the vessel wall and erythrocytes and leukocytes in the center. Circulating platelets are brought to the vascular surface by the processes of diffusion and convection. Diffusion is a directionless movement of platelets that depends on cell-cell collision caused by brownian motion and thus tends to distribute the platelets randomly in the fluid stream. Erythrocytes, the largest cell population in blood, play a critical role in platelet diffusion (8). It has been shown that changes in hematocrit from 0 to 40% result in an increase of two orders of magnitude in effective diffusion coefficient of platelets. Convection,

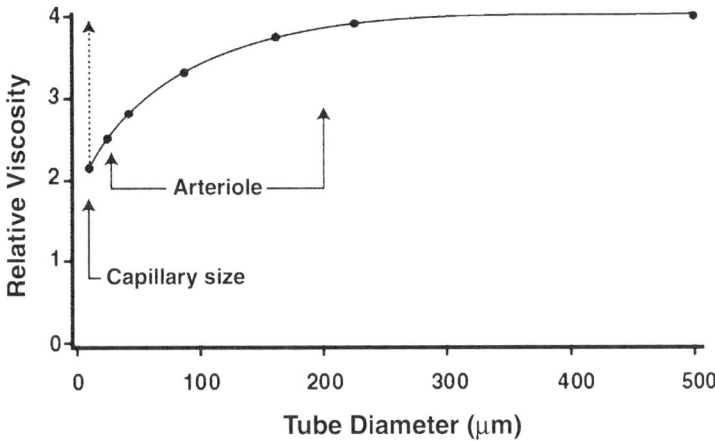

Fig. 3. Effect of vessel diameter on the relative viscosity of blood.

by contrast, is a much greater force that tends to move platelets toward the wall, with a magnitude related to the bulk flow of blood (8). Shear stress also enhances platelet diffusion in that an increase in wall shear rate from 10 to 1000 s^{-1} results in a greater than 10-fold increase in the rate of platelet diffusion (8).

Erythrocytes have another important effect on platelet behavior. As blood is pumped through ever smaller blood vessels, its apparent viscosity decreases—up to a point. This phenomenon is known as the Fåhraeus-Lindqvist effect and is caused by the axial accumulation and streaming of the erythrocytes, which stack in the smaller vessels in the center of the stream, leaving a plasma-rich margin a few microns thick along the wall of the blood vessel. In smaller vessels, the erythrocytes stack on each other in the center of the fluid stream, a process that facilitates their transit through these vessels. Thus, the relative viscosity of blood approaches that of plasma until the vessel diameter nears that of the red cell, or about 8 μm. At the capillary diameter of 4 μm, apparent viscosity increases because of the force required to push the deformable erythrocyte through the capillary (Fig. 3). Viscosity could increase even further with contraction of the precapillary sphincter, which can increase the viscosity owing to compression of the red cells to a point that flow ceases.

PLATELET ADHESION TO SITES OF INJURY

Although platelets circulate near the vessel wall, they are nevertheless faced with the daunting task of having to decelerate and stop at sites of vascular injury. To attach to the stationary surface from the rapidly flowing blood, platelets must form very rapid bonds between receptors

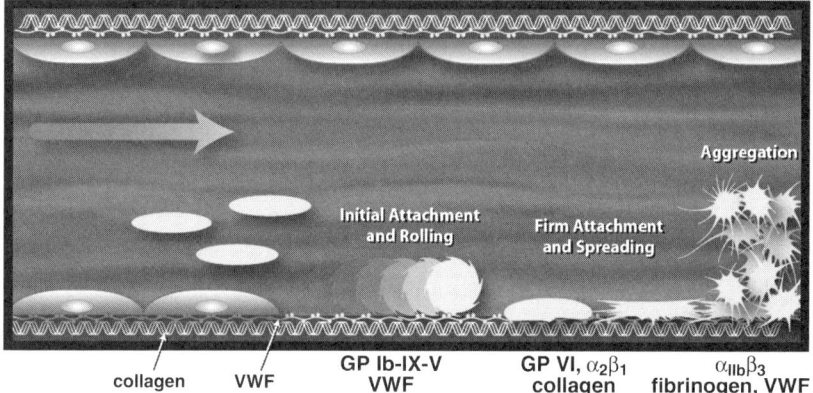

Fig. 4. Representation of the sequence of events in platelet-subendothelial interactions at a site of vascular injury. vWF, von Willebrand factor.

on their surfaces and ligands on the exposed vascular subendothelium. Because the shear stress is greatest at the vessel wall, the bonds experience tremendous torque, which they must be able to resist. The formation of a platelet plug at the site of vessel injury can be divided into three distinct and largely sequential steps: platelet attachment to the subendothelial matrix from the bulk flow, platelet activation and firm attachment, and platelet aggregation *(2)*. The process of platelet adhesion and the molecules involved are depicted in Fig. 4.

Glycoprotein Ib-IX-V Complex and von Willebrand Factor

Probably the most important ligand-receptor interaction in mediating platelet adhesion in regions of high shear stress is that between the platelet glycoprotein (GP)Ib-IX-V complex and von Willebrand factor (vWF). This interaction is the only one capable of capturing platelets from flowing blood at sites of vessel injury in the presence of elevated shear stress. It also enables the platelets to roll on the vWF-covered surface, in the process decelerating them and allowing for other ligand-receptor interactions that are characterized by slow on-rates, which on their own are inefficient in capturing platelets from rapidly flowing blood. In concert, the interactions of GPIb-IX-V with vWF and of the two collagen receptors, GPVI and $\alpha_2\beta_1$, with collagen send activation signals to the platelet interior. These signals have several consequences, including the secretion of granules (which amplifies platelet signals and also activates nearby platelets), the externalization of membrane anionic phospholipids and elaboration of platelet procoagulant activity, and conversion of the platelet integrins from quiescent to active forms. The activated integrins cause the platelets to adhere firmly to the surface, with $\alpha_2\beta_1$ mediating firm attachment to collagen and $\alpha_{IIb}\beta_3$ mediating attachment to surfaces containing vWF, fibrinogen, fibrin, or fibronectin (9).

The GPIb-IX-V complex is composed of four polypeptides, GPIbα, GPIbβ, GPIX, and GPV, with the entire ligand-binding function being carried out by the largest polypeptide, GPIbα (10). GPIbα interacts with immobilized vWF in the absence of modulators such as ristocetin or botrocetin, which are required for interaction between the complex and soluble vWF under static conditions (11). Under static conditions, the binding kinetics are very slow (12), suggesting that fluid shear stress plays an important role in promoting the interaction.

Shear stress has been reported to influence the conformations of both vWF and GPIbα to facilitate their interaction. Using atomic force microscopy, Siedlecki et al. (13) showed that vWF multimers attached to a hydrophobic surface are globular in the absence of flow and convert to an extended linear conformation after exposure to shear stress. In contrast, a recent study found no significant shear-induced changes in conformation of collagen-bound vWF (14), a form that more closely approximates that found in the vascular subendothelium. Evidence that shear might also induce an active conformation of the GPIb-IX-V complex was provided by Peterson et al. (15), who demonstrated that sheared platelets retained the ability to aggregate to added vWF for a short time after the shearing force was removed. The precise mechanism by which shear enhances GPIb-IX-V binding to vWF is yet to be determined.

On a surface of pure vWF, the velocity of rolling platelets increases with increasing shear stress until a plateau velocity is reached (16). This is an intrinsic characteristic of the GPIbα-vWF bond, as the same pattern is observed with the rolling of mammalian cells expressing the recombinant GPIb-IX-V complex (17). Gain- and loss-of-function mutations of either GPIbα or the vWF A1-domain manifest their phenotypes as reduced or increased rolling velocities, respectively (18). The decreased rolling velocity seen with the gain-of-function mutations results from a decrease in the off-rate of the bond between GPIbα and vWF (18), but gain-of-function mutations also increase the cellular on-rate considerably (that is, cells expressing GPIb-IX complexes with gain-of-function mutations of GPIbα attach more readily from bulk flow to a vWF-coated surface) (19).

Within the GPIb-IX-V complex, virtually all the regions known to be involved in the initial attachment of platelets and their subsequent rolling on a vWF surface reside within the largest polypeptide of the complex, GPIbα (10). This polypeptide contains the vWF-binding region within a domain encompassing the N-terminal 300 amino acids (of 623 in the most common of four polymorphic variants). In vWF, the entire GPIbα-binding region is contained in the first of three tandemly repeated A-domains with homology to the adhesive I-domains of integrins (20).

The GPIbα ligand-binding domain contains several subdomains that are worthy of note, each of which functions in the interaction with vWF (21–23). The structure is dominated by eight leucine-rich repeats (LRRs), which form a curved structure with the concave surface comprising a parallel β-sheet, each LRR contributing a strand to the structure. The LRR region is flanked by disulfide loops, one loop at the N terminus and two interdigitated loops at the C terminus. Downstream of the C-terminal loops is a region of extremely acidic character, containing 16 acidic side chains (including three sulfated tyrosines) in a stretch of 19 amino acids. Each of these subdomains is involved in the interaction of GPIbα with vWF.

The crystal structure of a complex between the N-terminal 290 amino acids of GPIbα and the vWF A1-domain reveals extended contacts between the two proteins, with two areas of tight contact (23). The most extensive contact involves GPIbα LRRs 5 through 8 and the C-terminal flanking loops, which interact with the A1-domain through A1-helix α_3, loop $\alpha_3\beta_4$, and strand β_3. Gain- and loss-of-function mutations of the first C-terminal disulfide loop of GPIbα function either to enhance or to diminish the interaction with vWF, but they rarely eliminate it (18). The gain-of-function mutations are postulated to stabilize a β-hairpin that aligns two β-strands in antiparallel fashion, contributing to a triple-stranded intermolecular β-sheet that includes as its third strand a sequence composed of vWF residues D560–Y565 from strand β_3 of the A1-domain (23).

The second, and smaller, site involves sequences in the N-terminal loop of GPIbα, the so-called β-finger region, with binds to the $\alpha_1\beta_2$ and $\beta_3\alpha_2$ loops of the A1-domain, near where the N and C termini of the A1-domain come together. Because both of these termini are attached to other globular domains in intact vWF, they are likely to be shielded in the plasma form of vWF, which has a much lower affinity for GPIbα than the isolated A1-domain. Of interest, the A1-domains in newly produced ultralarge forms of vWF bind to GPIbα with the same bond strength as does the isolated A1-domain, suggesting that in this form of vWF the A1-domain is exposed, becoming cryptic after processing in the plasma (24).

In addition to the two regions of direct tight contact, A1 and the N terminus of GPIbα have complementary surfaces of opposite charge that may mediate long-range electrostatic interactions between the two molecules (23); within GPIbα they involve most of the β-sheet surface.

The participation of the N- and C-terminal flanks of GPIbα and the first LLR in the interaction with the vWF A1-domain had previously been inferred from the mapping of inhibitory antibodies. Most of the antibodies that inhibit ristocetin- and shear-induced vWF binding map to the N-terminal flank and the first and second LRRs, although two inhibitory antibodies map to the C-terminal flank (25). Of interest, with respect to the potential importance of the long-range electrostatic interactions that involve the middle LRRs, the inhibitory GPIbα antibody 6D1 maps to LRR4.

The N-terminal 58 amino acids of human GPIbα also mediate the species-specific interaction with vWF, a conclusion based on the fact that GPIbα chimeras in which these amino acids have been replaced by the corresponding canine sequence lose their capacity for ristocetin-induced vWF binding (26).

Although the anionic sulfated region in the crystal structure of the complex of the GPIbα N terminus and the A1-domain was found to be disordered and therefore assumed to have no role in the interaction with GPIbα (23), substantial evidence exists that it does have a role in the adhesive interaction between the intact molecules. Suppression of sulfation in cells expressing the recombinant complex moderately reduces the ristocetin-induced interaction while completely eliminating the interaction induced by the other modulator, botrocetin (27–29). In addition, conversion of the three tyrosines to phenylalanines markedly disrupts both ristocetin- and botrocetin-induced interactions and the interaction of mutant-expressing cells with immobilized vWF under conditions of flow (30). By contrast, if the tyrosines are replaced by glutamates, which have a similar charge, the ristocetin-induced and shear-induced interactions are indistinguishable from those seen with wild-type GPIbα (30).

GPVI and $\alpha_2\beta_1$

Also important for adhesion under shear are the two collagen receptors, GPVI and integrin $\alpha_2\beta_1$, as well as integrin $\alpha_{IIb}\beta_3$. Collagen is the most abundant protein in the vascular matrix (31–33). Fibrillar collagens types I and III are major species in human arteries, along with types IV, V, and VI (34–38). Types I and III collagen are also abundant in atherosclerotic plaque (38–41). All of these collagens are able to bind platelets, albeit to different degrees. Of the major collagen receptors, GPVI appears to be more important for the early phases of platelet activation after the adhesion of platelets from flowing blood, acting primarily as a signaling molecule that works in concert with the GPIb-IX-V complex to activate the integrins and to induce granule secretion and thromboxane

A$_2$ formation *(42)*. Both integrins ($\alpha_2\beta_1$ and $\alpha_{IIb}\beta_3$) exist in quiescent states that are activated by signals produced by GPIb-IX-V and GPVI and by soluble agonists secreted by the platelets. They function to attach the platelets firmly to the subendothelial surface, $\alpha_2\beta_1$ by binding collagen and $\alpha_{IIb}\beta_3$ by binding vWF, fibrinogen, or fibronectin. $\alpha_{IIb}\beta_3$ also mediates platelet aggregation by binding soluble ligands, either fibrinogen or vWF.

GPVI belongs to a family of type I transmembrane proteins that include the family of natural killer receptors *(42)*. The polypeptide contains 339 amino acids, with two tandem extracellular Ig-C2 domains, each with a single disulfide loop. These domains are separated from the plasma membrane by a mucin-like domain predicted to contain several O-linked carbohydrate chains. Within the transmembrane domain, the polypeptide contains a single arginine residue, through which it associates noncovalently with Fcγ-chain homodimers, similar to the manner by which other receptors associate with the Fcγ-chain. The cytoplasmic domain is rather short (51 amino acids), with prominent features including a proline-rich domain that attracts the SH3 domain of the Src kinases Fyn and Lyn *(43)*, and a region rich in basic residues that binds calmodulin *(44)*.

GPVI binds collagen through a motif containing the sequence GPO (glycine-proline-hydroxyproline), which makes up approx 10% of the sequence of types I and III collagen and does not overlap the site bound by $\alpha_2\beta_1$ *(45)*. Crosslinked helical peptides composed of repeating GPO sequences (collagen-related peptide [CRP]) have been shown to be very potent platelet activators, a function that they carry out exclusively by binding GPVI *(45)*. CRP is up to 100 times more potent in activating platelets than collagen, possibly as a consequence of its high density of GPVI-binding motifs *(45)*. This finding indicates definitively that GPVI can transduce potent activation signals, but it remains an open question as to whether it is the only or primary mediator of platelet activation on native subendothelial matrix.

The other major collagen receptor, $\alpha_2\beta_1$, is a typical integrin, capable of binding not only collagen but also other ligands such as laminin, decorin, and fibronectin, depending on the cellular context *(46–49)*. Recent evidence suggests that like other integrins, $\alpha_2\beta_1$ only binds its ligands efficiently when activated by "inside-out" signals originating at other receptors, which induce a change in the integrin's extracellular conformation by modifying its intracellular domains *(47)*. Most of the collagen-binding properties of $\alpha_2\beta_1$ reside within an adhesive I-domain found in the α-chain, a motif homologous to the A-domains of vWF that mediate interactions with GPIbα and collagen *(50)*. The isolated I-domain has been crystallized in complex with a collagen peptide, revealing that the I-domain conformation is different when bound to ligand than when unbound *(51,52)*.

The involvement of $\alpha_2\beta_1$ in mediating platelet firm adhesion depends on the collagen substrate. For example, Savage et al. *(53)* found that inhibiting $\alpha_2\beta_1$ had no effect on the adhesion of human platelets to fibrillar type I collagen at either high or low shear stresses, but they noted a critical requirement for the integrin when the substrate was pepsin-solubilized type I collagen. Nieswandt and coworkers *(54)* observed similar requirements using mice lacking the β_1-subunit. These results have been interpreted as indicating that the fibrillar structure of the collagen is a critical determinant of its recognition by integrins, but they can also be explained by our recent observation that different commercial preparations of fibrillar collagen are substantially contaminated with vWF, whereas the acid-soluble forms are not *(55)*. This being the case, on fibrillar collagen containing bound vWF, the function of $\alpha_2\beta_1$ in firm adhesion could be replaced by $\alpha_{IIb}\beta_3$, which is able to bind an RGD-containing motif in vWF.

Signaling

Early activation signals following initial platelet adhesion are indispensable for subsequent thrombus growth, and it appears that both the GPIb-IX-V complex and GPVI cooperate in stimulating signaling pathways that activate both $\alpha_2\beta_1$ and $\alpha_{IIb}\beta_3$ and induce granule secretion and thromboxane A_2 production. Although in vivo the activation signals are very complex, it is clear that the GPIb-VWF interaction on its own is able to activate platelets. For example, binding of vWF to GPIb-IX expressed in Chinese hamster ovary (CHO) cells leads to phosphorylation of the tyrosine kinase Syk (normally not expressed in CHO cells) *(56)*. Even in the absence of Syk in these cells, engagement of vWF by GPIb is able to increase the strength of $\alpha_{IIb}\beta_3$-fibrinogen bonds by a similar degree as the addition of manganese ion, considered to induce the fully active conformation of $\alpha_{IIb}\beta_3$ *(57)*.

At lower shear stresses, the firm attachment of platelets to a vWF-coated surface (which requires tethering through GPIb-IX-V and firm attachment through $\alpha_{IIb}\beta_3$) requires primary signals from GPIb-IX-V and secondary signals from ADP released from the platelet granules *(58)*. At higher shear stresses (1800 s^{-1}, or about 70–80 dynes/cm^2), the full effect is seen even in the presence of ADP scavengers, indicating that the full signal produced by vWF binding to GPIbα is transmitted when stress is applied to the bond. Recent evidence from Rathore and colleagues *(59)* provides a potential explanation for this observation. These investigators found that vWF binding to the GPIb-IX-V complex induces phosphorylation and activation of platelet-endothelial cell adhesion molecule-1 (PECAM-1), a membrane protein containing an immunoreceptor tyrosine-based inhibitory motif (ITIM). Phosphorylation of this motif attracts the phosphatase SHP-2, which downmodulates signals by dephosphorylating immunoreceptor tyrosine-based activation motif (ITAM) phosphotyrosines. Three groups have shown a similar effect of PECAM-1 activation upon stimulation of GPVI-dependent signaling pathways $(60–62)$. Of interest with respect to the influence of shear, Rathore et al. (59) found increased thrombus formation on vWF in mice lacking PECAM-1 at shear rates of 600 s^{-1} and 800 s^{-1}, but not at 1200 s^{-1}, the highest shear rate tested.

It is generally appreciated that GPVI signals more potently than the GPIb-IX-V complex to activate platelets, especially given that platelets perfused over a surface of pure vWF rarely form thrombi and tend to roll continuously on the surface without becoming fixed. On collagen, on the other hand, platelets become fixed to the surface soon after adhering and rapidly bind other platelets to form thrombi. What seems likely is that the two receptors work in concert to produce the maximum effect. This is suggested by the fact that high levels of GPVI must be expressed in heterologous cells to transduce signals upon binding to collagen and by early studies showing that collagen-induced platelet aggregation is inhibited by antibodies against GPIbα (63). The latter finding is probably explained by contamination of the collagen preparations by vWF (55), but it nevertheless illustrates the cooperation of the two receptors.

Furthermore, several C-type lectin snake venom proteins activate platelets potently by binding both GPIbα and GPVI, including alboaggregin A (64), convulxin (65) (previously thought to be a GPVI–specific reagent), and alboluxin (66). Finally, Goto and coworkers (67) have demonstrated that many GPIb-IX-V complex-dependent functions can be negatively modulated by antibodies against GPVI that deplete the glycoprotein from the platelet surface.

Interestingly, the signaling pathways induced by the GPIb-IX-V complex and GPVI share many similarities. Both receptors, for example, have been shown to be localized to membrane microdomains called rafts that serve as signaling platforms, attracting numerous cytoplasmic signaling proteins $(68–70)$. The signals from both of these receptors appear to be dependent on their localization to these domains. In addition, the ability of the GPIb-IX-V complex to mediate adhesion efficiently to a vWF surface also depends on its localization to rafts (68). Critical steps in both signaling pathways include activation of kinases of the Src family, phosphorylation of Syk and phospholipase Cγ2, and activation of phosphoinositide 3 kinase $(45,71)$.

PLATELETS AND THE COAGULATION CASCADE

In addition to coating the exposed subendothelial surface at sites of vessel injury and heaping up to form thrombi, platelets associated with the vessel wall also facilitate the enzymatic reactions involved in generating thrombin and insoluble fibrin. For example, considerable recent evidence has surfaced showing that tissue factor (TF), the rate-limiting factor in the initiation of blood coagulation, is present in substantial quantities in blood in an encrypted form *(72,73)*. This blood-borne TF resides primarily on membrane-containing microvesicles (MVs) that arise from cells of the monocyte/macrophage lineage. Recent studies of in vivo thrombus formation indicate that TF becomes associated with the developing platelet thrombus before the appearance of fibrin *(74)*. The MVs dock to the activated platelets within the thrombus through the binding of P-selectin glycoprotein ligand-1 (PSGL-1) on the MV to platelet P-selectin, which appears on the platelet surface when the α-granules are released. This docking requirement may explain why inhibitors targeted against either counterreceptor have potent antithrombotic effects *(75–79)*. Recent evidence from our laboratory indicates that the MVs actually fuse with the platelet plasma membrane, in the process transferring their membranes and vesicle contents to the platelet *(80)*.

Full activation of the platelets also results in externalization of the anionic phospholipid phosphatidylserine, a critical requirement for assembly of the tenase and prothrombinase complexes on the platelet surface *(81)*. Finally, the reactions that allow feedback maintenance of blood coagulation also occur on the platelet surface, with thrombin produced in the initial round of reactions feeding back to activate factor XI to XIa, which will then activate factor IX and assembly of the intrinsic tenase *(82)*. This reaction involves a specialized subset of GPIb-IX-V complexes localized to lipid rafts on activated platelets *(83)*, the most likely mechanism involving the formation of a trimolecular complex among factor XI, thrombin, and GPIbα *(84)*. These reactions facilitate the formation and growth of platelet thrombi by producing thrombin, which not only activates newly arriving platelets but also stabilizes the developing thrombus by producing an insoluble fibrin mesh.

PLATELET INTERACTIONS WITH INTACT ENDOTHELIUM

Platelets can also bind endothelial cells, a prerequisite being prior activation of the endothelial cells and release of their Weibel-Palade bodies. This process externalizes two receptors for platelets, P-selectin and vWF *(85)*. Both bind platelet GPIbα, the former through a process similar to its recognition of PSGL-1, although the interaction is not inhibited by heparin *(86)*. GPIbα shares many features with PSGL-1, both receptors being heavily O-glycosylated elongated polypeptides with a highly anionic region containing tyrosine sulfates sitting atop a mucin-like stalk *(21)*. GPIbα binds P-selectin with low affinity and rapid bond kinetics, consistent with the interaction largely serving a surveillance function, that is, wherever platelets encounter P-selectin, they remain in loose contact with the endothelium *(87)*. This may serve as an additional mechanism facilitating efficient platelet recognition of sites of vessel wall injury or may contribute to the inflammatory role of platelets during systemic or local inflammation. Indeed, Katayama and coworkers *(87)* demonstrated that the periendothelial velocities of platelets in mice was markedly reduced with injection of endotoxin, a phenomenon that was prevented with antibodies against either GPIbα or P-selectin.

In addition to P-selectin, vWF also serves as an endothelial ligand for platelets. We recently demonstrated that histamine stimulation of cultured endothelial cells releases very large strands of vWF that remain attached to the endothelial surface and may reach lengths of several millimeters *(88)*. These ultralarge multimers of vWF are able to bind platelets efficiently, producing long beads-on-a-string structures. These structures are rapidly cleaved in the presence of normal plasma by the metalloprotease ADAMTS-13 (A disintegrin and metalloproteinase with thrombospondin motifs), a process deranged in the sometimes catastrophic condition thrombotic thrombocytopenic purpura, owing to absence of the protease *(89,90)* or its inhibition by antibodies *(91,92)*. Considerable evidence has emerged recently indicating that ADAMTS-13 activity varies substantially in the human population, as a consequence of both genetic polymorphism *(93)* and clinical condition *(94–98)*, raising the possibility that this mechanism of platelet attachment to the blood vessel wall may contribute to clinical thrombosis.

SHEAR-INDUCED PLATELET AGGREGATION

In addition to platelet adhesion to the subendothelium or stimulated endothelial cells, platelets can be induced to aggregate by soluble vWF under high fluid shear stress in the absence of any modulators *(99–104)*. This phenomenon is termed shear-induced platelet aggregation and is likely to be seen in areas of arterial stenosis, where fluid shear stresses are markedly elevated *(105)* (Table 1). Furthermore, ex vivo shear-induced platelet aggregation has been demonstrated to be enhanced in thrombotic diseases, such as myocardial infarction *(106)* and thrombotic thrombocytopenic purpura *(107)*.

Shear-induced platelet aggregation is a direct result of platelet-platelet collision and is thus affected by the frequency and efficiency of these collisions, the collision efficiency being defined as the faction of all collisions that result in binding. The collision frequency is determined by the level of applied shear stress and the total number of collisions and by the duration for which the shear stress is applied *(99,108)*. The collision efficiency, on the other hand, is determined by several factors, including the duration of contact between platelets and the concentration of soluble ligands that mediate the interaction between individual platelets. Obviously, another factor that will increase collision efficiency is the number of active adhesive receptors on the platelet surface. Thus, collision efficiency increases in the presence of chemical agonists *(99)* (which activate $\alpha_{IIb}\beta_3$ and increase the likelihood that it will bind fibrinogen) and with increasing size of vWF multimers, which bind more efficiently to both GPIbα and $\alpha_{IIb}\beta_3$ *(105,109)*. Erythrocytes increase the collision efficiency mechanically by prolonging the lifetime of platelet-platelet interaction *(110–114)* and chemically by releasing platelet agonists such as ADP *(113,115)*.

Although high shear stress is a major factor that induces platelet aggregation, the pattern and duration of shear stress are also important in determining the extent of shear-induced platelet aggregation. Local flow in the area of stenosis may be quite complex. Approaching a stenotic area, blood near the vessel wall first decelerates and then accelerates in proportion to the reduced cross-sectional area. For example, an 80% reduction in cross-sectional area of a vessel results in a more than 10-fold increase of the flow rate *(8)*. In addition, a region of flow perpendicular to the vessel wall develops, producing a local recirculation zone *(8,99)*. The flow profile in this recirculation zone is characterized by low shear and long residence time. Platelet-platelet collision and blood coagulation are both found to be increased in the recirculation zone *(8)*. Furthermore, factors secreted by platelets and other cells accumulate in this area, reaching concentrations sufficient to activate platelets. These facts suggest that, in addition to high shear stress, the low shear environment created by recirculation may also be important for inducing shear-induced platelet aggregation *(8,116)*. For example, Sutera *(117)* found that subjecting platelets to repeated short pulses of high shear stress resulted in more platelet aggregation than continuous exposure for the same period. We recently demonstrated that a pulse of high shear for as short as 2.5 s can lead to platelet aggregation, but only when it is followed by a period of low shear *(118)*. By contrast, significantly longer durations of constant high shear stress are required to induce a similar extent of aggregation *(100–104,106)*.

As in platelet adhesion to subendothelium, shear-induced platelet aggregation is also initiated by the GPIb-vWF interaction and requires platelet $\alpha_{IIb}\beta_3$ integrin *(109)*. In many respects, shear-induced platelet aggregation is mirrored closely by ristocetin-induced platelet aggregation. The two interactions involve the same sequences in the ligand and the receptor, and both activate similar signaling pathways *(119)*. The extent of platelet aggregation induced by both shear stress and ristocetin is proportional to the size of vWF, with the larger multimers of vWF being more potent *(105,109)*.

METHODS TO STUDY PLATELET FUNCTION UNDER SHEAR

Platelet function in flowing liquid under defined shear stresses is generally evaluated using two types of devices and their derivatives: viscometers and flow chamber systems.

Two types of viscometer are in general use. In the Couette viscometer, platelet samples are exposed to shear stress generated by rotating a co-axial cylinder around a stationary bob *(99,114,120)*. The cone and plate viscometer exposes platelet samples to shear stress generated by a rotating cone on a flat plate. In either case, shear stress is the measure of torque force required to rotate the cone or coaxial cylinder at defined speeds and is uniform throughout the shearing field. Viscometers are ideal for measuring shear-induced cell-cell interactions in the fluid phase and are often used to model conditions such as arterial stenosis. Recently, these devices have been modified to measure real-time shear-induced platelet aggregation and activation and to assess the interactions of platelets with adherent cells *(121,122)*.

As opposed to viscometers, flow chambers and their derivatives primarily measure the interaction of flowing cells with a surface coated with ligand or adherent cells. One of the most commonly used is the parallel-plate flow chamber system, which is composed of a polycarbonate stab, a silicon gasket that determines the height of the chamber, and a glass cover slip (or culture dish) coated with matrix proteins or adherent cells. Fluid is drawn through the chamber at a defined velocity, generating a known shear stress for a fluid with known viscosity. Interactions between platelets (or other cells) in flowing fluid and the immobilized matrix or cells can be monitored in real time with an inverted microscope and recorded optically.

A number of variations of the parallel-plate chamber rely on similar concepts, including the use of capillary tubes *(123)*. Shear stress is also taken into account in the clinical measurement of platelet function in the device called the Platelet Function Analyzer-100, or PFA-100, which applies the concepts of the parallel-plate flow chamber to the rapid analysis of clinical samples *(124,125)*. With this device, anticoagulated whole blood is aspirated through a capillary and then through an aperture of defined diameter in a membrane coated with collagen and ADP (or epinephrine). High shear stress, collagen, and ADP (or epinephrine) activate platelets as they near the membrane, leading to accumulation of a thrombus at the aperture, which gradually diminishes and finally arrests blood flow. The time to closure of the aperture is used as a measure of platelet activation and aggregation induced by a combination of high shear and chemical agonists *(124)*.

SUMMARY

Evaluation of platelet function is different from evaluation of the functions of any other cells, not only because platelets lack nuclei and are thus less amenable than virtually all other cell types to genetic manipulation (technically, or course, platelets are not cells at all, although they behave like them), but also because they are designed to function in rapidly flowing blood, a factor that must be considered carefully when evaluating platelet function. In this review, we have attempted to provide an overview of flow and the physical forces in flowing blood that affect platelet function, of the molecules involved specifically in platelet functions under flow, and of the means by which platelet function under flow is evaluated.

REFERENCES

1. Turitto VT. Blood viscosity, mass transport, and thrombogenesis. Prog Hemost Thromb 1982;6:139–177.
2. Rugger Z. Mechanisms initiating platelet thrombus formation. Thromb Haemost 1997;78:611–616.
3. Wootton DM, Ku DN. Fluid mechanics of vascular systems, diseases, and thrombosis. Annu Rev Biomed Eng 1999;1:299–329.
4. Kroll MH, Hellums JD, McIntire LV, Schafer AI, Moake JL. Platelets and shear stress. Blood 1996;88:1525–1541.
5. Langille BL. Morphologic responses of endothelium to shear stress: reorganization of the adherens junction. Microcirculation 2001;8:195–206.
6. Fujimura Y, Titani K, Holland LZ, et al. A heparin-binding domain of human von Willebrand factor. Characterization and localization to a tryptic fragment extending from amino acid residue Val-449 to Lys-728. J Biol Chem 1987;262:1734–1739.
7. Resnick N, Gimbrone MA Jr. Hemodynamic forces are complex regulators of endothelial gene expression. FASEB J 1995;9:874–882.
8. Turitto VT, Hall CL. Mechanical factors affecting hemostasis and thrombosis. Thromb Res 1998;92:S25–S31.
9. Du X, Ginsberg MH. Integrin $\alpha_{IIb}\beta_3$ and platelet function. Thromb Haemost 1997;78:96–100.
10. López JA. The platelet glycoprotein Ib-IX complex. Blood Coagul Fibrinolysis 1994;5:97–119.

11. Sakariassen KS, Bolhuis PA, Sixma JJ. Human blood platelet adhesion to artery subendothelium is mediated by factor VIII-von Willebrand factor bound to subendothelium. Nature 1979;279:636–638.

12. Olson JD, Moake JL, Collins MF, Michael BS. Adhesion of human platelets to purified solid-phase von Willebrand factor: studies of normal and Bernard-Soulier platelets. Thromb Res 1983;32:115–122.

13. Siedlecki CA, Lestini BJ, Kottke-Marchant KK, Eppell SJ, Wilson DL, Marchant RE. Shear-dependent changes in the three-dimensional structure of human von Willebrand factor. Blood 1996;88:2939–2950.

14. Novak L, Deckmyn H, Damjanovich S, Harsfalvi J. Shear-dependent morphology of von Willebrand factor bound to immobilized collagen. Blood 2002;99:2070–2076.

15. Peterson DM, Stathopoulos NA, Giorgio TD, Hellums JD, Moake JL. Shear-induced platelet aggregation requires von Willebrand factor and platelet membrane glycoproteins Ib and IIb-IIIa. Blood 1987;69:625–628.

16. Savage B, Saldivar E, Ruggeri ZM. Initiation of platelet adhesion by arrest onto fibrinogen or translocation on von Willebrand factor. Cell 1996;84:289–297.

17. Fredrickson BJ, Dong JF, McIntire LV, López JA. Shear-dependent rolling on von Willebrand factor of mammalian cells expressing the platelet glycoprotein Ib-IX-V complex. Blood 1998;92:3684–3693.

18. Dong J, Schade AJ, Romo GM, et al. Novel gain-of-function mutations of platelet glycoprotein Ibα by valine mutagenesis in the Cys–Cys248 disulfide loop. Functional analysis under static and dynamic conditions. J Biol Chem 2000; 275:27663–27670.

19. Kumar AR, Dong JF, Cruz M, López JA, McIntire LV. Kinetics of GP Ibα-VWF-A1 tether bond under flow: effect of GP Ibα mutations on the association and dissociation rates. Biophys J, 2003;85:4099–4109.

20. Andrews RK, Shen Y, Gardiner EE, Dong JF, López JA, Berndt MC. The glycoprotein Ib-IX-V complex in platelet adhesion and signaling. Thromb Haemost 1999;82:357–364.

21. López JA, Dong JF. Structure and function of the glycoprotein Ib-IX-V complex. Curr Opin Hematol 1997;4:323–329.

22. Uff S, Clemetson JM, Harrison T, Clemetson KJ, Emsley J. Crystal structure of the platelet glycoprotein Ib(alpha) N-terminal domain reveals an unmasking mechanism for receptor activation. J Biol Chem 2002;277:35657–35663.

23. Huizinga EG, Tsuji S, Romijn RA, et al. Structures of glycoprotein Ibalpha and its complex with von Willebrand factor A1 domain. Science 2002;297:1176–1179.

24. Arya M, Anvari B, Romo GM, et al. Ultralarge multimers of von Willebrand factor form spontaneous high-strength bonds with the platelet glycoprotein Ib-IX complex: studies using optical tweezers. Blood 2002;99:3971–3977.

25. Shen Y, Romo GM, Dong J, et al. Requirement of leucine-rich repeats of glycoprotein (GP) Ibα for shear-dependent and static binding of von Willebrand factor to the platelet membrane GP Ib-IX-V complex. Blood 2000;95:903–910.

26. Shen Y, Dong J, Romo GM, et al. Functional analysis of the C-terminal flanking sequence of platelet glycoprotein Iba using canine-human chimeras. Blood 2002;99:145–150.

27. Dong J-F, Li CQ, López JA. Tyrosine sulfation of the GP Ib-IX complex: identification of sulfated residues and effect on ligand binding. Biochemistry 1994;33:13946–13953.

28. Ward CM, Andrews RK, Smith AI, Berndt MC. Mocarhagin, a novel cobra venom metalloproteinase, cleaves the platelet von Willebrand factor receptor glycoprotein Ibα. Identification of the sulfated tyrosine/anionic sequence Tyr-276–Glu-282 of

glycoprotein Ibα as a binding site for von Willebrand factor and α-thrombin. Biochemistry 1996;35:4929–4938.

29. Marchese P, Murata M, Mazzucato M, et al. Identification of three tyrosine residues of glycoprotein Ibα with distinct roles in von Willebrand factor and α-thrombin binding. J Biol Chem 1995;270:9571–9578.

30. Dong J, Ye P, Schade AJ, et al. Tyrosine sulfation of glycoprotein Ibα. Role of electrostatic interactions in von Willebrand factor binding. J Biol Chem 2001;276:16690–16694.

31. Pareti FI, Niiya K, McPherson JM, Ruggeri ZM. Isolation and characterization of two domains of human von Willebrand factor that interact with fibrillar collagen types I and III. J Biol Chem 1987;262:13835–13841.

32. Pareti FI, Fujimura Y, Dent JA, Holland LZ, Zimmerman TS, Ruggeri ZM. Isolation and characterization of a collagen binding domain in human von Willebrand factor. J Biol Chem 1986;261:15310–15315.

33. Rand JH, Patel ND, Schwartz E, Zhou SL, Potter BJ. 150-kD von Willebrand factor binding protein extracted from human vascular subendothelium is type VI collagen. J Clin Invest 1991;88:253–259.

34. Murata K, Kotake C, Motoyama T. Collagen species in human aorta: with special reference to basement membrane-associated collagens in the intima and media and their alteration with atherosclerosis. Artery 1987;14:229–247.

35. Murata K, Motayama T, Kotake C. Collagen types in various layers of the human aorta and their changes with the atherosclerotic process. Atherosclerosis 1986;60:251–262.

36. Shekhonin BV, Domogatsky SP, Idelson GL, Koteliansky VE, Rukosuev VS. Relative distribution of fibronectin and type I, III, IV, V collagens in normal and atherosclerotic intima of human arteries. Atherosclerosis 1987;67:9–16.

37. Gay S, Balleisen L, Remberger K, Fietzek PP, Adelmann BC, Kuhn K. Immunohistochemical evidence for the presence of collagen type III in human arterial walls, arterial thrombi, and in leukocytes, incubated with collagen in vitro. Klin Wochenschr 1975;53:899–902.

38. McCullagh KG. Increased type I collagen in human atherosclerotic plaque. Atherosclerosis 1983;46:247–248.

39. McCullagh KG, Ehrhart LA. Increased arterial collagen synthesis in experimental canine atherosclerosis. Atherosclerosis 1974;19:13–28.

40. McCullagh KG, Duance VC, Bishop KA. The distribution of collagen types I, III and V (AB) in normal and atherosclerotic human aorta. J Pathol 1980;130:45–55.

41. McCullagh KG, Ehrhart LA. Enhanced synthesis and accumulation of collagen in cholesterol-aggravated pigeon atherosclerosis. Atherosclerosis 1977;26:341–352.

42. Clemetson KJ, Clemetson JM. Platelet collagen receptors. Thromb Haemost 2001;86:189–197.

43. Suzuki-Inoue K, Tulasne D, Shen Y, et al. Association of Fyn and Lyn with the proline-rich domain of glycoprotein VI regulates intracellular signaling. J Biol Chem 2002;277:21561–21566.

44. Andrews RK, Suzuki-Inoue K, Shen Y, Tulasne D, Watson SP, Berndt MC. Interaction of calmodulin with the cytoplasmic domain of platelet glycoprotein VI. Blood 2002;99:4219–4221.

45. Nieswandt B, Watson SP. Platelet-collagen interaction: is GPVI the central receptor? Blood 2003;102:449–461.

46. Elices MJ, Hemler ME. The human integrin VLA-2 is a collagen receptor on some cells and a collagen/laminin receptor on others. Proc Natl Acad Sci USA 1989;86:9906–9910.

47. Moroi M, Jung SM. Integrin-mediated platelet adhesion. Front Biosci 1998; 3:D719-D728.

48. Languino LR, Gehlsen KR, Wayner E, Carter WG, Engvall E, Ruoslahti E. Endothelial cells use α2β1 integrin as a laminin receptor. J Cell Biol 1989; 109:2455–2462.

49. Guidetti G, Bertoni A, Viola M, Tira E, Balduini C, Torti M. The small proteoglycan decorin supports adhesion and activation of human platelets. Blood 2002;100:1707–1714.

50. Smith C, Estavillo D, Emsley J, Bankston LA, Liddington RC, Cruz MA. Mapping the collagen-binding site in the I domain of the glycoprotein Ia/IIa (integrin alpha(2)beta(1)). J Biol Chem 2000;275:4205–4209.

51. Nolte M, Pepinsky RB, Venyaminov SY, Koteliansky V, Gotwals PJ, Karpusas M. Crystal structure of the alpha1beta1 integrin I-domain: insights into integrin I-domain function. FEBS Lett 1999;452:379–385.

52. Emsley J, Knight CG, Farndale RW, Barnes MJ, Liddington RC. Structural basis of collagen recognition by integrin alpha2beta1. Cell 2000;101:47–56.

53. Savage B, Ginsberg MH, Ruggeri ZM. Influence of fibrillar collagen structure on the mechanisms of platelet thrombus formation under flow. Blood 1999;94:2704–2715.

54. Nieswandt B, Brakebusch C, Bergmeier W, et al. Glycoprotein VI but not alpha2beta1 integrin is essential for platelet interaction with collagen. EMBO J 2001;20:2120–2130.

55. Bernardo A, Bergeron A, Sun CW, et al. Von Willebrand factor present in fibrillar collagen enhances platelet adhesion to collagen but also for collagen-induced platelet aggregation. J Thromb Haemost 2004;2:660–669.

56. Kasirer-Friede A, Ware J, Leng L, Marchese P, Ruggeri ZM, Shattil SJ. Lateral clustering of platelet GP Ib-IX complexes leads to up-regulation of the adhesive function of integrin alpha IIbbeta 3. J Biol Chem 2002;277:11949–11956.

57. Arya M, López JA, Romo GM, et al. Glycoprotein Ib-IX-mediated activation of integrin $\alpha_{IIb}\beta_3$: effects of receptor clustering and von Willebrand factor adhesion. J Thromb Haemost 2003;1:1150–1157.

58. Yap CL, Hughan SC, Cranmer SL, et al. Synergistic adhesive interactions and signaling mechanisms operating between platelet glycoprotein Ib/IX and integrin αIIbβ3. Studies in human platelets and transfected Chinese hamster ovary cells. J Biol Chem 2000;275:41377–41388.

59. Rathore V, Stapleton MA, Hillery CA, et al. PECAM-1 negatively regulates GPIb/V/IX signaling in murine platelets. Blood 2003;102:3658–3664.

60. Patil S, Newman DK, Newman PJ. Platelet endothelial cell adhesion molecule-1 serves as an inhibitory receptor that modulates platelet responses to collagen. Blood 2001;97:1727–1732.

61. Jones KL, Hughan SC, Dopheide SM, Farndale RW, Jackson SP, Jackson DE. Platelet endothelial cell adhesion molecule-1 is a negative regulator of platelet-collagen interactions. Blood 2001;98:1456–1463.

62. Cicmil M, Thomas JM, Leduc M, Bon C, Gibbins JM. Platelet endothelial cell adhesion molecule-1 signaling inhibits the activation of human platelets. Blood 2002;99:137–144.

63. Ruan C, Du X, Xi X, Castaldi PA, Berndt MC. A murine antiglycoprotein Ib complex monoclonal antibody, SZ 2, inhibits platelet aggregation induced by both ristocetin and collagen. Blood 1987;69:570–577.

64. Dormann D, Clemetson JM, Navdaev A, Kehrel BE, Clemetson KJ. Alboaggregin A activates platelets by a mechanism involving glycoprotein VI as well as glycoprotein Ib. Blood 2001;97:929–936.

65. Kanaji S, Kanaji T, Furihata K, Kato K, Ware JL, Kunicki TJ. Convulxin binds to native, human glycoprotein Ibalpha (GPIbalpha). J Biol Chem. 2003; 278:39452–39460.

66. Du X, Magnenat E, Wells TN, Clemetson KJ. Alboluxin, a snake C-type lectin from *Trimeresurus albolabris* venom is a potent platelet agonist acting via GPIb and GPVI. Thromb Haemost 2002;87:692–698.

67. Goto S, Tamura N, Handa S, Arai M, Kodama K, Takayama H. Involvement of glycoprotein VI in platelet thrombus formation on both collagen and von Willebrand factor surfaces under flow conditions. Circulation 2002;106:266–272.

68. Shrimpton CN, Borthakur G, Larrucea S, Cruz MA, Dong JF, López JA. Localization of the adhesion receptor glycoprotein Ib-IX-V complex to lipid rafts is required for platelet adhesion and activation. J Exp Med 2002;196:1057–1066.

69. Locke D, Chen H, Liu Y, Liu C, Kahn ML. Lipid rafts orchestrate signaling by the platelet receptor glycoprotein VI. J Biol Chem 2002;277:18801–18809.

70. Wonerow P, Obergfell A, Wilde JI, et al. Differential role of glycolipid-enriched membrane domains in glycoprotein VI- and integrin-mediated phospholipase Cgamma2 regulation in platelets. Biochem J 2002;364:755–765.

71. Andrews RK, Gardiner EE, Shen Y, Whisstock JC, Berndt MC. Glycoprotein Ib-IX-V. Int J Biochem Cell Biol 2003;35:1170–1174.

72. Koyama T, Nishida K, Ohdama S, et al. Determination of plasma tissue factor antigen and its clinical significance. Br J Haematol 1994;87:343–347.

73. Giesen PL, Rauch U, Bohrmann B, et al. Blood-borne tissue factor: another view of thrombosis. Proc Natl Acad Sci USA 1999;96:2311–2315.

74. Falati S, Liu Q, Gross P, et al. Accumulation of tissue factor into developing thrombi in vivo is dependent upon microparticle P-selectin glycoprotein ligand 1 and platelet P-selectin. J Exp Med 2003;197:1585–1598.

75. Palabrica T, Lobb R, Furie BC, et al. Leukocyte accumulation promoting fibrin deposition is mediated in vivo by P-selectin on adherent platelets. Nature 1992;359:848–851.

76. Myers D, Wrobleski S, Londy F, et al. New and effective treatment of experimentally induced venous thrombosis with anti-inflammatory rPSGL-Ig. Thromb Haemost 2002;87:374–382.

77. Myers DD Jr, Schaub R, Wrobleski SK, et al. P-selectin antagonism causes dose-dependent venous thrombosis inhibition. Thromb Haemost 2001;85:423–429.

78. Eppihimer MJ, Schaub RG. P-Selectin-dependent inhibition of thrombosis during venous stasis. Arterioscler Thromb Vasc Biol 2000;20:2483–2488.

79. Kumar A, Villani MP, Patel UK, Keith JC Jr, Schaub RG. Recombinant soluble form of PSGL-1 accelerates thrombolysis and prevents reocclusion in a porcine model. Circulation 1999;99:1363–1369.

80. del Conde I, Shrimpton CN, Thiagarajan P, Lopez JA. Tissue factor-bearing microvesicles arise from lipid rafts and fuse with activated platelets to initiate coagulation. Blood 2005; Mar, 1 [ePub].

81. Nesheim ME, Taswell JB, Mann KG. The contribution of bovine factor V and factor Va to the activity of prothrombinase. J Biol Chem 1979;254:10952–10962.

82. Baglia FA, Badellino KO, Li CQ, Lopez JA, Walsh PN. Factor XI binding to the platelet glycoprotein Ib-IX-V complex promotes factor XI activation by thrombin. J Biol Chem 2002;277:1662–1668.

83. Baglia FA, Shrimpton CN, Lopez JA, Walsh PN. The glycoprotein Ib-IX-V complex mediates localization of factor XI to lipid rafts on the platelet membrane. J Biol Chem 2003;278:21744–21750.

84. Yun TH, Baglia FA, Myles T, et al. Thrombin activation of factor XI on activated platelets requires the interaction of factor XI and platelet glycoprotein Ibalpha with

thrombin anion binding exosites I and II respectively. J Biol Chem 2003;278:48112–48119.

85. Wagner DD. The Weibel-Palade body: the storage granule for von Willebrand factor and P-selectin. Thromb Haemost 1993;70:105–110.

86. Romo GM, Dong JF, Schade AJ, et al. The glycoprotein Ib-IX-V complex is a platelet counter-receptor for P-selectin. J Exp Med 1999;190:803–813.

87. Katayama T, Ikeda Y, Handa M, et al. Immunoneutralization of glycoprotein Ibα attenuates endotoxin-induced interactions of platelets and leukocytes with rat venular endothelium in vivo. Circ Res 2000;86:1031–1037.

88. Dong JF, Moake JL, Nolasco L, et al. ADAMTS-13 rapidly cleaves newly secreted ultralarge von Willebrand factor multimers on the endothelial surface under flowing conditions. Blood 2002;100:4033–4039.

89. Levy GG, Nichols WC, Lian EC, et al. Mutations in a member of the ADAMTS gene family cause thrombotic thrombocytopenic purpura. Nature 2001;413:488–494.

90. Savasan S, Lee SK, Ginsburg D, Tsai HM. ADAMTS13 gene mutation in congenital thrombotic thrombocytopenic purpura with previously reported normal VWF cleaving protease activity. Blood 2003;101:4449–4451.

91. Moake JL. Thrombotic microangiopathies. N Engl J Med 2002;347:589–600.

92. Zheng X, Majerus EM, Sadler JE. ADAMTS13 and TTP. Curr Opin Hematol 2002;9:389–394.

93. Kokame K, Matsumoto M, Soejima K, et al. Mutations and common polymorphisms in ADAMTS13 gene responsible for von Willebrand factor-cleaving protease activity. Proc Natl Acad Sci USA 2002;99:11902–11907.

94. George JN. The association of pregnancy with thrombotic thrombocytopenic purpura-hemolytic uremic syndrome. Curr Opin Hematol 2003;10:339–344.

95. Park YD, Yoshioka A, Kawa K, et al. Impaired activity of plasma von Willebrand factor-cleaving protease may predict the occurrence of hepatic veno-occlusive disease after stem cell transplantation. Bone Marrow Transplant 2002;29:789–794.

96. Lattuada A, Rossi E, Calzarossa C, Candolfi R, Mannucci PM. Mild to moderate reduction of a von Willebrand factor cleaving protease (ADAMTS-13) in pregnant women with HELLP microangiopathic syndrome. Haematologica 2003;88:1029–1034.

97. Mannucci PM, Vanoli M, Forza I, Canciani MT, Scorza R. Von Willebrand factor cleaving protease (ADAMTS-13) in 123 patients with connective tissue diseases (systemic lupus erythematosus and systemic sclerosis). Haematologica 2003;88:914–918.

98. Kavakli K, Canciani MT, Mannucci PM. Plasma levels of the von Willebrand factor-cleaving protease in physiological and pathological conditions in children. Pediatr Hematol Oncol 2002;19:467–473.

99. Hellums JD. 1993 Whitaker lecture: biorheology in thrombosis research. Ann Biomed Eng 1994;22:445–455.

100. Feng S, Resendiz JC, Christodoulides N, et al. Pathological shear stress stimulates the tyrosine phosphorylation of alpha-actinin associated with the glycoprotein Ib-IX complex. Biochemistry 2002;41:1100–1108.

101. Razdan K, Hellums JD, Kroll MH. Shear-stress-induced von Willebrand factor binding to platelets causes the activation of tyrosine kinase(s). Biochem J 1994;302:681–686.

102. Nomura S, Nakamura T, Cone J, Tandon NN, Kambayashi J. Cytometric analysis of high shear-induced platelet microparticles and effect of cytokines on microparticle generation. Cytometry 2000;40:173–181.

103. Nomura S, Tandon NN, Nakamura T, Kambayashi J. Morphological differences between GPIb antibody-induced and shear stress-induced platelet aggregates. Haemostasis 2000;30:174–188.

104. Merten M, Chow T, Hellums JD, Thiagarajan P. A new role for P-selectin in shear-induced platelet aggregation. Circulation 2000;102:2045–2050.

105. Kawano K, Yoshino H, Aoki N, et al. Shear-induced platelet aggregation increases in patients with proximal and severe coronary artery stenosis. Clin Cardiol 2002;25:154–160.

106. Tanigawa T, Nishikawa M, Kitai T, et al. Increased platelet aggregability in response to shear stress in acute myocardial infarction and its inhibition by combined therapy with aspirin and cilostazol after coronary intervention. Am J Cardiol 2000;85:1054–1059.

107. Ajzenberg N, Denis CV, Veyradier A, Girma JP, Meyer D, Baruch D. Complete defect in vWF-cleaving protease activity associated with increased shear-induced platelet aggregation in thrombotic microangiopathy. Thromb Haemost 2002;87:808–811.

108. Jen CJ, McIntire LV. Characteristics of shear-induced aggregation in whole blood. J Lab Clin Med 1984;103:115–124.

109. Moake JL, Turner NA, Stathopoulos NA, Nolasco LH, Hellums JD. Involvement of large plasma von Willebrand factor (vWF) multimers and unusually large vWF forms derived from endothelial cells in shear stress-induced platelet aggregation. J Clin Invest 1986;78:1456–1461.

110. Alkhamis TM, Beissinger RL, Chedian JR. Effect of red blood cells on platelet adhesion and aggregation in low-stress shear flow. ASAIO Trans 1987;33:636–642.

111. Alkhamis TM, Beissinger RL, Chediak JR. Artificial surface effect on red blood cells and platelets in laminar shear flow. Blood 1990;75:1568–1575.

112. Reimers RC, Sutera SP, Joist JH. Potentiation by red blood cells of shear-induced platelet aggregation: relative importance of chemical and physical mechanisms. Blood 1984;64:1200–1206.

113. Goldsmith HL, Bell DN, Braovac S, Steinberg A, McIntosh F. Physical and chemical effects of red cells in the shear-induced aggregation of human platelets. Biophys J 1995;69:1584–1595.

114. Goldsmith HL, Yu SS, Marlow J. Fluid mechanical stress and the platelet. Thromb Diath Haemorrh 1975;34:32–41.

115. Turitto VT, Weiss HJ. Red blood cells: their dual role in thrombus formation. Science 1980;207:541–543.

116. Glaumann H, Bergstrand A, Ericsson JLE. Studies on the synthesis and intracellular transport of lipoprotein particles in rat liver. J Cell Biol 1975;64:356–377.

117. Sutera SP, Nowak MD, Joist JH, Zeffren DJ, Bauman JE. A programmable, computer-controlled cone-plate viscometer for the application of pulsatile shear stress to platelet suspensions. Biorheology 1988;25:449–459.

118. Zhang JN, Bergeron AL, Yu Q, et al. Platelet aggregation and activation under complex patterns of shear stress. Thromb Haemost 2002;88:817–821.

119. Dong JF, Berndt MC, Schade A, McIntire LV, Andrews RK, López JA. Ristocetin-dependent, but not botrocetin-dependent, binding of von Willebrand factor to the platelet glycoprotein Ib-IX-V complex correlates with shear-dependent interactions. Blood 2001;97:162–168.

120. Heuser G, Opitz R. A Couette viscometer for short time shearing of blood. Biorheology 1980;17:17–24.

121. Ikeda Y, Handa M, Kamata T, et al. Transmembrane calcium influx associated with von Willebrand factor binding to GP Ib in the initiation of shear-induced platelet aggregation. Thromb Haemost 1993;69:496–502.

122. Ikeda Y, Handa M, Kawano K, et al. The role of von Willebrand factor and fibrinogen in platelet aggregation under varying shear stress. J Clin Invest 1991;87:1234–1240.

123. Cooke BM, Usami S, Perry I, Nash GB. A simplified method for culture of endothelial cells and analysis of adhesion of blood cells under conditions of flow. Microvasc Res 1993;45:33–45.

124. Kundu SK, Heilmann EJ, Sio R, Garcia C, Davidson RM, Ostgaard RA. Description of an in vitro platelet function analyzer—PFA-100. Semin Thromb Hemost 1995;21(suppl 2):106–112.

125. Heilmann EJ, Kundu SK, Sio R, Garcia C, Gomez R, Christie DJ. Comparison of four commercial citrate blood collection systems for platelet function analysis by the PFA-100 system. Thromb Res 1997;87:159–164.

10 Pharmacodynamics of GPIIb-IIIa Receptor Blockade

*Lisa K. Jennings, PhD,
and Melanie M. White, BS*

Contents

INTRODUCTION

Platelet activation and aggregation are implicated in the pathophysiology of unstable angina, myocardial infarction, transient ischemic at-

From: *Contemporary Cardiology:*
Platelet Function: Assessment, Diagnosis, and Treatment
Edited by: M. Quinn and D. Fitzgerald © Humana Press Inc., Totowa, NJ

tacks, and stroke *(1–3)*. Currently available oral antiplatelet agents (aspirin, ticlopidine, and clopidogrel) suppress arachidonic acid or adenosine diphosphate (ADP)-mediated platelet aggregation and have proven clinical benefit in reducing the adverse outcomes from these vascular events *(4–7)*. More complete blockade of platelet function could potentially achieve even greater reductions of acute and secondary vascular events. In fact, the more potent antiplatelet agents, such as platelet glycoprotein (GP)IIb-IIIa receptor antagonists, have shown additional clinical benefit beyond that conferred by aspirin, especially in intermediate-to-high risk patients *(8–14)*. Data have suggested that combination therapies targeting multiple thrombotic pathways are superior to single-agent use *(11,13,15–17)*. The understanding of the pharmacodynamics of all agents—singly or in combination—is critically important to the treatment of patients presenting with vascular disease.

PLATELET FUNCTION

GPIIb-IIIa is a platelet-specific membrane glycoprotein that has a primary role in platelet function *(18,19)*. Specifically, it serves as the primary cell surface receptor that mediates platelet aggregation and clot retraction. Ligand occupied GPIIb-IIIa transmits outside-in signals that include activation of phosphokinases, inositol phosphate generation, and transient calcium increases. Postligand binding events regulated by GPIIb-IIIa include the stabilization of large platelet aggregates, platelet spreading, granule release, clot retraction, and perhaps procoagulant activity *(20)*. Platelet activation induces a calcium-dependent conversion of the platelet GPIIb-IIIa complex into an active receptor for fibrinogen and von Willebrand factor (vWF) *(18–20)*. These multivalent adhesion molecules crosslink platelets into aggregates by binding to other GPIIb-IIIa receptors on adjacent platelets. The conversion of the GPIIb-IIIa complex into an active receptor for fibrinogen and vWF is the final common pathway for all physiologic mediators of platelet aggregation, as these bound multivalent molecules crosslink nearby platelets to form the thrombus. An inhibitor of this pathway should, therefore, be an effective therapeutic agent, and this has been the case with the parenteral GPIIb-IIIa receptor antagonists in the acute setting *(21)*.

UNDERSTANDING THE BIOLOGICAL EFFECTS OF ANTITHROMBOTIC THERAPY

In the development of anticoagulant or antiplatelet agents, there are significant benefits to measuring their biological effects. With either type of agent, a balance must be achieved between efficacy of inhibition

Table 1
Platelet Aggregometry for Pharmacodynamic
Evaluation of Antiplatelet Therapy

Advantages	Disadvantages
Established normal range of response to most agonists	Analysis must be completed within 3 hr of blood collection
Flexibility of anticoagulant and agonist choice and concentration for assay	Requires approx 1.5 h to carry out assay
Visual assessment of platelet aggregation response	Demands technical expertise
Multiple assays can be run concurrently via two or four channel aggregometer	Assay conditions must be standardized
Capability of measuring platelet secretion and aggregation response simultaneously	Assessment of platelet inhibition requires predrug sample

of function (either platelet or procoagulant) and risk of bleeding. The effect of antiplatelet therapies has been more difficult to assess than most anticoagulant therapies because of the intrinsic difficulty of measuring platelet function (22). Historically, platelet function has been evaluated by the bleeding time and ex vivo platelet aggregation response using light transmission aggregometry (LTA). With antiplatelet therapy becoming the cornerstone of treatment for patients with atherosclerotic vascular disease and with the advent of new, more potent platelet single-agent and combination therapies, there is a need for laboratory studies that provide reliable markers of safety and efficacy. Platelet aggregometry using the platelet-rich plasma photooptical (turbidometric) method is frequently employed for evaluating the pharmacodynamic effects of novel antiplatelet agents in clinical development (22).

Using platelet aggregation testing in this fashion requires an understanding of its advantages and disadvantages (Table 1). A clear advantage of platelet aggregation assessment is that one can evaluate ex vivo platelet function inhibition in the background of or in combination with other platelet-inhibitory medications. These data can be analyzed in comparison with documented normal ranges of platelet response. In addition, the effectiveness of, or resistance to, a particular antiplatelet therapy can be assessed depending on the type and strength of agonists chosen for the platelet aggregation assay (Table 2). For example, aspirin-induced inhibition of platelet function can be evaluated by platelet aggregation response to arachidonic acid. Clopidogrel effectiveness can

Table 2
Agonist of Choice for the Evaluation of Platelet Aggregation
Inhibition by Antiplatelet Therapies

Agent	Agonist	Mechanism of drug action
Aspirin	Arachidonic acid	Cyclooxygenase
Clopidogrel, ticlopidine	ADP	PGY12 antagonist
Heparins, direct thrombin inhibitors	Thrombin	Blocks thrombin protease activity
GPIIb-IIIa antagonists	ADP, TRAP	Blocks binding of fibrinogen and von Willebrand factor

be assessed by measuring aggregation response to ADP, whereas inhibition of thrombin activity by antithrombins such as the heparins or direct thrombin inhibitors can be measured by platelet response to the addition of human α-thrombin.

QUALITY ASSURANCE PROCEDURES
FOR EVALUATION OF PLATELET FUNCTION

In utilizing LTA as a surrogate marker of drug effect, a significant concern is the lack of quality assurance procedures for this methodology as it is performed from site to site. Without a method to assess and reduce interlaboratory variation in quantitative platelet aggregometry testing, there is the potential for confounded results in multicentered phase II and phase III clinical trials. An additional limitation is that with any platelet function testing, a predrug sample must be collected in order to assess a subject's threshold for platelet activation. This predrug sample is also critical if the therapy will be assessed in the background of other concomitant medications. The extent of platelet function inhibition upon addition of an antiplatelet agent or anticoagulant must be considered relative to this baseline measurement. Raw platelet aggregation data provide little insight into the pharmacodynamic effects of a particular dosing regimen.

GPIIb-IIIa antagonists have significant clinical benefits in the treatment of acute coronary syndromes (*see* refs. *8–14* and references therein). The use of inhibitors of the GPIIb-IIIa receptor for the management of patients undergoing percutaneous coronary intervention (PCI) and for those with unstable angina and non-Q-wave myocardial infarction (MI) has resulted in a dramatic reduction in the combined incidence of death or MI during treatment and with continued benefit up to 1 yr. Data from the TACTICS-TIMI 18 trial (Treat Angina with Aggrastat and Deter-

Table 3
Standardization of Platelet Function Assessment: Practical Considerations

Anticoagulant choice
Venipuncture technique
Blood processing technique
A report mechanism in place for notifying sponsor or core laboratory of
  unacceptable samples (clotted, grossly hemolyzed, outside analysis time
  frame—late arrival to a laboratory, etc.)
Instrumentation certification: centrifuge, cell counter, aggregometer, and
  refrigerator/freezer
Agonist selection, preparation, and storage
Assay conditions and procedure
Labeling aggregometer tracings and reporting results

mine Cost of Therapy with an Invasive or Conservative Strategy) suggest that longer treatment periods with a GPIIb-IIIa antagonist prior to PCI resulted in additional benefit in improving myocardial perfusion, TIMI grade III flow, and minimal lumen diameter (23).

To assess fully the clinical and biologic effects of GPIIb-IIIa antagonists, it is important to understand variability in platelet function as described above as well as differences in the biologic activity of specific receptor blockers. In order to make appropriate conclusions, ex vivo testing conditions must be standardized (Table 3). In addition, the criteria for platelet function evaluation must be well understood. Variation in the test parameters without clear justification will confound whether treatment regimens for specific indications are in fact providing projected and desired pharmacodynamic effects and how these effects compare to other agents. Only after standardization is achieved can we begin to assess which ex vivo test may be useful in predicting the desired clinical outcome.

In the context of platelet function, we have previously reported that GPIIb-IIIa antagonists can have different pharmacodynamic effects depending on the anticoagulant used for blood collection (24,25). These data suggest that citrate anticoagulant removes calcium from the GPIIb-IIIa complex and enhances the apparent inhibitory activity of the GPIIb-IIIa blockers. GPIIb-IIIa binds Ca^{2+} at its five identified cation binding sites (26). Reductions in the divalent cation binding to GPIIb-IIIa markedly alter GPIIb-IIIa structure and function, resulting in a decrease in fibrinogen binding. Initial work by D'Souza et al. (27) suggested that divalent cations and competitive antagonists may compete for binding to GPIIb-IIIa. Studies by Phillips et al. (24) and by Jennings et al. (25) demonstrated that the extent of platelet inhibition by the three currently approved parenteral agents (abciximab, eptifibatide, and tirofiban) is affected by the collection of blood samples into citrate and that collection of blood samples into this traditional anticoagulant will overestimate drug effect, particularly at drug levels that have less than the desired target of platelet aggregation inhibition.

It is also important to note that there have not yet been any direct, large interagent comparative trials to determine whether apparent differences in drug efficacy or clinical outcomes are related to specific drug properties or the extent of platelet GPIIb-IIIa receptor blockade. However, one study did show that higher levels of platelet inhibition resulted in lower cardiac event rates compared with subjects with less platelet inhibition *(28)*. Furthermore, there are a variety of reports to suggest that certain GPIIb-IIIa antagonists at lower levels of receptor occupancy may have an agonist effect on platelets and this effect may be, in part, responsible for the failed trials of the oral GPIIb-IIIa inhibitors. Because of the obvious implications of platelet inhibition extent in regard to improving patient outcomes, we have attempted to address the methods and rationale of pharmacodynamic evaluation of GPIIb-IIIa receptor antagonists.

GPIIb-IIIa CONFORMATIONAL STATES
AND LIGAND-INDUCED BINDING SITES

GPIIb-IIIa, a member of the integrin family of adhesive protein receptors, binds soluble adhesive proteins fibrinogen and vWF as well as other adhesive proteins, vitronectin and fibronectin *(18)*. GPIIb-IIIa does not bind these ligands in the soluble phase when the receptor is in a low-affinity state; however, upon platelet activation and subsequent activation of the GPIIb-IIIa receptor, binding occurs and facilitates platelet adhesion and platelet aggregation *(29,30)*. Activation of the receptor results in a conformational change that permits ligand interaction. This conformation has been identified through the binding of monoclonal antibodies that recognize activated GPIIb-IIIa complex. One widely used antibody, PAC-1, was originally described by Shattil et al. *(31)*. This antibody competes for fibrinogen binding and recognizes activated but not ligand-occupied GPIIb-IIIa.

Once ligand has bound, another shift in GPIIb-IIIa conformation is detected by antibodies called anti-LIBS (ligand-induced binding sites). These antibodies do not bind well to either inactivated or activated GPIIb-IIIa without bound ligand but bind with increased affinity to the ligand-occupied receptor. LIBS antibodies have been characterized by the laboratories of Ginsberg *(32,33)*, Jennings *(34,35)*, and others *(36)* and have proved extremely useful in characterizing the dynamic nature of GPIIb-IIIa and its response to inside-out and outside-in platelet signaling.

Studies by Jennings et al. *(37)* demonstrated that interactions of platelet antagonists with GPIIb-IIIa caused differential expression of high-affinity LIBS, suggesting that each antagonist has a specific signature and consequence on the receptor. For example, abciximab binding caused no detectable increase in binding of either D3 or LIBS6, whereas eptifibatide, tirofiban, and the ligand recognition sequences RGDS and H12 induced differential expression of the high-affinity binding sites. As previously shown, the binding of abciximab reduced the binding of both D3 and LIBS6. Since abciximab is 50–90 times greater in molecular mass compared with the small-molecule antagonists, it is possible that this reduction in binding is owing to abciximab-mediated steric hindrance of D3 binding, as agents with less mass such as the peptides and nonpeptides elicit LIBS upon binding to GPIIb-IIIa. Once the drug is eluted from the receptor on the intact platelet, LIBS sites are no longer detected, indicating that upon dissociation of the bound ligand, the GPIIb-IIIa reverts to a resting conformation rather than maintaining an irreversible GPIIb-IIIa-activated state *(38)*.

LIBS and Consequences of Expression

It has been documented that GPIIb-IIIa antagonists can illicit thrombocytopenia in about 2% of patients via production of drug-dependent antibodies *(39,40)*. These antibodies appear to bind to neoepitopes or LIBS that are induced upon antagonist binding. The functional relevance of LIBS is not clear, although it has been demonstrated that antibodies that bind to LIBS sites can effect full-scale platelet aggregation response and clot retraction. Interestingly, Murphy et al. *(41)* showed that a GPIIb-IIIa antagonist that failed to induce previously identified LIBS, D3, resulted in a greater suppression of thromboxane A_2 (TXA_2) formation in an in vivo model of coronary thrombolysis compared with another antagonist that induced LIBS. The mechanism for this variability in response is unknown, but the hypothesis that differential exposure of neoepitopes could regulate the extent of TXA_2 formation may be pertinent to the design of future platelet receptor antagonists and serve as one criterion for monitoring for agonist activity. Other experiments by Honda et al. *(42)* found that only compounds that induced conformational change in the GPIIIa subunit caused an increase in platelet ionized calcium concentrations and in platelet aggregation response.

CLINICAL OUTCOMES IN RELATIONSHIP
TO GPIIb-IIIa RECEPTOR BLOCKADE

Recent trial data suggested that there were differences in the currently approved agents in terms of their platelet pharmacodynamics, as comparison trials have not demonstrated equivalent results in terms of reduction of event rates. For example, the Global Use of Streptokinase and Tissue Plasminogen Activator for Occluded Arteries (GUSTO)-IV trial actually showed a negative trend for abciximab vs placebo in the setting of pure medical management of acute coronary syndromes *(43)*. The fact that abciximab has not resulted in outcomes as good as the other GPIIb-IIIa antagonists in the unstable angina population is not well understood and could be owing to a number of factors: (1) differences in the patient population studied compared with other unstable angina trials, (2) the level of platelet inhibition obtained in view of new pharmacodynamic information, or (3) the possibility that the trial was underpowered owing to lower event rates than predicted.

The effects of abciximab on platelet function have been monitored by ex vivo LTA and GPIIb-IIIa receptor blockade by flow cytometry. Interestingly, data suggest that the bolus dose of abciximab, although variable, achieved a mean platelet inhibition of 80%, whereas the infusion regimen resulted in less than the 80% desired target *(44)*. These new data may be explained by the rapid clearance of free drug in the circulating plasma. In addition, the extent of receptor occupancy by abciximab during an activation event is more dependent on platelet count and GPIIb-IIIa receptor density compared with the small molecules (eptifibatide and tirofiban), which have a longer circulating half-life in the plasma *(44,45)*. Thus, owing to the rapid clearance of plasma abciximab, some internal GPIIb-IIIa receptors expressed on the platelet surface in response to strong agonists are not blocked *(45)*. In addition, the dose of abciximab was derived prior to the understanding that the extent of pharmacodynamic effect is overestimated in blood anticoagulated by citrate *(25)*. Thus, all three factors may have some bearing on the fact that not all patients receiving the currently approved abciximab infusion dose will achieve 80% or greater platelet inhibition to 20 μM ADP in D-phenylalanyl-L-propyl-L-arginine chloromethylketone (PPACK) anticoagulant (Fig 1).

The results from the Tirofiban and Reopro Give Similar Efficacy Outcomes Trial (TARGET), one of the first head-to-head comparisons of the GPIIb-IIIa antagonists abciximab and tirofiban in patients undergoing PCI with stenting, showed superiority for abciximab on the com-

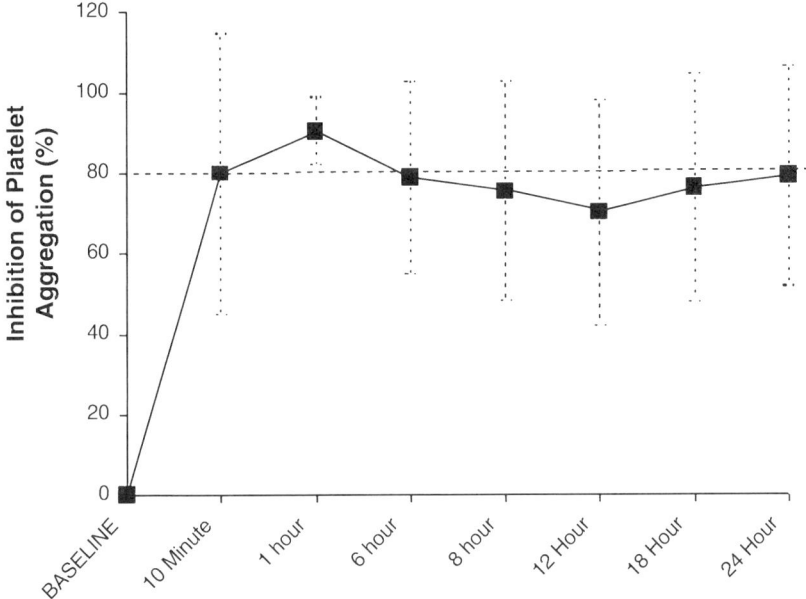

Fig. 1. Mean inhibition of platelet aggregation (IPA) with abciximab (0.25 µg/kg bolus, followed by a 0.125 µg/kg/min (maximum of 10 µg/min) infusion for at least 24 h) in unstable angina patients. Platelet aggregation was evaluated in light transmission aggregometry assays using D-phenylalanyl-L-propyl-L-arginine chloromethylketone (PPACK) as the anticoagulant and 20 µmol adenosine diphosphate (ADP) as the agonist. Vertical lines indicate standard deviation; $N = 20$.

posite end point of death, MI, and urgent target vessel revascularization at 30 d *(46)*. Although not powered to examine mortality at 1 yr, there was no evidence that abciximab had a long-term benefit over tirofiban. These results suggest that abciximab is superior to tirofiban for early outcome events primarily by reduction in the occurrence of periprocedural MI with abciximab. These data point toward the potential importance of high and consistent levels of platelet inhibition when mechanical injury is taking place within the artery, as with stent placement. Comparison studies have shown that the bolus dose of tirofiban would have to be significantly increased to achieve the levels of inhibition currently seen with the bolus dose of abciximab or eptifibatide *(44,47)*. A recently completed study, the TAM 1 trial, showed that the mean level of platelet inhibition of patients receiving tirofiban was significantly less than that observed with the other small molecule, eptifibatide (Fig. 2).

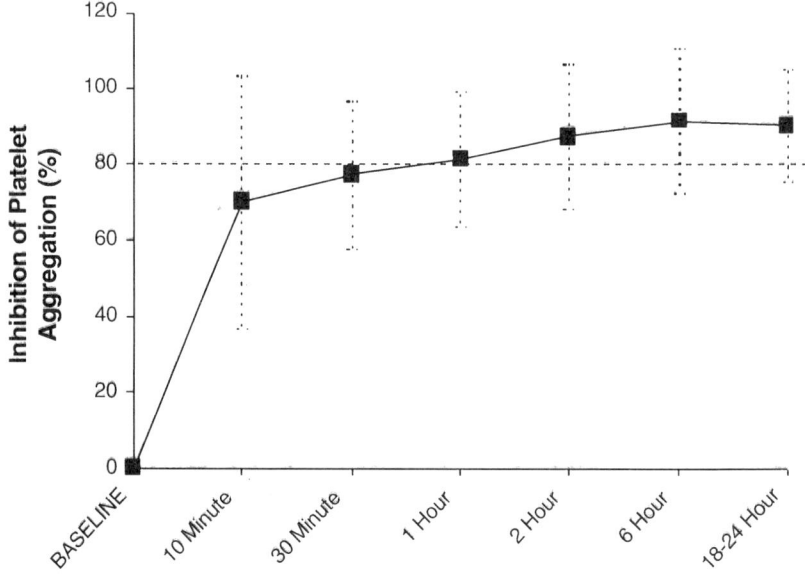

Fig. 2. Mean platelet aggregation inhibition (PAI) with tirofiban HCl (10 µg/kg bolus plus 0.15 µg/kg/min infusion for 18–24 h) in PCI patients. Platelet aggregation was evaluated in light transmission aggregometry assays using D-phenylalanyl-L-propyl-L-arginine chloromethylketone (PPACK) as the anticoagulant and 20 µmol adenosine diphosphate (ADP) as the agonist. Vertical lines indicate standard deviation; $N = 19$.

GPIIb-IIIa: A MULTIFUNCTIONAL PROTEIN

An inherited bleeding disorder called Glanzmann's thrombasthenia is a gene mutation(s) in either GPIIb or GPIIIa *(48)*. These mutations may result in altered mRNA splicing or mRNA stability, altered GPIIb-IIIa subunit expression or association, or defective cation binding. Interestingly, platelet adhesion and/or clot retraction in Glanzmann's thrombasthenia variants can be preserved, and these results demonstrate that the GPIIb-IIIa-mediated aggregation function can be independent of adhesion and postreceptor occupancy events such as clot retraction. It has been documented that occupancy by the three parenteral GPIIb-IIIa antagonists has different effects on platelet-mediated clot retraction. Abciximab at 100% receptor occupancy totally blocks clot retraction, whereas the small molecules eptifibatide and tirofiban, at maximum receptor occupancy, block clot retraction by about 45% *(25)*. The implications of these pharmacodynamic differences are not clear. However, although it is evident that the GPIIb-IIIa antagonists as a drug class have an overall positive impact on the reduction of MI and death in the acute coronary syndromes, there are interagent differences that may affect outcomes and are dependent on the patient population.

Fullard et al. *(49)* described a mutation in GPIIIa that resulted in increased adhesion to immobilized fibrinogen and binding affinity for a nonpeptide GPIIb-IIIa antagonist, SC52012. Despite this altered adhesion phenotype, the patient still had a bleeding diathesis, pointing toward the importance of platelet aggregation rather than platelet adhesion in bleeding risk.

LOW LEVELS OF GPIIb-IIIa BLOCKADE
MAY HAVE A PARTIAL AGONIST EFFECT

Thus far, oral GPIIb-IIIa antagonists, compared with placebo, have not proved efficacious in reducing death and MI in large clinical trials of patients with acute coronary syndromes. In fact, at least three trials (Orbofiban in Patients With Unstable Coronary Syndromes-Thrombolysis in Myocardial Infarction 16 [OPUS-TIMI16] and Sibrafaban vs Aspirin to Yield Maximum Protection from Ischemic Heart Events Postacute Coronary Syndromes [SYMPHONY] I and II) reported an increase in death and MI of patients in the active treatment arm compared with placebo. The explanation for this result is still unknown; however, studies have shown that low levels of antagonists chronically administered may have initiated platelet activation. For example, Cox et al. *(50)* found that the expression of CD63, a marker for platelet activation, was increased throughout the treatment period in patients receiving orbofiban. The underlying contributing factor appears to be that partial receptor occupancy by specific peptides or nonpeptides may induce outside-in signaling via GPIIb-IIIa that results in activated platelets or platelets primed for response. Under these circumstances, platelet activation may have elicited release or shedding of proinflammatory mediators that exacerbated vascular injury response. This point is supported by recent studies demonstrating that concentrations of GPIIb-IIIa parenteral inhibitors that result in less than 80% platelet inhibition encourage the release of the platelet proinflammatory molecule sCD40L *(51)*. CD40L has been demonstrated to have a role in atherosclerotic lesion progression and plaque stability. Whether doses of oral GPIIb-IIIa antagonists that gave less than 80% platelet aggregation inhibition caused increased levels of sCD40L and potentiated secondary reactions such as thrombosis and the enhancement of atherosclerosis remains to be proven.

GPIIb-IIIa RECEPTOR ANTAGONISTS:
INTERAGENT COMPARISONS

The GPIIb-IIIa complex was first identified as an early target for regulation of platelet aggregate formation when abciximab, the human/ murine chimera Fab fragment of the monoclonal antibody 7E3, was introduced into clinical trials (10). Subsequently, several agents (peptides, nonpeptides, and chimeric Fab fragments) have been generated as potential clinical therapies for the treatment of acute coronary syndromes. Three such agents, eptifibatide, tirofiban, and abciximab, have been approved for use in the treatment of non-ST-segment evaluation (NSTE) acute coronary syndromes. Of the three, eptifibatide is the only agent in this class approved for use in both PCI and NSTE acute coronary syndrome patient populations, whereas tirofiban is approved for patients with NSTE acute coronary syndromes. Abciximab is approved only for patients undergoing PCI (21).

Whether the antiplatelet activity of these agents should be monitored to obtain a consistent and high level of platelet inhibition especially during the time of coronary intervention, remains debatable. Demonstrated high and consistent levels of platelet inhibition appear to be important for the reduction of thrombosis and inflammatory response; therefore, in the acute setting, maximum platelet inhibition with appropriate anticoagulation may be ideal. In the current era, we are faced with combination therapies resulting in different levels of platelet function inhibition depending on the dose of antiplatelet therapy administered and inherent patient platelet function differences. For example, it is likely that an individual's platelet activation threshold, platelet count, drug target receptor density, and drug resistance/sensitivity will all have a bearing on the pharmacodynamic effects of the anticoagulant and antiplatelet therapies. Thus, an appreciation of the effects of these therapies in terms of platelet biology is critical in order to provide the ideal treatment for each patient. Of keen interest is how the level of anticoagulation and platelet inhibition translates into reduction of events such as MI and death while minimizing adverse events such as serious bleeding. More data are needed to address this issue.

METHODS FOR EVALUATING GPIIb-IIIa ANTAGONISTS

Historically, platelet function inhibition has been utilized for the evaluation of the GPIIb-IIIa receptor antagonists. The gold standard continues to be LTA, as normal ranges of response are documented for a variety of agonists and concentrations (22). In addition, this method

Table 4
Methods Available for Assessing Antiplatelet Therapy

Assay system	Agonist/agent choice	Labor required
Platelet aggregation	Investigator's discretion	1.5–2 h
Accumetrics Ultegra®	Iso-TRAP	minutes
Helena PlateletWorks®	Investigator's discretion	minutes
Dade Behring PFA-100®	Collagen/epinephrine or collagen/ADP	minutes
Xylum Clot Signature Analyzer (CSA®)	Shear stress/no anticoagulant used	minutes
Receptor occupancy	Monoclonal antibodies, anti-LIBS	15–30 min

has provided an acceptable means for investigating the relationship, if any, of the level of platelet inhibition with drug dose administered, plasma drug levels, or safety issues. These pharmacodynamic evaluations have proved useful for dose evaluation studies, as the target inhibition for GPIIb-IIIa receptor antagonists has been 80% or higher *(52)*. Point-of-care instruments have been evaluated as surrogates for LTA, and these approaches have provided some useful information (Table 4). One pharmacodynamic study using the Accumetric Ultegra® demonstrated that a readout of more than 95% resulted in fewer cardiac events than patients having less than 95% *(28)*. Although it initially showed promise, the Ultegra instrument has not yet proven to be as accurate as anticipated for monitoring all anti-GPIIb-IIIa therapy in the critical dosing range. Results reported by Kereiakes et al. *(44)* suggest that values obtained by the Ultegra overestimated the level of platelet inhibition and did not mirror LTA results. Simon et al. *(53)* compared standard LTA and two bedside platelet function assays, the Ultegra and Xylum Clot Signature Analyzer®. Their results showed that Ultegra measurements were similar to those obtained with LTA for abciximab but overestimated platelet inhibition achieved by the small molecules eptifibatide and tirofiban.

Another study, using the anticoagulant sodium citrate, previously shown to overestimate GPIIb-IIIa antagonist effects, showed high correlations of Ultegra results with LTA slope (rate of aggregation); however, data comparing Ultegra results with inhibition of LTA extent were not reported *(54)*. In regard to the Plateletworks® system, Lakkis et al. *(55)* showed a correlation of $r = 0.83$ when comparing platelet aggregation results using Plateletworks with LTA in 225 paired samples. In addition, a small acute coronary syndrome patient cohort receiving either abciximab or tirofiban was evaluated for platelet aggregation inhibition using Plateletworks, and the results confirmed previously reported levels of platelet inhibition achieved with these two agents. Recent data suggest that Plateletworks may serve as a surrogate for LTA in the evaluation of GPIIb-IIIa antagonists provided modifications are made in the manufacturer's instructions (56). The advantage of the Plateletworks system is that a predrug sample is not necessary to determine pharmacodynamic effects of the GPIIb-IIIa antagonists.

The PFA-100, although proven useful for the diagnosis of von Willebrand's disease and for aspirin resistance, has not been routinely used for triage or for dose monitoring of antiplatelet therapies such as clopidogrel or GPIIb-IIIa receptor blockers (57). Continued analyses of these and newer point-of-care instruments will identify the optimal conditions and assays required to monitor antiplatelet therapy in both acute and long-term patient care.

The increased use of GPIIb-IIIa antagonists and clopidogrel has mandated the development of standardized methods to assess platelet inhibition and predict subsequent efficacy as a result of treatment. Furthermore, recent data suggest that high levels of platelet function inhibition by GPIIb-IIIa antagonists also reduce the release of proinflammatory mediators such as platelet-soluble CD40L that may promote coagulation and facilitate high shear platelet thrombus formation (58,59). Thus, the extent of platelet GPIIb-IIIa receptor blockade may not only affect acute platelet thrombus formation but may also modulate vascular inflammatory response. For these reasons, confirmation of the levels of platelet aggregation inhibition becomes increasingly important.

RECEPTOR OCCUPANCY MEASUREMENTS
Specific Antibody Probes

Another method for evaluating receptor antagonists is a flow cytometric technique that measures drug bound to the targeted receptor. Several methods have been utilized to report the percent of total surface receptors with bound drug at the various study time points of drug administration. One method utilizes the binding of a specific antibody targeted to the human/mouse chimera Fab fragment, abciximab, to report the number of bound abciximab molecules per platelet (60). The utilization of a targeted antibody to the specific antagonist requires a specialized reagent that will bind with high affinity to the drug-GPIIb-IIIa receptor complex. This approach has limited utility for assessing the pharmacodynamics of any agent other than the specific target.

Dual Antibody Detection Methods

A second method employs the use of a GPIIb-IIIa receptor occupancy kit developed by Biocytex (Marseille, France), which contains two anti-GPIIb-IIIa antibodies, MAb 1 (LYP18) and MAb 2 (4F8), and calibration beads. This methodology was used to determine GPIIb-IIIa receptor number and occupancy during the Evaluation of Oral Xemilofiban in Controlling Thrombotic Events (EXCITE) trial, a multicenter study of xemilofiban in 7232 patients undergoing PCI. In one report, the effect of SC-54701, the active metabolite of xemilofiban, on MAb1 and MAb2 binding was evaluated, and results showed that the inhibition of MAb2 binding in platelet-rich plasma (PRP) correlated with SC-54701 inhibition of 20 μM ADP induced platelet aggregation *(61)*. MAb2 binding was inhibited at a concentration that would inhibit platelet aggregation by 50% (IC_{50}) of $0.8 \times 10^{-8} M$ in PRP. Curiously, the dose response for aggregation inhibition was steeper than that measured for inhibition of MAb2 binding. Maximum inhibition of ADP-induced platelet aggregation was observed at only a 60% reduction in MAb2 binding or 60% SC54701 occupancy. The correlation coefficient (r^2) was 0.81.

D3 Monoclonal Antibody

A third method utilizes the D3 monoclonal antibody. This antibody has been well characterized as a LIBS located on the GPIIIa β_3-subunit of the GPIIb-IIIa complex *(34,35,52,62)*. Data have been published showing that D3 receptor occupancy tracks the level of platelet inhibition and also correlates with plasma drug levels *(52,62)*. For example, in TIMI15A and 15B trials, a strong correlation was observed between the mean inhibition of platelet aggregation and mean receptor occupancy with both intravenous and oral formulations of RPR 109891 *(63)*. This MAb has been used extensively to measure receptor occupancy by all three approved parenteral antagonists as well as new agents undergoing evaluation in preclinical studies and phase I and phase II trials. When evaluating the D3 occupancy assay using the antagonist SC-54701, it was observed that the RO_{50} (dose of drug necessary to saturate 50% of the total surface receptors) was $4.8 \times 10^{-8} M$ and corresponded to a measured IC_{50} of $4.0 \times 10^{-8} M$. This assay was further evaluated by determining the correlation between SC54701 induction of the D3 epitope and inhibition of 20 μM ADP-induced aggregation (Fig 3). The correlation coefficient (r^2) was 0.90.

When the antagonist blocks D3 binding or the agent does not elicit the high-affinity D3 binding site, surrogate assays have been devised. For example, when RO is determined for abciximab-treated platelets, a competitive inhibition-type assay must be used. In this assay, unlike the

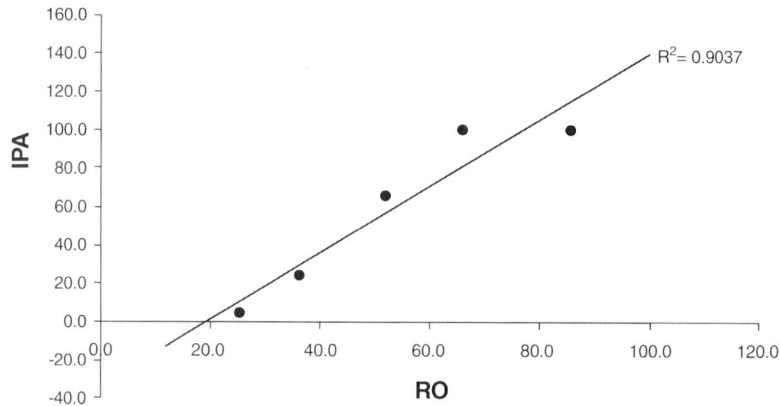

Fig. 3. Correlation of xemilofiban receptor occupancy (RO) with inhibition of platelet aggregation inhibition (IPA) to 20 μ*M* ADP. Platelets in autologous plasma were treated with increasing concentrations of xemilofiban, and the extent of receptor occupancy was measured by the D3 MAb. Treated platelets were also assessed for platelet aggregation inhibition using light transmission aggregometry and 20 μ*M* ADP. Three individuals were evaluated and the mean of the three determinations plotted. *y*-axis, mean IPA; *x*-axis, mean RO. The correlation coefficient, r^2, was 0.90.

direct D3 RO method that does not require a predrug sample, a baseline sample must be drawn before the initiation of treatment. Maximum D3 binding is measured in this baseline sample after the addition of an RGD peptide. When a sample is obtained after initiation of abciximab treatment, the amount of D3 binding is inhibited by the presence of abciximab where the more abciximab is bound, the less D3 binding. The percent D3 binding relative to the baseline maximum sample is the reciprocal of the amount of receptor occupancy by abciximab. To avoid the requirement of a predrug sample, another antibody may be used for determining the total receptor value, and the decreased binding of D3 in the presence of antagonist can be used to determine the level of receptor occupancy, similar to that described above for the MAb1/MAb2 binding assays.

Fibrinogen Binding as Readout for Receptor Blockade

A fourth method is the measured binding of plasma fibrinogen to the activated platelets in the presence of antagonist. This assay format has limitations since the platelets must be evaluated within the same time frame as platelet aggregation assays. Accurate measurements require familiarity with cell binding assays, and the samples cannot be shipped overnight to a core laboratory for evaluation unless an appropriate fixation method has been identified.

SUMMARY

The goal of receptor blockade measurements is twofold: (1) to determine how much drug is bound to the platelet, and (2) to determine the specific contribution of the GPIIb-IIIa antagonist to the overall pharmacodynamic effect. The ultimate goal is to have a reliable method available in the acute or outpatient setting to monitor drug effect and to ensure that the results may be translated into improving patient outcomes.

In summary, many factors enter into the pharmacodynamic evaluation of GPIIb-IIIa receptor antagonists. Once these factors are defined within the setting of phase II and III clinical trial designs, then an understanding of the biology of these compounds in the context of clinical outcomes can be satisfactorily addressed.

REFERENCES

1. Anti-Platelet Trialists' Collaboration. Collaborative overview of randomized trials of anti-platelet therapy-I: prevention of death, myocardial infarction, and stroke by prolonged anti-platelet therapy in various categories of patients. Br Med J 1994;308:81–106.
2. Quinn MJ, Plow EF, Topol EJ. Platelet glycoprotein IIb/IIIa inhibitors. Circulation 2002;106:379–385.
3. Bhatt DL, Topol EJ. Scientific and therapeutic advances in antiplatelet therapy. Nat Rev Drug Discov 2003;2:15–28.
4. ISIS-2 (Secondary International Study of Infarct Survival) Collaborative Group. Randomized trial of intravenous streptokinase, oral aspirin, both, or neither among 17,187 cases of suspected acute myocardial infarction: ISIS-2. Lancet 1988;2:349–360.
5. Gent M, Blakely JA, Easton JD, et al. The Canadian/American Ticlopidine Study (CATS) in thromboembolic stroke. Lancet 1989;1:1215–1220.
6. Hass WK, Easton JD, Adams HP Jr, et al. A randomized trial comparing ticlopidine hydrochloride with aspirin for the prevention of stroke in high-risk patients: Ticlopidine, Aspirin, Stroke, Study Group. N Engl J Med 1989;321:501–507.
7. CAPRIE Steering Committee. A randomised, blinded, trial of clopidogrel versus aspirin in patients at risk of ischaemic events (CAPRIE). Lancet 1996;348:1329–1339.
8. Kong DF, Califf RM, Miller DP, et al. Clinical outcomes of therapeutic agents that block the platelet glycoprotein IIb/IIIa integrin in ischaemic heart disease. Circulation 1998;98:2829–2835.
9. Chong PH. Glycoprotein IIb/IIIa receptor antagonists in the management of cardiovascular diseases. Am J Health Syst Pharm 1998;55:2363–2386.
10. EPIC Investigators. Use of a monoclonal antibody directed against the platelet glycoprotein IIb/IIIa receptor in high-risk coronary angioplasty. N Engl J Med 1994;330:956–961.
11. The CAPTURE investigators. Randomised placebo-controlled trial of abciximab before and during coronary intervention in refractory unstable angina: the CAPTURE study. Lancet 1997;349:1429–1435.
12. The Platelet Receptor Inhibition in Ischaemic Syndrome Management (PRISM) Study Investigators. A comparison of aspirin plus tirofiban with aspirin plus heparin for unstable angina. N Engl J Med 1998;338:1498–1505.

13. The PURSUIT trial investigators. Inhibition of platelet glycoprotein IIb/IIIa with eptifibatide in patients with acute coronary syndromes. N Engl J Med 1998; 339:436–443.

14. O'Shea C, for the ESPIRIT Investigators. Long-term efficacy of platelet glycoprotein IIb/IIIa integrin blockade with eptifibatide in coronary stent intervention. JAMA 2003;287:618–621.

15. Mehta SR, Yusuf S, Peters RJG, et al. Effects of pretreatment with clopidogrel and aspirin followed by long-term therapy in patients undergoing percutaneous coronary intervention: the PCI-CURE study. Lancet 2001;358:527–533.

16. The Platelet Receptor Inhibition for Ischemic Syndrome Management in Patients Limited by Unstable Signs and Symptoms (PRISM-Plus) Study Investigators. Inhibition of the platelet glycoprotein IIb/IIIa receptor with tirofiban in unstable angina and non Q-wave myocardial infarction. N Engl J Med 1998;339:436–443.

17. Ferguson JJ, Antman EM, Bates ER, et al. Combining enoxaparin and glycoprotein IIb/IIIa antagonists for the treatment of acute coronary syndromes: final results of the National Investigators Collaborating on Enoxaparin-3 (NICE-3) study. Am Heart J 2003;146:628–634.

18. Phillips DR, Charo IF, Parise LV, Fitzgerald LA. The platelet membrane glycoprotein IIb-IIIa complex. Blood 1988;71:831–843.

19. Hato T, Ginsberg MH, Shattil SJ. Integrin $\alpha_{IIb}\beta3$. In: Michelson AD, ed. Platelets. Academic, San Diego, 2002, pp. 105–116.

20. Shattil S, Kashiwagi H, Pampori N. Integrin signaling: the platelet paradigm. Blood 1998;91:2645–2657.

21. Jennings LK. Clinical trials of the parenteral glycoprotein IIb-IIIa inhibitors. Health Sciences Center for Continuing Medical Education, June 2001.

22. White MM, Jennings LK, eds. Platelet Protocols: Research and Clinical Laboratory Procedures. Academic, San Diego, 1999.

23. Cannon CP, Weintraub WS, Demopoulos LA, et al. Comparison of early invasive to conservative strategies in patients with unstable coronary syndromes treated with the glycoprotein Iib/IIIa inhibitor tirofiban. N Engl J Med 2001;344:1879–1887.

24. Phillips DR, Teng W, Affsten A, et al. Effect of Ca^{2+} on GpIIb-IIIa interactions with Integrilin. Circulation 1997;96:1488–1494.

25. Jennings LK, Jacoski MV, White MM. The pharmacodynamics of parenteral glycoprotein IIb/IIIa inhibitors. J Interven Cardiol 2002;15:45–60.

26. Cierniewski CS, Haas TA, Smith JW, et al. Characterization of cation-binding sequences in the platelet integrin GPIIb-IIIa ($\alpha_{IIb}\beta3$) by terbium luminescence. Biochemistry 1994;33:12238–12246.

27. D'Souza SE, Haas TA, Piotrowicz RS, et al. Ligand and cation binding are dual functions of a discrete segment of the integrin $\beta3$ subunit: cation displacement is involved in ligand binding. Cell 194;79:659–667.

28. Steinhubl SR, the GOLD Multicenter Study. Point-of-care measured platelet inhibition correlates with a reduced risk of an adverse cardiac event after percutaneous coronary intervention. Circulation 2001;103:2572–2578.

29. Marguerie GA, Edgington TS, Plow EF. Interaction of fibrinogen wih its platelet receptor as part of a multistep reaction in ADP-induced platelet aggregation. J Biol Chem 1985;260:11366–11374.

30. Sims PJ, Ginsberg MH, Plow EF, Shattill SJ. Effect of platelet activation on the conformation of the plasma membrane glycoprotein Iib-IIIa complex. J Biol Chem 1991;266:7347–7352.

31. Shattil SJ, Hoxie JA, Cunningham M, et al. Changes in the platelet membrane glycoprotein IIb-IIIa complex during platelet aggregation. J Biol Chem 1985;20:11107–11114.

32. Frelinger AL, Cohen I, Plow EF, et al. Selective inhibition of integrin function by antibodies specific for ligand-occupied receptor conformers. J Biol Chem 1990;265:6346–6352.

33. Frelinger AL, Du XP, Plow EF, et al. Monoclonal antibodies to ligand-occupied conformers of integrin alpha IIb beta 3 (glycoprotein IIb-IIIa) alter receptor affinity, specificity, and function. J Biol Chem 1991;266:17106–17111.

34. Kouns WC, Wall CD, White MM, et al. A conformation-dependent epitope of human platelet glycoprotein IIIa. J Biol Chem 1990;265:2059–20601.

35. Mondoro TH, Wall CD, White MM, et al. Selective induction of a GPIIIa LIBS by fibrinogen and von Willebrand factor. Blood 1996;88:3824–3830.

36. Honda S, Tomiyama Y, Pelletier AJ, et al. Topography of ligand-induced binding sites, including a novel cation-sensitive epitope (AP5) at the amino terminus, of the human integrin beta 3 subunit. J Biol Chem 1995;270:11947–11954.

37. Jennings LK, Haga JH, Slack SM. Differential expression of a ligand induced binding site (LIBS) by GPIIb-IIIa ligand recognition peptides and parenteral antagonists. Thromb Haemost 2000;84:1095–1102.

38. Kouns WC, Kirchhofer D, Hadvary P, et al. Reversible conformational changes induced in glycoprotein IIb-IIIa by a potent and selective peptidomimetic inhibitor. Blood 1992;80:2539–2547.

39. Giugliano RP. Drug-induced thrombocytopenia: is it a serious concern for glycoprotein IIb/IIIa receptor inhibitors? J Thromb Thrombol 1998;5:191–202.

40. Berkowitz SD, Harrington RA, Rund MM, et al. Acute profound thrombocytopenia after c7E3 Fab (abciximab) therapy. Circulation 2000;95:809–815.

41. Murphy NP, Pratico D, Fitzgerald DJ. Functional relevance of the expression of ligand-induced binding sites in the response to platelet GP IIb/IIIa antagonists *in vivo*. JPET 1998;286:945–951.

42. Honda S, Tomiyama Y, Aoki T, et al. Association between ligand-induced conformational changes of integrin IIbβ 3 and IIbβ3-mediated intracellular Ca^{2+} signaling. Blood 1998;92:3675–3683.

43. Simoons ML; The GUSTO IV-ACS Investigators. Effect of glycoprotein IIb/IIIa receptor blocker abciximab on outcome in patients with acute coronary syndromes without early coronary revascularization: the GUSTO IV-ACS randomized trial. Lancet 2001;357:1915–1924.

44. Kereiakes DJ, Broderick TM, Roth EM, et al. Time course magnitude, and consistency of platelet inhibition by abciximab, tirofiban, or eptifibatide in patients with unstable angina pectoris undergoing percutaneous coronary intervention. Am J Cardiol 1999;84:391–395.

45. Quinn MJ, Murphy RT, Dooley M, Foley JB, Fitzgerald DJ. Occupancy of the internal and external pools of glycoprotein IIb/IIIa following abciximab bolus and infusion. JPET 2001;297:496–500.

46. Stone GW, Moliterno DJ, Bertrand M, et al. Impact of clinical syndrome acuity on the differential response to 2 glycoprotein IIb/IIIa inhibitors in patients undergoing coronary stenting: the TARGET trial Circulation 2002;105:2347–2354.

47. Batchelor WB, Tolleson TR, Huang Y, et al. Randomized COMparison of platelet inhibition with Abciximab, TiRofiban and Eptifibatide during percutaneous coronary intervention in acute coronary symdromes. Circulation 2002;106:1470–1476.

48. Coller BS, Seligsohn U, Peretz H, et al. Glanzmann thrombasthenia: new insights from an historical perspective. Semin Hematol 1994;31:301–311.

49. Fullard J, Murphy R, O'Neill S, Moran N, Ottridge B, Fitzgerald DJ. A Val193Met mutation in GPIIIa results in a GPIIb/IIIa receptor with a constitutively high affinity for a small ligand. B J Haematol 2001;115:113–139.

50. Cox D, Smith R, Quinn M, Theroux P, Crean P, Fitzgerald DJ. Evidence of platelet activation during treatment with a GPIIb/IIIa antagonist in patients presenting with acute coronary syndromes. J Am Coll Cardiol 2000;36:1514–1519.

51. Nannizzi-Alaimo L, Alves VL, Prasad KS, Stockett DE, Phillips DR. GPIIb-IIIa antagonists demonstrate a dose-dependent inhibition and potentiation of soluble CD40L (CD154) release during platelet stimulation. Circulation 2001;104(suppl II):II-318, abstract no. 1533.

52. Gilchrist IC, O'Shea JC, Kosoglou T, et al. Pharmacodynamics and pharmacokinetics of higher-dose, double-bolus eptifibatide in percutaneous intervention. Circulation 2001;104:406–411.

53. Simon DI, Liu CB, Ganz P, et al. A comparative study of light transmission aggregometry and automated bedside platelet function assays in patients undergoing percutaneous coronary intervention and receiving abciximab, eptifibatide, or tirofiban. Cathet Cardiovasc Intervent 2001;52:425–432.

54. Wheeler, GL, Braden, GA, Steinhubl, SR, et al. The Ultegra rapid platelet-function assay: comparison to standard platelet function assays in patients undergoing percutaneous coronary intervention with abciximab therapy. Am Heart J 2002;143:602–61111.

55. Lakkis NM, George S, Thomas E, Ali M, Guyer K, Carville D. Use of ICHOR-Plateletworks to assess platelet function in patients treated with GP IIb/IIIa inhibitors. Cathet Cardiovasc Intervent 2001;53:346–351.

56. White MM, Krishnan R, Jacoski MV, et al. Evaluation of the point of care Helena ICHOR/Plateletworks® and the Accumetrics Ultegra® RPFA for assessment of platelet function with small molecule GPIIb-IIIa antagonists. J Thromb Haemost 2003;1(suppl 1):P1821.

57. Madan M, Berkowitz SD, Christie DJ, et al. Rapid assessment of glycoprotein IIb/IIIa blockade with the platelet function analyzer (PFA-100) during percutaneous coronary intervention. Am Heart J 2001;141:226–233.

58. Andre P, Nannizzi-Alaimo L, Srinivasa K, Prasad KS, Philips DR. Platelet-derived CD40L: the switch-hitting player of cardiovascular disease. Circulation 2002;106:896–899.

59. Nannizzi-Alaimo L, Alves VL, Phillips DR. Inhibitory effects of glycoprotein IIb/IIIa antagonists and aspirin on release of soluble CD40 ligand during platelet stimulation. Circulation 2003;107:1123–1128.

60. Mascelli MA, Lance ET, Damaraju L, et al. Pharmacodynamic profile of short-term abciximab treatment demonstrates prolonged platelet inhibition with gradual recovery from GPIIb/IIIa receptor blockade. Circulation 1998;97:1680–1688.

61. Quinn MJ, Cox D, Foley JB, Fitzgerald DJ. Glycoprotein IIb/IIIa receptor number and occupancy during chronic administration of an oral antagonist. JEPT 2000;295:670–676.

62. Tardiff BE, Jennings LK, Harrington RA, et al. Pharmacodynamics and pharmacokinetics of eptifibatide in patients with acute coronary syndromes: prospective analysis from PURSUIT. Circulation 2001;104:399–405.

63. Giugliano RP, McCabe CH, Sequeira RF, et al. First report of an intravenous and oral glycoprotein IIb/IIIa inhibitor (RPR 109891) in patients with recent acute coronary syndromes: results of the TIMI 15A and 15B trials. Am Heart J 2000;140:81–93.

11 Prostanoid Generation in Platelet Function
Assessment and Clinical Relevance

Bianca Rocca, MD, and Carlo Patrono, MD

CONTENTS

INTRODUCTION
Arachidonic Acid Metabolism in Platelets
ENZYMATIC AND NONENZYMATIC PATHWAYS, BIOACTIVE PROSTANOIDS, AND RECEPTORS

In response to a variety of proaggregatory stimuli such as thrombin, adenosine diphosphate (ADP), or collagen, platelets synthesize eicosanoids, biologically active metabolites derived from arachidonic acid (Fig. 1).

Upon activation, intraplatelet Ca^{2+} increases, rapidly activating cytosolic phospholipase A$_2$ (PLA$_2$), which mobilizes arachidonic acid from the membrane phospholipid bilayer. Arachidonic acid is then converted to prostaglandin H$_2$ (PGH$_2$) by PGH synthase-1 or -2, also referred to as cyclooxygenase (COX)-1 or -2, and to 12-(S)-hydroxyeicosatetraenoic acid (HETE) by 12-lipoxygenase. Downstream isomerases or reduc-

From: *Contemporary Cardiology:*
Platelet Function: Assessment, Diagnosis, and Treatment
Edited by: M. Quinn and D. Fitzgerald © Humana Press Inc., Totowa, NJ

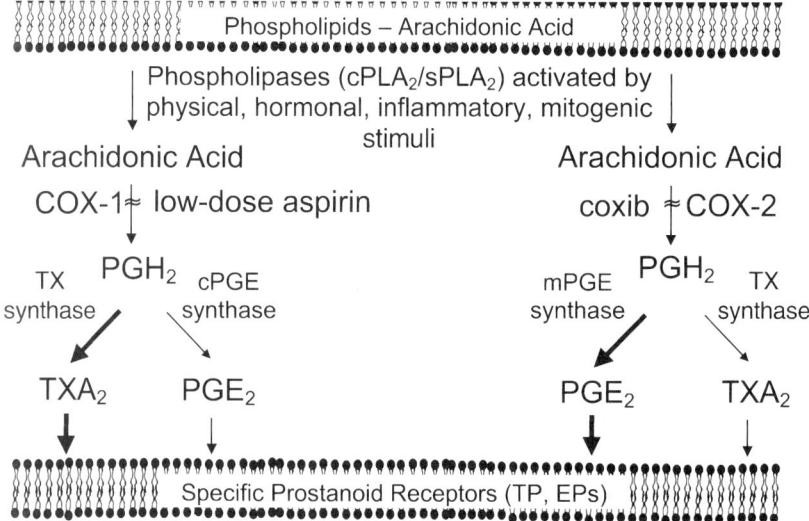

Fig. 1. Platelet arachidonic acid metabolism catalyzed by cyclooxygenases (COX). The arachidonic acid cascade through COX isozymes is depicted in the figure. ≈, inhibition; cPLA₂, cytosolic phospholipase A₂; sPLA₂, secretory phospholipase A₂; coxib, selective COX-2 inhibitor; mPGES, microsomal PGE₂ synthase; cPGES, cytosolic PGE₂ synthase; TX, thromboxane; TP, thromboxane receptor; EP, PGE₂ receptor. Bold arrows indicate a preferential metabolic path.

tases, differentially expressed in a cell-specific fashion, catalyze the conversion of the PGH_2 intermediate to biologically active end products including PGE_2, $PGF_{2\alpha}$, PGD_2, PGI_2, and thromboxane A_2 (TXA_2), known collectively as prostanoids (1) (Fig. 1).

COX isozymes are integral membrane proteins, and they catalyze the same two-step reaction, first cyclizing arachidonic acid to form PGG_2, and then reducing the 15-hydroperoxy group to form PGH_2. They share approx 60% homology within a given species and exhibit remarkable structural homology at the atomic level (1). Nevertheless, they are encoded by different genes, located on distinct chromosomes, and, most importantly, may be coupled to different prostanoid synthases, even within the same cell type (2). COX-1 is the prevalent isoform expressed by mature platelets, whereas COX-2 expression (3–5) has been observed only in the youngest platelet population and is carried over from the parent megakaryocytes (5) (Fig. 2). Therefore, COX-2 expression is physiologically present only in a small portion (<8%) of the entire circulating platelet pool (5). However, COX-2-expressing platelets increase substantially in clinical settings associated with high platelet regenera-

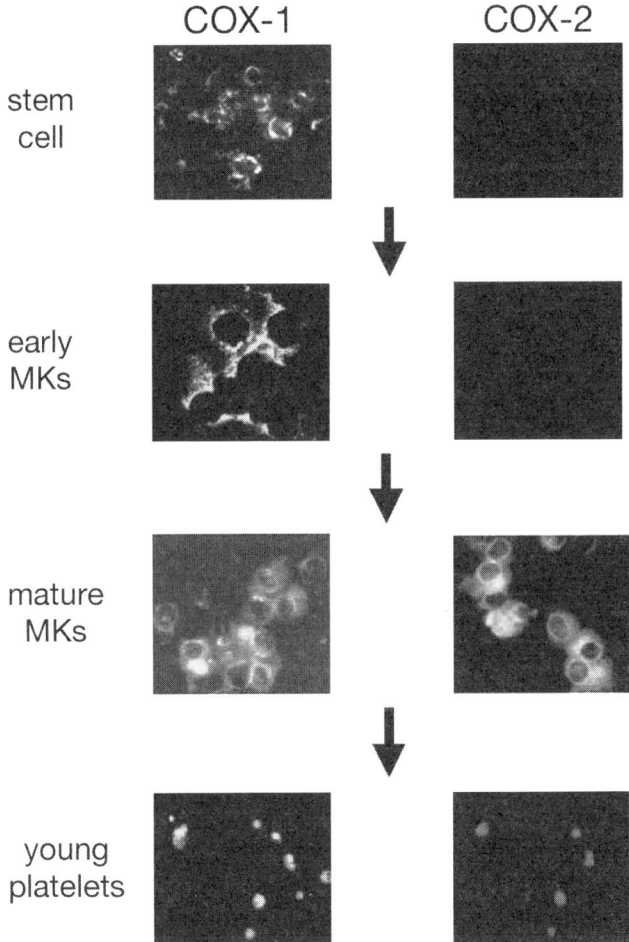

Fig. 2. Pattern of cyclooxygenase (COX)-1 and COX-2 expression during platelet formation. The differential expression of COX-1 and COX-2 along megakaryopoiesis is indicated in the figure, at different stages of development. The upper panels depict immunofluorescent staining for COX-1 or COX-2 of purified human stem cells differentiated toward megakaryocytes (MKs) in culture, with thrombopoietin. The bottom panels depict immunofluorescent stainings of washed peripheral platelets from a patient in the regenerative phase following stem cell transplantation.

tion *(5)*. Whereas COX-1 is primarily a constitutive enzyme, COX-2 is both constitutively expressed in some tissues (e.g., kidney and brain) and inducible in many different cell types. It has recently been shown that human platelets can synthesize new proteins such as bcl-3 and interleukin-1β (IL-1β) from preformed mRNAs in an activation-dependent fashion *(6,7)*. Whether this regulated translation applies to platelet COX-2 mRNA at sites of inflammation or hemostatic response is presently unknown.

Platelet COX-1 activity is predominant and is mainly coupled to TX synthase, although a smaller but consistent amount of COX-1-derived PGE_2 is also released during platelet activation. At variance with COX-1, COX-2-dependent TXA_2 synthesis from thrombin-stimulated platelets seems negligible under physiological circumstances *(5,8)*. COX-2 activity appears to be mainly coupled with PGE synthase(s), although under conditions of high platelet turnover a detectable, albeit small, amount of TXA_2 is COX-2 derived *(5)*.

TXA_2 is synthesized and released in response to a variety of platelet agonists and provides a strong signal that amplifies platelet activation, by inducing irreversible platelet aggregation. TXA_2 exerts its biological actions by binding specific receptors (TP). One gene and two alternative splicing isoforms of TP have been identified so far in humans: the α-isoform is a heptahelical transmembrane G-protein-coupled receptor, preferentially expressed on the platelet membrane. It couples Gq, inhibiting adenyl cyclase activity, thus leading to intraplatelet activatory signals *(9)*. The TPβ-isoform has been cloned from an umbilical endothelial cell library, and its presence and function in platelets remain controversial. Furthermore, on the basis of ligand/binding studies, two different types of PGH_2/TXA_2 receptors have been pharmacologically defined on human platelets, characterized by high and low affinity states *(10)*. Whether they correspond to the two cloned isoforms of TP is presently uncertain.

In addition to TXA_2, activated platelets release PGE_2, although at much lower concentrations compared with TXA_2. PGE_2 at low (nM) or high (μM) concentrations can increase platelet aggregation in response to subthreshold concentrations of different agonists or can inhibit the platelet response, respectively *(11–15)*. mRNAs for PGE_2 receptors (EP) of the EP3 and EP4 subtypes have been located on human platelets *(16)*. Studies in genetically modified mice showed that EP3 activation potentiates platelet aggregation in vitro in response to low-dose agonists, and EP3 gene deletion results in increased bleeding time and decreased incidence of thrombosis induced by arachidonic acid infusion *(14,17)*. Whether EP3 is activatory in human platelets and what is the role of EP4 during aggregation is presently unknown.

Although platelets cannot synthesize prostacyclin (PGI_2), they express its receptor (IP). PGI_2 triggers inhibitory signals in platelets. Consistently, IP-gene-deleted mice showed increased incidence of thrombosis induced in vivo by different experimental stimuli *(18)*. In addition, PGE_2 at μM concentrations decreases platelet aggregation by heterologous binding to the IP *(14)*.

Arachidonic acid can also be enzymatically converted by the platelet-type 12-lipoxygenases (P-12-LO) to 12-(S)-HETE. Mice lacking the P-12-LO gene showed increased sensitivity to ADP-induced aggregation, implying an inhibitory modulation exerted by 12-HETE on platelet activation *(19)*. A human P-12-LO has been cloned *(20)*, although its physiological role is less defined compared with the murine enzyme.

In addition to the above enzymatic pathways, arachidonic acid can be converted nonenzymatically to isomeric eicosanoid species called the *isoeicosanoids* (reviewed in ref. *21*), through a process of free radical-catalyzed lipid peroxidation *(22)*. Among this class of compounds, the most extensively studied are the F_2 isoprostanes, isomers of $PGF_{2\alpha}$, in particular 8-iso-$PGF_{2\alpha}$. Nanomolar concentrations of the latter compound cause vasoconstriction and activate platelets, causing shape change or potentiating the platelet response to subthreshold concentrations of other agonists *(22)*. Pharmacological studies in vitro or using genetically manipulated mice, either lacking or overexpressing the TP gene, strongly suggest that 8-iso-$PGF_{2\alpha}$ acts as a TP agonist *(23)*, although some data suggest that other, currently unknown, receptors may bind 8-iso-$PGF_{2\alpha}$ in platelets *(24)*. Importantly, F_2 isoprostanes can be measured in both plasma and urine *(22)* and can therefore provide a noninvasive index of lipid peroxidation in vivo.

Constitutive and Inducible Transcellular Arachidonic Acid Metabolism

Platelets and neighboring cells such as circulating leukocytes and/or endothelial cells, which also express phospholipases and COX isozymes, can cooperate in synthesizing various prostanoids *(21)*. This transcellular metabolism of arachidonic acid may have pharmacological and clinical implications (*see* TXA_2 Biosynthesis in Health and Disease section below).

In particular, it has been demonstrated that endothelial cells stimulated by thrombin in vitro can restore the capacity of aspirin-inactivated platelets to synthesize TXA_2, by providing biosynthetic intermediates that overcome the pharmacological blockade of platelet COX-1 *(25)*. On the other hand, platelet microparticles, shed from platelets into the extracellular space following activation, have been shown to upregulate COX-2 and PGI_2 synthesis in human endothelial cells in coculture systems *(26)*. COX-2-dependent PGI_2 synthesis is likely to represent a physiological antithrombotic mechanism that limits platelet activation, counteracting the proaggregatory action of TXA_2. Nevertheless, the pathophysiological relevance of the endothelial, COX-2-derived PGI_2 synthesis in humans is largely unknown *(27)*.

A bidirectional cross-talk might operate between platelets and leukocytes, although less direct evidence is available in this respect. Neutrophils upregulate COX-2 when exposed to inflammatory stimuli such as cytokines or lipopolysaccharide (LPS), and, as a consequence, PGE_2 and TXA_2 production increases in parallel, TXA_2 being the most abundant product *(28)*. Moreover, once activated, monocytes upregulate COX-2-dependent PGE_2 production *(28)*. Therefore, neutrophils, and possibly monocytes, express enzymatically active TX synthase. Owing to the capacity of nucleated leukocytes to resynthesize new enzyme, the irreversible inactivation of COX-1 by aspirin (*see* following sections) can be overcome in these cells, in contrast to the life-long defect in anucleated platelets. As a result, activated leukocytes might either provide PGH_2 to the platelet TX synthase or produce TXA_2, which may in turn activate adjacent, aspirinated platelets. Several studies indicate leukocytosis as an independent cardiovascular risk factor *(29)*, but whether this involves arachidonid acid metabolism is currently unknown.

Aside from using or responding to leukocyte-derived biosynthetic intermediates or prostanoids, platelets can also actively stimulate leukocytes. It has been demonstrated that adhesion of human monocytes to P-selectin via the P-selectin glycoprotein ligand-1 (PSGL-1) rapidly induces different mRNAs in the same cells, including COX-2 *(30,31)*. Indeed activated platelets express P-selectin, thus providing an excitatory signal to adjacent leukocytes. The same P-selectin-dependent activation has been demonstrated for tumor cells bearing PSGL-1. This mechanism may therefore induce COX-2 expression in tumor cells via activated platelets. Interestingly, the pharmacoepidemiology of colorectal cancer suggests a protective effect of low doses of aspirin, which presumably do not inhibit COX-2 in nucleated cells while permanently blocking platelet COX-1 activity *(32,33)*. Such a mechanism may link platelet activation to COX-2 induction in intestinal epithelial cells.

Finally, erythrocytes represent the vast majority of circulating blood cells. Their active role in hemostasis has been hypothesized *(34–36)*, based on studies showing that preincubation with erythrocytes facilitates platelet activation and recruitment in vitro *(35,36)*. This effect can be completely suppressed by administration of a single, high dose of aspirin (500 mg) in vivo, whereas a lower dose (50 mg/d) for up to 15 d only incompletely inhibits this phenomenon. The biochemical basis and clinical significance of these observations are presently unknown.

In conclusion, transcellular metabolism of arachidonic acid may involve multidirectional interactions between the different cellular players of hemostasis and thrombosis capable of processing biosynthetic intermediates to prostanoids, such as platelets, neutrophils, monocyte/

macrophages, and possibly erythrocytes. These interactions might lead to different net effects depending on several variables such as the vascular district (venous vs arterial, coronary vs cerebral), cardiovascular risk factors, and shear stress. These interactions may also affect the effectiveness of antithrombotic prophylaxis with low-dose aspirin, possibly through mechanism(s) that overcome the pharmacological blockade of platelet COX-1.

ANALYTICAL TOOLS FOR ASSESSING COX-1 AND -2 ACTIVITIES IN PLATELETS

The analytical tools for investigating platelet-derived TXA_2 metabolism in vivo and ex vivo is largely based on the knowledge of the catabolic pathways of TXA_2 and on the unique physiological features of platelets, with survival spanning 7–10 d. The lack of nucleus implies that these particles cannot transcribe new mRNAs and therefore have a limited, although not completely absent, capacity for translating new proteins. In the case of platelet COX-1, its irreversible inactivation by aspirin (*see* also Drugs Inhibiting Platelet Prostanoid Synthesis section below) lasts for the entire life span of the platelet, which cannot translate *de novo* COX-1 enzyme.

TXA_2 is a chemically unstable prostanoid that undergoes a rapid (half-life, 30 s), nonenzymatic hydration to TXB_2, a biologically inactive but chemically stable compound. Therefore, measurement of TXB_2 produced in vitro during whole blood clotting reflects the maximal, largely COX-1-dependent, biosynthetic capacity of circulating platelets activated by thrombin generated during clot formation *(37)*. The whole blood clotting assay has been used extensively both in vitro and ex vivo, to measure platelet-derived prostanoids (e.g., TXB_2 and PGE_2) and their pharmacological inhibition *(38)*.

Measurement of the actual rate of TXA_2 biosynthesis in vivo is based on characterization of the metabolic disposition of systemically infused TXB_2 in humans *(39,40)*. TXB_2 undergoes two major enzymatic degradation pathways, β-oxidation, which results in the formation of 2,3-dinor-TXB_2, and transformation through 11-OH-dehydrogenase into 11-dehydro-TXB_2. Both metabolites are chemically stable, have an extended plasma half-life, and are excreted in the urine of many mammalian species, including humans *(39,40)*. Compared with 2,3-dinor-TXB_2, 11-dehydro-TXB_2 a has longer half-life in plasma and is a more abundant metabolite of TXB_2 in human urine *(40)*. Measurement of thromboxane metabolite (TXM) excretion provides a reliable index of the actual rate of TXA_2 biosynthesis in vivo *(39)*.

Human studies assessing the effects of low-dose aspirin administration on TXM excretion suggest that in healthy subjects TXA_2 largely derives from platelets *(38)*. Therefore, measurement of urinary TXM and its pharmacological inhibition is currently the most reliable and widely used tool for studying TXA_2-dependent platelet activation in various clinical conditions.

On the other hand, the intrinsic capacity of platelets to generate TXA_2 when challenged ex vivo, as reflected by measurements of serum TXB_2, represents the maximal biosynthetic capacity and exceeds the endogenous rate of production of TXA_2 in vivo by several thousand fold in humans *(39)*. Therefore, serum TXB_2 represents a capacity index, whereas urinary TXM reflects—in a time-integrated fashion—the actual rate of TXA_2 production.

Other tests of platelet function, such as platelet aggregometry according to Born's method, assessment of platelet function using the Platelet Function Analyzer (PFA)-100, or cytofluorimetric studies of different platelet antigens, are far less sensitive and less specific for assessing platelet arachidonic acid metabolism and can be biased by several methodological factors compared with the assays described above *(41)*. Thus, platelet aggregation as measured by conventional methods ex vivo has less than ideal intra- and intersubject variability and displays limited sensitivity to the effect of aspirin, often considered a "weak" antiplatelet agent based on such measurements. In addition to technical variables, platelet aggregation responses among normal persons can vary with mental stress, age, gender, race, diet, and hematocrit level, and a person may have different responses on repeat determinations *(42)*. Moreover, the relevance of changes in this index of capacity to the actual occurrence of platelet activation and inhibition in vivo is largely unknown. It is perhaps important to remember that platelet aggregation measurements have not been particularly useful in describing the human pharmacology of aspirin. In fact, the development of low-dose aspirin as an antiplatelet agent was largely based on measurements of serum TXB_2, i.e., a mechanism-based biochemical end point *(38)*.

DRUGS INHIBITING PLATELET PROSTANOID SYNTHESIS

Aspirin

Aspirin and nonsteroidal antiinflammatory drugs (NSAIDs) are among the most widely used drugs worldwide. These drugs act through the inhibition of COX activity and consequently prevent the formation of prostanoids, although with different mechanisms and with variable COX-isozyme selectivity *(27)*.

Aspirin irreversibly acetylates Ser529 in the COX channel of human COX-1, thus hampering the access of substrate to the active site of the enzyme *(42)*. Aspirin acetylates Ser516 of human COX-2 as well, although it is approx 50–100-fold more potent in inhibiting platelet COX-1 than monocyte COX-2 *(43)*. The unique pharmacological features of aspirin, such as its short plasma half-life (15–20 min) and its efficiency in permanently inactivating COX-1 at low concentrations, as well as the unique biological features of anucleated platelets, such as their lack of substantial new protein synthesis, together result in complete and persistent blockade of platelet COX-1-dependent TXA_2 biosynthesis upon administration of low-dose aspirin in vivo *(42)*. Single oral doses of aspirin ranging from 5 to 100 mg, dose-dependently reduce platelet TXB_2 production in normal subjects, as measured by the whole blood assay ex vivo *(44)*.

Furthermore, the inhibitory effect of doses of aspirin less than 100 mg is cumulative upon repeated daily dosing, reaching a plateau within 3–10 d, depending on the dose and platelet turnover *(44,45)*. After aspirin withdrawal, the kinetics of TXA_2 synthesis recovery are consistent with the rate of platelet turnover, reflecting the entrance into the peripheral circulation of new platelets bearing nonacetylated COX-1 enzyme *(44)*. Thus, aspirin pharmacodynamics are completely dissociated from their pharmacokinetics.

The consistency of dose requirements and saturability of the effects of aspirin in acetylating platelet COX-1, inhibiting TXA_2 production, and preventing atherothrombotic complications constitutes the best evidence that aspirin prevents thrombosis through inhibition of platelet TXA_2 biosynthesis *(42)*.

Reversible Cyclooxygenase Inhibitors

A variety of NSAIDs can inhibit TXA_2-dependent platelet function through competitive, reversible inhibition of platelet COX-1. In general, these drugs, when used at conventional analgesic dosage, inhibit reversibly platelet COX activity by 70–90% *(42,45)*. This level of inhibition may be insufficient to block platelet aggregation adequately in vivo, because of the very substantial biosynthetic capacity of human platelets to produce TXA_2. Population-based observational studies have failed to detect an association between nonaspirin NSAID use and risk of myocardial infarction, although it is debated whether individual pharmacokinetic/pharmacodynamic features may explain conflicting results on naproxen *(42,46)*. Unfortunately, such case-control studies involve inherent biases that may be difficult or impossible to identify and adjust for, so they cannot detect moderate treatment effects reliably.

Coxibs were developed in an attempt to prevent the adverse gastrointestinal effects of nonselective NSAIDs (by avoiding inhibition of COX-1) while maintaining equivalent antiinflammatory efficacy (by inhibiting COX-2) *(27)*. Several large randomized trials have demonstrated that coxibs are associated with lower risk of serious gastrointestinal events than nonselective NSAIDs. However, the Vioxx Gastrointestinal Outcomes Research (VIGOR) Study of around 8000 patients with rheumatoid arthritis showed that those allocated to rofecoxib 50 mg daily experienced a higher risk of vascular events than those allocated to naproxen 500 mg twice daily *(47)*. This excess was almost entirely accounted for by a difference in the incidence of myocardial infarction (20 in 2699 person-years of follow-up among rofecoxib-allocated patients vs 4 in 2699 person-years among naproxen-allocated patients [relative risk 0.20, 95% CI 0.07–0.58]). There were no significant differences in stroke (11 rofecoxib vs 9 naproxen) or vascular deaths (7 rofecoxib vs 7 naproxen) *(47)*. Although the cause of the apparent excess risk of myocardial infarction in the VIGOR trial could not be conclusively established, a combination of some cardioprotective effect of naproxen and the play of chance did seem to offer a plausible explanation for these unexpected findings *(46)*. More recently, the results of two distinct long-term, placebo-controlled trials of rofecoxib and celecoxib for the prevention of colorectal polyp recurrence have raised a broader cardiovascular safety concern over COX-2 inhibitors *(48)*. However, given the relatively limited amount of information from placebo-controlled studies, both the size and mechanism(s) of the increased cardiovascular risk associated with this class of drugs remain uncertain.

TXA$_2$ BIOSYNTHESIS IN HEALTH AND DISEASE

TXM excretion reflects the actual rate of TXA$_2$ biosynthesis, largely derived from platelet COX-1 activity under physiological circumstances. Thus, TXM measurements have been used extensively to monitor platelet activation in vivo, in a variety of clinical settings in which platelet function is transiently or persistently enhanced in responses to pathophysiologic stimuli.

Persistently enhanced TXM excretion has been reported in association with major cardiovascular risk factors, such as cigarette smoking *(49)*, type IIa hypercholesterolemia *(50)*, type 2 diabetes mellitus *(51)*, severe hyperhomocysteinemia *(52)*, and visceral obesity *(53)*. Moreover, myeloproliferative disorders such as polycythemia vera *(54)* and essential thrombocythemia *(55)* are also characterized by markedly enhanced TXM excretion. Abnormal platelet activation in response to stimuli operating in vivo in the setting of myeloproliferative disorders is not reflected by capacity indexes of platelet function, as measured ex vivo, and is unrelated to the abnormal platelet count *(54,55)*.

Episodic increases in TXM excretion have been reported in patients with acute coronary syndromes *(56,57)* and in the acute phase of ischemic stroke *(58)*. These are likely to reflect episodes of platelet activation in response to acute vascular injury and are largely although not completely suppressed by low-dose aspirin *(57)*.

At least three potential mechanisms may underlie the occurrence of aspirin-resistant TXA_2 biosynthesis *(42)*. The transient expression of COX-2 in newly formed platelets *(5)* in clinical settings of enhanced platelet turnover is a potentially important mechanism that deserves further investigation. Extraplatelet sources of TXA_2 (e.g., monocyte/macrophage COX-2) may contribute to aspirin-insensitive TXA_2 biosynthesis in acute coronary syndromes *(58)*. Furthermore, Catella-Lawson et al. *(60)* have recently reported that concomitant administration of NSAIDs (e.g., ibuprofen) may interfere with the irreversible inactivation of platelet COX-1 by aspirin. This is owing to competition for a common docking site within the COX channel (arginine-120), which aspirin binds to with weak affinity prior to irreversible acetylation of Serine-529. This pharmacodynamic interaction does not occur with rofecoxib, or diclofenac, drugs endowed with variable COX-2 selectivity *(27)*. Thus, concomitant treatment with readily available over-the-counter NSAIDs may limit the cardioprotective effects of aspirin and contribute to aspirin "resistance." A recent observational study in patients with established cardiovascular disease lends support to the hypothesis of a clinically relevant interaction of ibuprofen and aspirin resulting in increased risk of cardiovascular mortality *(61)*.

The clinical relevance of aspirin-resistant TXA_2 biosynthesis has been explored by Eikelboom et al. *(62)*, who performed a nested case-control study of baseline urinary TXM excretion in relation to the occurrence of major vascular events in aspirin-treated high-risk patients enrolled in the Health, Osteoporosis, Progestin, Estrogen (HOPE) trial. After adjustment for baseline differences, the odds for the composite outcome of myocardial infarction, stroke, or cardiovascular death increased with each increasing quartile of 11-dehydro-TXB_2 excretion, with patients in the upper quartile having a 1.8-times higher risk than those in the lower quartile *(62)*. These interesting findings provide a rationale for testing the efficacy and safety of additional treatments (e.g., highly selective COX-2 inhibitors or TP antagonists) that more effectively block in vivo TXA_2 biosynthesis or action in a subset of high-risk patients displaying aspirin-resistant TXA_2 biosynthesis.

REFERENCES

1. Smith WL, Langenbach R. Why there are two cyclooxygenase isozymes. J Clin Invest 2001;107:1491–1495.
2. Ueno N, Murakami M, Tanioka T, et al. Coupling between cyclooxygenase, terminal prostanoid synthase, and phospholipase A_2. J Biol Chem 2001;276:34918–34927.
3. Matijevic-Aleksic N, Sanduja SK, Wang LH, Wu KK. Differential expression of thromboxane A synthase and prostaglandin H synthase in megakaryocytic cell line. Biochim Biophys Acta 1995;1269:167–175.
4. Weber AA, Zimmermann KC, Meyer-Kirchrath J, Schror K. Cyclooxygenase-2 in human platelets as a possible factor in aspirin resistance. Lancet 1999;353:900.
5. Rocca B, Secchiero P, Ciabattoni G, et al. Cyclooxygenase-2 is induced during human megakaryopoiesis and characterizes newly formed platelets. Proc Natl Acad Sci USA 2002;99:7634–7639.
6. Pabla R, Weyrich AS, Dixon DA, et al. Integrin-dependent control of translation: engagement of integrin alphaIIb beta3 regulates synthesis of proteins in activated human platelets. J Cell Biol 1999;144:175–184.
7. Lindemann S, Tolley ND, Dixon DA, et al. Activated platelets mediate inflammatory signaling by regulated interleukin 1beta synthesis. J Cell Biol 2001;154:485–490.
8. Patrignani P, Sciulli MG, Manarini S, et al. Patrignani COX-2 is not involved in thromboxane biosynthesis by activated human platelets. J Physiol Pharmacol 1999;50:661–667.
9. Raychowdhury MK, Yukawa M, Collins LJ, et al. Alternative splicing produces a divergent cytoplasmic tail in the human endothelial thromboxane A_2 receptor. J Biol Chem 1994;269:19256–19261.
10. Furci L, Fitzgerald DJ, FitzGerald GA. Heterogeneity of prostaglandin H_2/thromboxane A_2 receptors: distinct subtypes mediate vascular smooth muscle contraction and platelet aggregation. J Pharmacol Exp Ther 1991;258:74–81.
11. MacIntyre DE, Gordon JL. Calcium-dependent stimulation of platelet aggregation by PGE_2. Nature 1975;258:337–339.
12. Gray SJ, Heptinstall S. Interactions between prostaglandin E_2 and inhibitors of platelet aggregation which act through cyclic AMP. Eur J Pharmacol 1991;194:63–70.
13. Vezza R, Roberti R, Nenci GG, Gresele P. Prostaglandin E_2 potentiates platelet aggregation by priming protein kinase C. Blood 1993;82:2704–2713.
14. Fabre JE, Nguyen M, Athirakul K, et al. Activation of the murine EP3 receptor for PGE_2 inhibits cAMP production and promotes platelet aggregation. J Clin Invest 2001;107:603–610.
15. Matthews JS, Jones RL. Potentiation of aggregation and inhibition of adenylate cyclase in human platelets by prostaglandin E analogues. Br J Pharmacol 1993;108:363–369.
16. Paul BZ, Ashby B, Sheth SB. Distribution of prostaglandin IP and EP receptor subtypes and isoforms in platelets and human umbilical artery smooth muscle cells. Br J Haematol 1998;102:1204–1211.
17. Ma H, Hara A, Xiao CY, et al. Increased bleeding tendency and decreased susceptibility to thromboembolism in mice lacking the prostaglandin E receptor subtype EP(3). Circulation 2001;104:1176–1180.
18. Murata T Ushikubi F, Matsuoka T, et al. Altered pain perception and inflammatory response in mice lacking prostacyclin receptor. Nature 1997;388:678–682.
19. Johnson E, Brass LF, Funk CD. Increased platelet sensitivity to ADP in mice lacking platelet-type 12-lipoxygenase. Proc Natl Acad Sci USA 1998;95:3100–3105.

20. Funk CD, Furci L, FitzGerald GA. Molecular cloning, primary structure, and expression of the human platelet/erythroleukemia cell 12-lipoxygenase. Proc Natl Acad Sci USA 1990;87:5638–5642.

21. Maclouf J, Folco G, Patrono C. Eicosanoids and iso-eicosanoids: constitutive, inducible and transcellular biosynthesis in vascular disease. Thromb Haemost 1998;79:691–705.

22. Patrono C, FitzGerald GA. Isoprostanes: potential markers of oxidant stress in atherothrombotic disease. Arterioscler Thromb Vasc Biol 1997;17:2309–2315.

23. Audoly LP, Rocca B, Loeb AL, Coffman TM, FitzGerald GA. Cardiovascular responses to the isoprostanes iPF(2alpha)-III and iPE(2)-III are mediated via the thromboxane A(2) receptor in vivo. Circulation 2000;101:2833–2840.

24. Pratico D, Smyth EM, Violi F, FitzGerald GA. Local amplification of platelet function by 8-Epi prostaglandin F2alpha is not mediated by thromboxane receptor isoforms. J Biol Chem 1996;271:14916–14924.

25. Karim S, Habib A, Levy-Toledano S, Maclouf J. Cyclooxygenase-1 and -2 of endothelial cells utilize exogenous or endogenous arachidonic acid for transcellular production of thromboxane. J Biol Chem 1996;271:12042–12048.

26. Barry OP, FitzGerald GA. Mechanisms of cellular activation by platelet microparticles. Thromb Haemost 1999;82:794–800.

27. FitzGerald GA, Patrono C. The coxibs, selective inhibitors of cyclooxygenase-2. N Engl J Med 2001;345:433–442.

28. Rocca B, FitzGerald GA. Cyclooxygenases and prostaglandins: shaping up the immune response. Int Immunopharmacol 2002;2:603–630.

29. Brown DW, Giles WH, Croft JB. White blood cell count: an independent predictor of coronary heart disease mortality among a national cohort. J Clin Epidemiol 2001;54:316–322.

30. Mahoney TS Weyrich AS, Dixon DA, McIntyre T, Prescott SM, Zimmerman GA. Cell adhesion regulates gene expression at translational checkpoints in human myeloid leukocytes. Proc Natl Acad Sci USA 2001;98:10284–10289.

31. Zimmerman GA. Two by two: the pairings of P-selectin and P-selectin glycoprotein ligand 1. Proc Natl Acad Sci USA 2001;98:10023–10024.

32. Thun MJ, Henly SJ, Patrono C. Nonsteroidal antiinflammatory drugs as anticancer agents: mechanistic, pharmacological and clinical issues. J Natl Cancer Inst 2002;94:252–262.

33. Baron JA, Cole BF, Sandler RS, et al. A randomized trial of aspirin to prevent colorectal adenomas. N Engl J Med 2003;348:891–899.

34. Andrew DA, Low PS. Role of red blood cells in thrombosis. Curr Opin Hematol 1999;6:76–82.

35. Rocca B, FitzGerald GA. Simply read: erythrocytes modulate platelet function. Should we rethink the way we give aspirin? Circulation 1997;95:11–13.

36. Santos MT, Valles J, Aznar J, Marcus AJ, Broekman MJ, Safier LB. Prothrombotic effects of erythrocytes on platelet reactivity. Reduction by aspirin. Circulation 1997;95:63–68.

37. Patrono C, Ciabattoni G, Pinca E, et al. Low dose aspirin and inhibition of thromboxane B_2 production in healthy subjects. Thromb Res 1980;17:317–327.

38. Patrono C. Aspirin as an antiplatelet drug. N Engl J Med 1994; 330:1287–1294.

39. Patrono C, Ciabattoni G, Pugliese F, Pierucci A, Blair IA, FitzGerald GA. Estimated rate thromboxane secretion into the circulation of normal man. J Clin Invest 1986;77:590–594.

40. Ciabattoni G, Pugliese F, Davi G, Pierucci A, Simonetti BM, Patrono C. Fractional conversion of thromboxane B_2 to urinary 11-dehydrothromboxane B_2 in man. Biochim Biophys Acta 1989;992:66–70.

41. Patrono C, Patrignani P, Rocca B, Landolfi R. Characterization of biochemical and functional effects of antiplatelet drugs as a key to their clinical development. Thromb Haemost 1995;74:396–400.

42. Patrono C, Coller B, FitzGerald GA, Hirsh J, Roth G. Platelet-active drugs: the relationships among dose, effectiveness, and side effects: the Seventh ACCP Conference on Antithrombotic and Thrombolytic Therapy. Chest 2004;126(suppl 3):234S–264S.

43. Cipollone F, Patrignani P, Greco A, et al. Differential suppression of thromboxane biosynthesis by indobufen and aspirin in patients with unstable angina. Circulation 1997;96:1109–1116.

44. Patrignani P, Filabozzi P, Patrono C. Selective cumulative inhibition of platelet thromboxane production by low-dose aspirin in healthy subjects. J Clin Invest 1982;69:1366–1372.

45. Patrono C, Ciabattoni G, Patrignani P, et al. Clinical pharmacology of platelet cyclooxygenase inhibition. Circulation 1985;72:1177–1184.

46. Baigent C, Patrono C. Selective cyclooxygenase-2 inhibitors, aspirin and cardiovascular disease: a re-appraisal. Arthritis Rheum 2003;48:12–20.

47. Bombardier C, Laine L, Reicin A, et al.; VIGOR Study Group. Comparison of upper gastrointestinal toxicity of rofecoxib and naproxen in patients with rheumatoid arthritis. N Engl J Med 2000;343:1520–1528.

48. FitzGerald GA. Coxibs and cardiovascular disease. New Engl J Med. 2004; 351:1709–1711.

49. Nowak J, Murray JJ, Oates JA, FitzGerald GA. Biochemical evidence of a chronic abnormality in platelet and vascular function in healthy individuals who smoke cigarettes. Circulation 1987;76:6–14.

50. Davì G, Averna M, Catalano I, et al. Increased thromboxane biosynthesis in type IIa hypercholesterolemia. Circulation 1992;85:1792–1798.

51. Davì G, Catalano I, Averna M, et al. Thromboxane biosynthesis and platelet function in type II diabetes mellitus. N Engl J Med 1990;322:1769–1774.

52. Di Minno G, Davi G, Margaglione M, et al. Abnormally high thromboxane biosynthesis in homozygous homocystinuria. Evidence for platelet involvement and probucol-sensitive mechanism. J Clin Invest 1993;92:1400–1406.

53. Davi G, Guagnano MT, Ciabattoni G, et al. Platelet activation in obese women: role of inflammation and oxidant stress. JAMA 2002;288:2008–2014.

54. Landolfi R, Ciabattoni G, Patrignani P, et al. Increased thromboxane biosynthesis in patients with polycythemia vera. Evidence for aspirin-suppressable platelet activation in vivo. Blood 1992;80:1965–1971.

55. Rocca B, Ciabattoni G, Tartaglione R, et al. Increased thromboxane biosynthesis in essential thrombocythemia. Thromb Haemost 1995;74:1225–1230.

56. Fitzgerald DJ, Roy L, Catella F, FitzGerald GA. Platelet activation in unstable coronary disease. N Engl J Med 1986;315:983–989.

57. Vejar M, Fragasso G, Hackett D, et al. Dissociation of platelet activation and spontaneous myocardial ischemia in unstable angina. Thromb Haemost 1990;63:163–168.

58. Koudstaal PJ, Ciabattoni G, van Gijn J, et al. Increased thromboxane biosynthesis in patients with acute cerebral ischemia. Stroke 1993;24:219–223.

59. Cipollone F, Ciabattoni G, Patrignani P, et al. Oxidant stress and aspirin-insensitive thromboxane biosynthesis in severe unstable angina. Circulation 2000;102:1007–1013.

60. Catella-Lawson F, Reilly MP, Kapoor SC, et al. Cyclooxygenase inhibitors and the antiplatelet effects of aspirin. N Engl J Med 2001;345:1809–1817.

61. MacDonald TM, Wei L. Effect of ibuprofen on cardioprotective effect of aspirin. Lancet 2003;361:573–574.
62. Eikelboom Hirsh J, Weitz JI, Johnston M, Yi Q, Yusuf S. Aspirin-resistant thromboxane biosynthesis and the risk of myocardial infarction, stroke, or cardiovascular death in patients at high risk for cardiovascular events. Circulation 2002;105:1650–1655.

12 Platelets and Prothrombin

Michael Kalafatis, PhD,
Emil Negrescu, MD, PhD,
Tatiana Byzova, PhD,
and Edward F. Plow, PhD

INTRODUCTION

Blood coagulation is initiated following injury to the blood vessel wall through the exposure of tissue factor, which mediates the activation of circulating factor VII. Activated factor VIIa forms a complex with tissue factor and triggers the subsequent steps in the activation of the coagulation system, ultimately culminating in the conversion of prothrombin to thrombin *(1–5)*. The platelet membrane surface is crucial for this process, providing a milieu, referred to as the prothrombinase complex, for efficient assembly of the coagulation complexes and localization of the procoagulant response. Indeed, recent data have even implicated platelets in the initiation of coagulation as they acquire cir-

From: *Contemporary Cardiology:*
Platelet Function: Assessment, Diagnosis, and Treatment
Edited by: M. Quinn and D. Fitzgerald © Humana Press Inc., Totowa, NJ

culating forms of tissue factor, generated from other cells, on their surface *(6,7)*. Thrombin mediates fibrin formation and plays a critical role in the inflammatory responses *(8)*; thus, the regulation of prothrombin activation by the platelet membrane has broad physiological and pathophysiological implications.

The kinetic constants controlling the interactions between platelets and proteins of the coagulation cascade have been studied intensively for many years (reviewed in ref. 9). The accumulated data have demonstrated that most, if not all, of the coagulation factors interact with the phospholipid surface or with specific receptors on the platelet membrane. Direct comparisons between platelets and synthetic phospholipids vesicles have suggested that the activities of the different procoagulant complexes on the platelet surface cannot be fully recapitulated by phospholipid vesicles. These observations have stimulated the search for platelet surface receptors that facilitate, amplify, and localize the activity of the blood clotting factors. The present review focuses on the principle mechanisms for platelet interaction with specific coagulation proteins and the consequences of these interactions. We begin with a brief consideration of the molecular participants in these interactions.

COMPONENTS OF THE PROTHROMBINASE COMPLEX

The Platelet Membrane

Platelets circulate in a quiescent state. In resting platelets, a lipid asymmetry is maintained *(10)* with negatively charged phospholipids (phosphatidyl serine [PS] and phosphatidyl inositol [PI]) almost exclusively positioned on the inside leaflet of the membrane, with their polar headgroups oriented toward the cytosol. Platelet agonists alter this asymmetry. Such agonists include ADP, epinephrine, serotonin, and thrombin in the fluid phase and collagen or von Willebrand factor in the subendothelial matrix, at sites of vascular damage. An aminophospholipid translocase moves PS and phosphatidyl ethanolamine (PE) rapidly from the outer surface to the inner membrane in an energy-dependent process *(11)*. Neutral choline lipids (i.e., phosphatidyl choline [PC]) are moved negligibly or very slowly by this enzyme *(12–14)*. This movement is attenuated by increased cytosolic calcium levels *(15,16)*.

Another enzyme, a floppase, transports both aminophospholipids (PS and PE) and PC from the inner to the outer leaflet *(17)*. A lipid scramblase has also been characterized in platelets, which reorients phospholipids and requires the presence of cytosolic calcium *(18–20)*. In unactivated platelets, cytosolic calcium is low, and the opposing activities of the translocase and floppase result in a dynamic phospholipid distribution process, wherein the negative aminophospholipids (PS and PE) accumulate mostly on the inner monolayer. Activation of the platelets by any of several agonists (thrombin, ADP, and others) causes calcium release from internal stores, which inhibits the translocase but upregulates the scramblase. Hence, there is a redistribution of PS to the outer surface, where it can support prothrombin activation. If activation is not prolonged, a reversal of the calcium-inhibited translocase activity can be observed such that the outer membrane again becomes PS poor *(21)*. A strong phospholipid redistribution of the membrane lipids is observed upon treatment of platelets with calcium ionophores (such as A23817) and a combination of thrombin and collagen, whereas weaker effects are detected following treatment with thrombin or collagen alone. Differences among all these platelet activators have been reported to correlate with prothrombin-activating activity of the stimulated platelets *(22)*. An additional mechanism by which the platelet membrane influences prothrombin activation is through the release of procoagulant microvesicles, which occurs over time following initial activation of platelets *(23)*. This process depends on the activation of calpain, an intracellular protease, which may induce cytoskeletal rearrangements leading to microparticle extrusion *(23)*.

Factor X

Factor X is encoded by a 27-kb gene located on chromosome 13 *(24,25)*. Transcription of this gene results in formation of a 1.5-kb mRNA, which encodes for the factor X zymogen of M_r 59,000 *(26)*. The concentration of factor X in plasma is 170 nM *(27)*. Factor X is composed of a heavy chain (M_r 42,000) and a light chain (M_r 16,500) covalently associated through a disulfide bond. The light chain contains the γ-carboxyglutamate residues required for the proper interaction of the molecule with the membrane surface. Factor X is converted to its active form, factor Xa, following cleavage of the heavy chain at Arg194. This cleavage is catalyzed either by the *intrinsic tenase* (factor IXa/factor VIIIa) *(28)* or the *extrinsic tenase* (factor VIIa/TF) *(29)* and results in the release of a peptide of M_r 12,000.

Factor V

The factor V gene is located on chromosome 1, is 80 kb in length, and contains 24 introns; its transcription gives rise to a 6.9-kb mRNA *(30–32)*. Human factor V circulates in plasma at a concentration of 20 nM *(33)*, as a large, single-chain procofactor with an M_r of 330,000 *(34)*. Factor V is synthesized by the liver and by megakaryocytes. Platelet factor V, which accounts for 20% of the circulating factor V, is packaged in the secretory α-granules *(33)*. There are suggestions that platelet factor V is different from the plasma forms, based on experiments using a

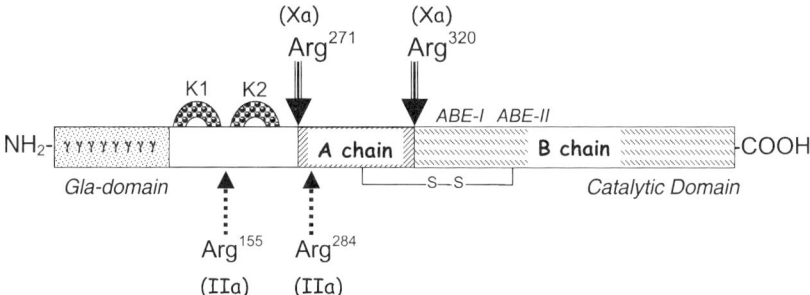

Fig. 1. Schematic representation of the prothrombin molecule. Prothrombin contains several specific features: a Gla domain with 10 γ-carboxyglutamic acids, 2 kringle domains, 2 anionic binding exosites (anionic binding exosite [ABE] I and II), and a catalytic domain. The activation cleavage sites by factor Xa are indicated on the top and the feedback cleavage sites by thrombin are indicated at the bottom.

mutant form of factor V and samples from a patient who underwent liver transplantation *(35)*. Factor V is cleaved by α-thrombin at Arg709, Arg1018, and Arg1545 to generate the active cofactor and two activation polypeptides *(32,34)*. The factor Va molecule is a heterodimer composed of a heavy chain of M_r 105,000 and a light chain of M_r 74,000. The two subunits are noncovalently associated via divalent metal ions.

Prothrombin

Prothrombin is encoded by a 21-kb gene located on chromosome 11 *(36,37)*. The gene is transcribed in the liver and gives rise to a 2-kb mRNA *(38)*. Prothrombin circulates in plasma at a concentration of approx 1.4 μM as an inactive zymogen of M_r 72,000 *(39,40)*. Prothrombin levels in plasma can vary, and a single-nucleotide polymorphism can give rise to increased prothrombin levels and is associated with an increased risk of venous thrombosis *(41)*. The 10 γ-carboxyglutamate residues that are involved in the Ca^{2+} and membrane binding properties of the protein (Gla domain) are located at the NH_2-terminal portion of the molecule (Fig. 1). This Gla domain is followed by two kringle domains. The Gla domain as well as the two kringle domains are released followed activation of the molecule by the factor Xa/Va complex (Fig. 1). Factor Xa in the presence of its cofactor, factor Va, and Ca^{2+} ions, activates membrane-bound prothrombin following proteolysis at two positions to yield thrombin. A first cleavage at Arg320 generates a two-chain intermediate of M_r 72,000 (meizothrombin), which is highly unstable *(42–44)* (Fig. 2). Meizothrombin is cleaved at Arg271 to generate α-thrombin and fragment 1•2. The latter is further cleaved by α-thrombin to pro-

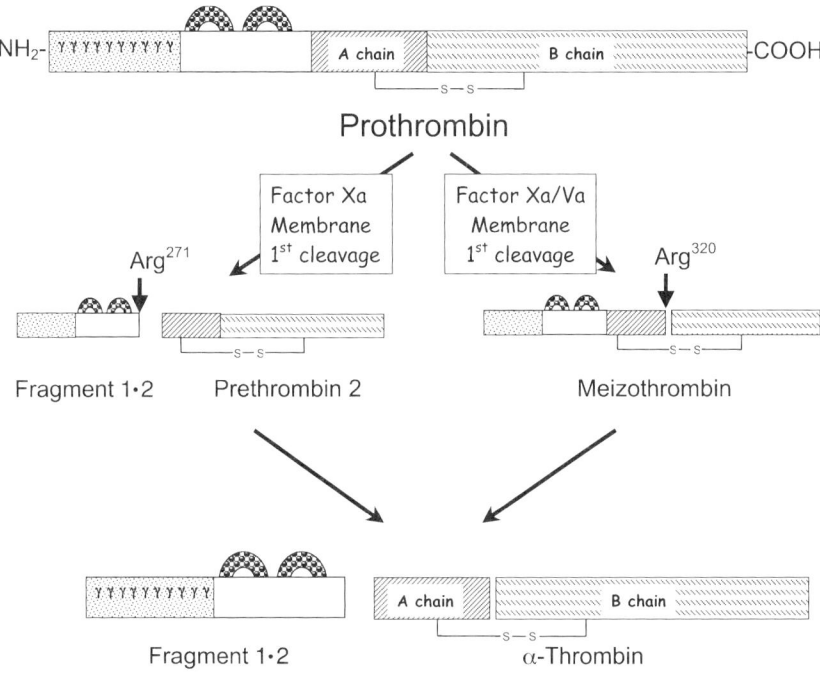

Fig. 2. Diagram of the pathways for activation of prothrombin and the effect of the cofactor. Cleavage of prothrombin by membrane-bound factor Xa is sequential, with the first cleavage at Arg271 generating fragment 1•2 and prothrombin 2 followed by cleavage at Arg320 and formation of α-thrombin. Binding of the nonenzymatic cofactor, factor Va, to cell-bound factor Xa reverses the order of cleavage and considerably increases the rate of thrombin formation. A first cleavage at Arg320 generates an enzymatically active intermediate, called meizothrombin, with the second cleavage at Arg271 producing fragment 1•2 and α-thrombin. α-Thrombin is a heterodimer composed of a light chain (α-chain) and a heavy chain (β-chain) associated through disulfide bonds.

thrombin fragment 1 plus prothrombin fragment 2 *(43,44)*. In the absence of factor Va, factor Xa cleaves prothrombin at Arg271 first, followed by cleavage at Arg320 (Fig. 2). The rate of thrombin formation by this pathway is approx 600 times slower than the alternative pathway for thrombin formation in the presence of factor Va *(43–45)*.

ASSEMBLY OF PROTHROMBINASE ON THE PLATELET MEMBRANE

The prothrombinase complex is composed of factor Va, the activated cofactor, factor Xa, the activated coagulation enzyme, and prothrombin, the substrate. These proteins associate in the presence of Ca^{2+} ions on the platelet membrane and catalyze the timely activation of prothrombin at sites of vascular injury. Human factor Va binds to platelets, and this interaction is independent of platelet activation. However, comparison of the interaction factor V and factor Va with activated platelets indicates that factor Va binds to the platelet surface with higher affinity *(46)*. This observation can be taken as evidence for a more complex interaction of factor V/Va with platelets than mediated exclusively phospholipid binding, and other evidence also supports this hypothesis. For example, the affinity of factor Va for the platelet membrane is an order of magnitude higher than the affinity of factor Va for phospholipid vesicles, i.e., the dissociation constant (K_d) of factor Va for binding to phospholipid vesicles is 2.9 nM *(47,48)* whereas the K_d for factor Va binding to human platelets is 0.1 nM. These data can be most readily explained by postulating a separate class of binding sites for factor Va on the platelet surface. The number of factor V/Va binding sites on platelets was estimated to be approx 2700–3000/platelet *(49)*. Data from several investigators *(48–51)* have established the existence of prothrombinase binding sites on the platelet surface. The kinetic parameters for prothrombin activation on platelets are similar to those obtained with synthetic phospholipids vesicles: a K_m of 0.5–1 μM and k_{cat} of 8–32 s^{-1}.

Platelet activation also plays a regulatory role in the activation of the prothrombinase complex. The factor Va/factor Xa complex binds equivalently to unstimulated and thrombin-stimulated platelets in suspension; however, platelet activation is required for optimal prothrombinase activation. When bound to thrombin-stimulated platelets, the complex mediates immediate prothrombin activation, whereas a lag is observed with resting platelets. Prothrombin, the substrate of the prothrombinase complex, and factor X can both bind to negatively charged phospholipid upon activation of platelets; however, the data again suggest that more complex receptors may exist on the platelet surface than can be accounted for by phospholipid alone *(50–52)*, as suggested by patients with bleeding disorders who have decreased binding sites for prothrombinbase on platelets *(50)*. A factor Xa receptor has been hypothesized, and a specific protein, named effector protein receptor-1 (EPR-1), that may function as such a receptor was identified *(53)* and shown to be present on platelets *(54)*. However, recent data have brought these claims into question *(55,56)*.

REGULATION OF PROTHROMBINASE ASSEMBLY AND FUNCTION

Assembly of enzyme complexes on a surface during tissue factor-induced coagulation presents opportunities for regulation of enzyme activity. Regulation is a process whereby the function or activity of each component in the complex is modulated. The binding of calcium to a number of sites in the Gla domain stabilizes the structure in this region of the prothrombin molecule *(57–60)*.

Whereas prothrombin is synthesized and processed almost exclusively in the liver, the tissue sources of cofactor molecule, which are limiting and are required for efficient complex assembly, are quite disparate. Significant stores of factor V are found in platelets *(33)*. In addition, regulation of the cell-associated binding sites occurs at several levels. Subsequent to early findings correlating the upregulation of procoagulant surface activity and redistribution of phospholipids within the inner and outer leaflets of the platelet membrane *(18,19,22)*, understanding of the role of the lipid membrane in hemostasis and thrombosis has progressed significantly. Currently, in a variety of cell types, common mechanisms are thought to exist that regulate the asymmetric distribution of lipids between the inner and outer leaflets of the bilayer. Activation of the cell during a hemostatic response results in a loss of membrane asymmetry and the redistribution of the lipids between the inner and outer surfaces of the membrane, providing a procoagulant surface on the exterior, which supports the assembly of complexes during the coagulation reaction.

Defects in platelet scramblase activity have been noted in a bleeding disorder known as Scott's syndrome *(61,62)*. This disease has been found in a French family and was considered hereditary in nature *(63)*. Scott's syndrome is characterized by a failure to accumulate PS at the platelet surface. Poor binding of the cofactors results in impaired prothrombinase activity *(50,51)*. It was also shown that hyperglycemia induces a loss in the phospholipid asymmetry of human erythrocytes *(64)*. Although it is evident that the defect affects Ca^{2+}-dependent lipid scrambling, the exact molecular cause of the defect remains unknown despite intensive study *(65,66)*. This defect was also demonstrated in erythrocytes, suggesting a common genetic origin in various cell types *(67)*. Finally, it must be noted that whereas calcium ionophores induce loss of lipid asymmetry on red cells, leukocytes, and endothelium, thrombin and other platelet activators do not universally cause loss of lipid asymmetry. For example, apoptosis is accompanied by a loss of lipid asymmetry in a variety of cell types, including lymphocytes, vascular smooth muscle cells *(68)*, and endothelium *(69)*.

INTEGRIN $\alpha_{IIb}\beta3$: AN ALTERNATIVE PROTHROMBINASE

The above synopsis indicates the importance of the platelet membrane, its phospholipid distribution, and the contributions of specific membrane receptors in the assembly and activation of the prothrombinase complex. In the context of the prothrombinase complex, the prothrombin "receptor" is factorVa/Xa/PL. Over the years, there have been suggestions that platelets might express specific binding sites for prothrombin that can influence thrombin generation and are unrelated to the "classic" prothrombinase. One such alternative prothrombinase is integrin $\alpha_{IIb}\beta_3$.

Interaction of $\alpha_{IIb}\beta_3$ With Prothrombin

$\alpha_{IIb}\beta_3$, glycoprotein (GP)IIb-IIIa, is a member of the integrin family of cell adhesion receptors (70,71). Each integrin is composed of an α- and a β-subunit, and each subunit is composed of a short cytoplasmic tail containing the C terminus of the polypeptide chain, a transmembrane segment, and a large extracellular domain composed of several hundred amino acids. Noncovalent interactions between the extracellular domains maintain the heterodimeric structure of each integrin. $\alpha_V\beta_3$, which is discussed in the Integrin-Mediated Recognition of Prothrombin on Vascular Cells section below, has the same β-subunit as $\alpha_{IIb}\beta_3$ (72). Whereas $\alpha_{IIb}\beta_3$ is restricted primarily to platelets and megakaryocytes, $\alpha_V\beta_3$ is expressed more broadly but is present at only low density on platelets (40,000–80,000 copies of $\alpha_{IIb}\beta_3$ per platelet vs 100–400 copies of $\alpha_V\beta_3$ (73,74). The two β_3-integrins recognize many ligands; some ligands interact with both integrins, and others are specific for either $\alpha_{IIb}\beta_3$ or $\alpha_V\beta_3$ (75,76). $\alpha_{IIb}\beta_3$ and $\alpha_V\beta_3$ belong to the class of integrins that recognize the RGD tripeptide sequence with high affinity (77): peptides containing RGD sequences inhibit the binding of many ligands to these integrins, and RGD sequences in ligands may but do not necessarily serve as recognition sequences. The structure and function of $\alpha_{IIb}\beta_3$ are discussed in many reviews (e.g., refs. 72, 78, and 79) and within several contributions to this volume.

One of the first inklings that $\alpha_{IIb}\beta_3$ may be involved in regulating prothrombin activation on platelets was derived from studies of patients with Glanzmann's thrombasthenia. This bleeding disorder is a consequence of a lack of functional $\alpha_{IIb}\beta_3$ on platelets. In the 1960s, it was reported that prothrombin activation was decreased with thrombasthenic compared with normal platelets (80–82), and this finding was corroborated in 1997 (83). Almost 30 yr after the initial observation, Reverter et al. (84) demonstrated that the combination of blocking monoclonal antibodies (MAbs) to $\alpha_{IIb}\beta_3$ and $\alpha_V\beta_3$ inhibited thrombin generation by platelets by approx 30–50% and that RGD peptides were also suppressive. Also relevant were the observations of Bar-Shavit et al. (85,86), who showed that endothelial cells adhered to altered forms of thrombin but not to native α-thrombin.

Based on these observations, we undertook an analysis of the direct interaction of prothrombin with platelets and the β_3-integrins. Utilizing ^{125}I-prothrombin, specific and saturable binding of this ligand to platelets was demonstrated. Saturation was observed at physiologic prothrombin concentrations, and approx 8000 prothrombin molecules were bound per platelet. The binding was inhibited by MAbs to $\alpha_{IIb}\beta_3$ and by RGD peptides, and the interaction was divalent ion dependent. Platelet activation did not affect the extent of prothrombin binding but did alter the susceptibility of its binding to physiological competitors. Fibrinogen, which binds only the activated $\alpha_{IIb}\beta_3$ on stimulated platelets, only inhibited prothrombin binding to the activated integrin and was unable to inhibit prothrombin binding to resting $\alpha_{IIb}\beta_3$. This reaction of prothrombin with resting $\alpha_{IIb}\beta_3$ distinguishes it from most of the other physiological RGD ligands of the receptors. Thrombin was not an inhibitor of prothrombin binding to either resting or stimulated platelets (87,88). We have also been able to detect prothrombin binding to $\alpha_{IIb}\beta_3$ on platelets by fluorescence-activated cell sorting analyses.

Binding of prothrombin to purified $\alpha_{IIb}\beta_3$ was also demonstrable, and the features of the interaction mirrored those for its interaction with platelets (87). More recently, platelets also were shown to adhere to prothrombin through an $\alpha_{IIb}\beta_3$ interaction (89). The candidate site for prothrombin recognition by $\alpha_{IIb}\beta_3$ is its RGD sequence, which resides at positions 187–189 in the thrombin region of the molecule in close proximity to the active site serine at position 195. Crystal structural data indicate that this sequence is not at the hydrated surface of thrombin (90) but might be available in prothrombin (91). Hence, there is a structural explanation for the selectivity of $\alpha_{IIb}\beta_3$ for prothrombin vs thrombin.

Influence of $\alpha_{IIb}\beta_3$ on Prothrombin Activation

A functional role of the interaction of prothrombin with $\alpha_{IIb}\beta_3$ was demonstrable. Binding to the integrin accelerated prothrombin activation by either factor Xa or factorXa/Va. This was shown by the ability of a MAb to $\alpha_{IIb}\beta_3$ to inhibit thrombin generation in an assay in which prothrombin was added to the immobilized integrin followed by the addition of the activators and a chromogenic thrombin substrate. The extent of inhibition by the $\alpha_{IIb}\beta_3$ MAb (Fab fragment) in this assay system was approx 25–30%. The best estimate of the accelerating effect of $\alpha_{IIb}\beta_3$ in this system was several hundred fold, a far cry from the several hundred thousand fold obtained with the assembled prothrombinase complex on platelets. However, as described in the next section, there is a rationale to suggest that the activation of prothrombin on $\alpha_{IIb}\beta_3$ may be of physiological importance. Fab inhibition was also used to demonstrate a role of $\alpha_{IIb}\beta_3$ on prothrombin activation with intact

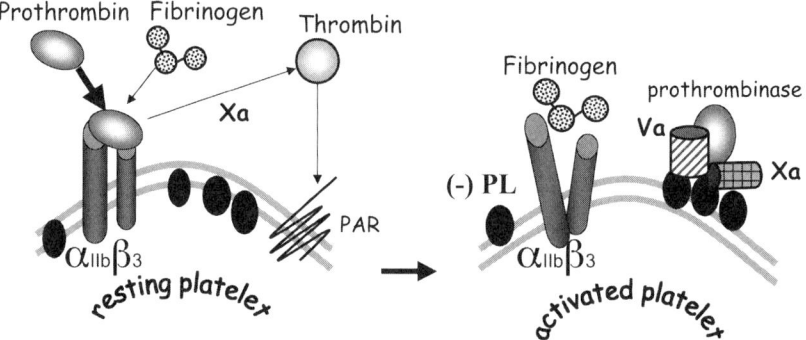

Fig. 3. Model for the role of $\alpha_{IIb}\beta_3$ in prothrombin activation. $\alpha_{IIb}\beta_3$ in its nonactivated state is capable of binding prothrombin but not fibrinogen. A source of factor Xa (or factor Xa/Va) can activate the prothrombin bound to $\alpha_{IIb}\beta_3$, and thrombin is released from the receptor. The thrombin can mediate platelet activation through the protease-activated receptors (PARs), leading to activation of $\alpha_{IIb}\beta_3$. Fibrinogen (or other ligands) "outcompetes" prothrombin for binding to the activated receptor.

platelets. Prothrombin activation by factor Xa or factor Va/Xa was suppressed by the Fab fragments on both resting and activated platelets, particularly at early time points. The fact that this accelerating effect can be observed with resting platelets, with no capacity to assemble to prothrombinase complex, i.e., no PS is exposed, implies a potentially unique role for $\alpha_{IIb}\beta_3$ as a prothrombinase.

Role of $\alpha_{IIb}\beta_3$ in Prothrombin Activation on Platelets

A model can be envisioned in which platelets circulate in blood with prothrombin on their surface bound to $\alpha_{IIb}\beta_3$ (Fig. 3). Generation of factor Xa, either on the platelet or on another cell type, can trigger activation of the integrin-bound prothrombin. Activation of this prothrombin leads to release of the thrombin from the integrin as its RGD sequence, which anchors it to $\alpha_{IIb}\beta_3$, undergoes a conformational rearrangement. The released thrombin in the vicinity of the platelet may activate the platelets by binding and cleaving PARs on the platelet surface *(92)*. The released thrombin also may bind to GPIb, a high-affinity site *(93)*, and this interaction can regulate its capacity to activate platelets and initiate formation of the prothrombinase complex by inducing PL translocation reactions *(94)*. Consequently, there is an explosive amplication of prothrombin activation. Thrombin generation will also lead to activation of $\alpha_{IIb}\beta_3$. The activated integrin is capable of binding any one of a number of adhesive proteins, which readily compete with plasma prothrombin for the activated integrin and support platelet aggregation and thrombus formation.

Pharmacological Implications of Involvement of $\alpha_{IIb}\beta_3$ in Prothrombin Activation

As noted above, Fab fragments reactive with $\alpha_{IIb}\beta_3$ can inhibit prothrombin activation by platelets. The Fab fragments used in these experiments was abciximab, one of the three intravenous $\alpha_{IIb}\beta_3$ antagonists in broad clinical use as antithrombotic drugs (95–97). As shown in Fig. 4, not only abciximab but also the two other Food and Drug Administration approved intravenous agents, eptifibatide, a cyclic peptide, and tirofiban, an RGD-based nonpeptidomimetic, suppressed prothrombin binding to platelets (Fig. 4A) and thrombin generation (Fig. 4B). Inhibition of prothrombin binding and thrombin generation was maximal with abciximab. The concentration of each agent used gave full inhibition of fibrinogen binding. Suppression of procoagulant activity has been noted in vitro and in vivo upon treatment with the $\alpha_{IIb}\beta_3$ antagonists (98–100). It has been suggested that this effect might arise from a suppression of PS expression by the drugs (101,102). However, under conditions in which the $\alpha_{IIb}\beta_3$ antagonists inhibited prothrombin, we did not detect PS expression, as assessed by annexin V, a probe for PS binding. On the contrary, it has been suggested that partial occupancy of $\alpha_{IIb}\beta_3$ may stimulate activation of the receptor, platelet activation, and, consequently, platelet procoagulant activity (103). This has been suggested as a basis for lower than anticipated efficacy to the negative effect of certain $\alpha_{IIb}\beta_3$ antagonists, particularly of the oral variety, in the treatment of acute coronary syndromes. It has been further suggested that, although all the $\alpha_{IIb}\beta_3$ antagonists are potent inhibitors of platelet aggregation and fibrinogen binding to the receptor, the inhibitors may differ in other functional activities, such as inhibition of platelet procoagulant activity, and this could account for differences in the efficacy of these drugs. However, the induction of platelet activation by $\alpha_{IIb}\beta_3$ antagonists remains controversial (104). With the contraction of the field of $\alpha_{IIb}\beta_3$ antagonists to a relatively small number, the three intravenous agents, and the cessation of programs to develop orally active $\alpha_{IIb}\beta_3$ antagonists, the importance that the inhibition of prothrombin binding and activation plays in their antithrombotic functions may not be resolved.

INTEGRIN-MEDIATED RECOGNITION OF PROTHROMBIN ON VASCULAR CELLS

On vascular endothelial and smooth muscle cells, integrin-mediated recognition of prothrombin can also be demonstrated (105). Binding is

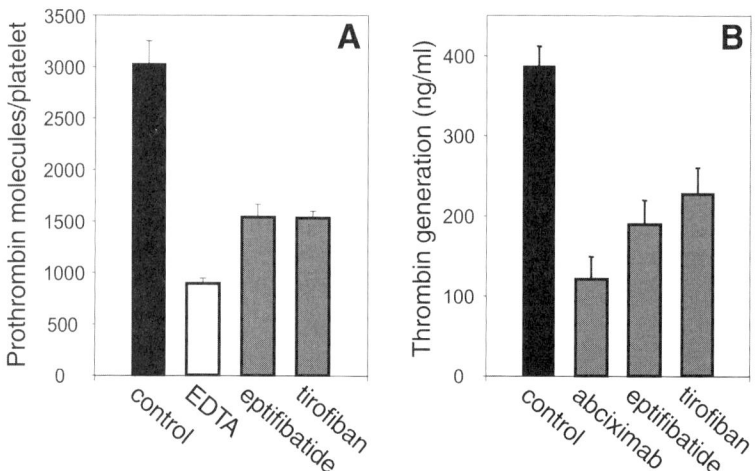

Fig. 4. (A) Inhibition of prothrombin binding to platelets by $\alpha_{IIb}\beta_3$ antagonists. Isolated platelets (5×10^8/mL) in Tyrode's buffer containing 1 mM CaCl$_2$ and 1 mM MgCl$_2$ were preincubated for 15 min at 37°C with the $\alpha_{IIb}\beta_3$ antagonists eptifibatide (5 μM) or tirofiban (20 nM), or with EDTA (20 mM), concentrations of these agents that fully blocked fibrinogen binding to platelets, and then ^{125}I-prothrombin, 100 μg/mL, was added. After 1 h at room temperature, platelet-bound ligand was separated by centrifugation through 20% sucrose, and the bound ligand was quantified. The data are means ± SD of quadruplicates and are representative of three separate experiments. **(B)** Effect of $\alpha_{IIb}\beta_3$ antagonists on thrombin generation by platelets. Platelets at 5×10^8/mL were incubated at 37°C with abciximab, 10 μg/mL; eptifibatide, 5 μM; or tirofiban, 20 nM). Then prothrombin at 100 μg/mL was added, and its activation was initiated by 1 μg/mL factor Xa and 1 μg/mL factor Va. Samples (15 μL) were removed after 2 min from the incubation mixtures and added to 200 μL of cold (4°C) buffer containing recombinant tick anticoagulant peptide at 1 μM in 0.1 M NaCl, 0.05 M Tris-HCl, 0.05% bovine serum albumin (w/v), 20 mM EDTA, pH 7.9. Then, samples (10 μL) were added to a prewarmed thrombin chromogenic substrate, Spectrozyme TH (75 μL), at a final concentration of 0.5 mM. The release of free chromophore was measured at 405 nm, and thrombin, at known concentration, was used for calibration. The data are means ± SD of triplicates and are representative of three separate experiments.

mediated primarily by $\alpha_V\beta_3$, although recognition by other integrins is not excluded. Interaction with $\alpha_V\beta_3$ requires activation of the integrin, and activation can be induced by model agonists, such as phorbol 12-myristate 13-acetate (PMA) or Mn^{2+}, or by physiological agonists, such as ADP or vascular endothelial growth factor *(106,107)*. Recognition can manifest as cell adhesion and migration to prothrombin or its binding as a soluble ligand. Although we know that binding of prothrombin to $\alpha_V\beta_3$ can enhance thrombin generation, critical comparison of this function by the two β_3-integrins has not been conducted. The recognition of prothrombin by vascular integrins may contribute to its localization in the vessel wall *(108,109)* and its enrichment in injured vessel walls *(110)*.

REFERENCES

1. Davie EW, Ratnoff OD. Waterfall sequence for intrinsic blood clotting. Science 1964;145:1310–1312.
2. MacFarlane RG. An enzyme cascade in the blood clotting mechanism, and its function as a biochemical amplifier. Nature 1964;202:498–499.
3. Mann KG, Krishnaswamy S, Lawson JH. Surface-dependent hemostasis. Semin Hematol 1992;29:213–226.
4. Kalafatis M, Swords NA, Rand MD, Mann KG. Membrane-dependent reactions in blood coagulation: role of the vitamin K-dependent enzyme complexes. Biochim Biophys Acta 1994;1227:113–129.
5. Broze, GJ Jr. Tissue factor pathway inhibitor and the revised theory of coagulation. Annu Rev Med 1995;46:103–112.
6. Giesen PLA, Rauch U, Bohrmann B, et al. Blood-borne tissue factor: another view of thrombosis. Proc Natl Acad Sci USA 1999;96:2311–2315.
7. Balasubramanian V, Grabowski E, Bini A, Nemerson Y. Platelets, circulating tissue factor, and fibrin colocalize in ex vivo thrombi: real-time fluorescence images of thrombus formation and propagation under defined flow conditions. Blood 2002;100:2787–2792.
8. Coughlin SR. Thrombin signalling and protease-activated receptors. Nature 2000;407:258–264.
9. Kalafatis M, Egan JO, van't Veer C, Cawthern KM, Mann KG. The regulation of clotting factors. Crit Rev Eukaryot Gene Expr 1997;7:241–280.
10. Zwaal RFA, Bevers EM, Comfurius P, Rosing J, Tilly RHJ, Verhallen PFJ. Loss of membrane phospholipid assymetry during activation of blood platelets and sickled red cells; mechanisms and physiological significance. Mol Cell Biochem 1989;91:23–31.
11. Bennett MR, Gibson DF, Schwartz SM, Tait JF. Binding and phagocytosis of apoptotic vascular smooth muscle cells is mediated in part by exposure of phosphatidylserine. Circ Res 1995;77:1136–1142.
12. Daleke DL, Huestis WH. Incorporation and translocation of aminophospholipids in human erythrocytes. Biochemistry 1985;24:5406–5416.
13. Sune A, Bette-Bobillo P, Bienvenue A, Fellman P, Devaux PF. Selective outside-inside translocation of aminophospholipids in human platelets. Biochemistry 1987;26:2972–2978.
14. Zimmerman ML, Daleke DL. Regulation of a candidate aminophospholipid-transporting ATPase by lipid. Biochemistry 1993;32:12257–12263.
15. Bitbol M, Fellman P, Zachowski A, Devaux PF. Ion regulation of phosphatidylserine and phosphatidylethanolamine outside-inside translocation in human erythrocytes. Biochim Biophys Acta 1987;904:268–282.
16. Tilly RHJ, Senden JMG, Comfurius P, Bevers EM, Zwaal RFA. Increased aminophospholipid translocase activity in human platelets during secretion. Biochim Biophys Acta 1990;1029:188–190.
17. Connor J, Pak CH, Zwaal PF, Schroit AJ. Bidirectional transbilayer movement of phospholipid analogs in human red blood cells. J Biol Chem 1992;267:19412–19417.
18. Bevers EM, Comfurius P, Zwaal RFA. Changes in membrane phospholipid distribution during platelet activation. Biochim Biophys Acta 1983;736:57–66.

19. Bevers EM, Tilly RH, Senden JM, Comfurius P, Zwaal RFA. Exposure of endogenous phosphatidylserine at the outer surface of stimulated platelets is reversed by restoration of aminophospholipid tranlocase activity. Biochemistry 1989;28:2382–2387.

20. Williamson P, Bevers EM, Smeets EF, Comfurius P, Schlegel RA, Zwaal RFA. Continuous analysis of the mechanism of activated transbilayer movement lipid movement in platelets. Biochemistry 1995;34:10448–10455.

21. Bevers EM, Comfurius P, VanRijn JLML, Hemker HC, Zwaal RFA. Generation of prothrombin-converting activity and the exposure of phosphatidylserine at the outer surface of platelets. Eur J Biochem 1982;122:429–436.

22. Rosing J, VanRijn JLML, Bevers EM, VanDiejen G, Comfurius P, Zwaal RFA. The role of activated human platelets in prothrombin and factor X activation. Blood 1985;65:319–322.

23. Dachary-Prigent J, Pasquet JM, Freyssinet JM, Nurden AT. Calcium involvement in aminophospholipid exposure and microparticle formation during platelet activation: a study using Ca^{2+}-ATPase inhibitors. Biochemistry 1995;34:11625–11634.

24. Royle NJ, Fung MR, MacGillivray RTA, Hamerton JL. The gene for clotting factor X is mapped to 13q32:qter. Cytogenet Cell Genet 1986;41:185–188.

25. Leytus SP, Chung DW, Kisiel W, Kurachi K, Davie EW. Characterization of a cDNA coding for human factor X. Proc Natl Acad Sci USA 1984;81:3699–3702.

26. Fujikawa K, Legaz ME, Davie EW. Bovine factors X_1 and X_2 (Stuart factor). Isolation and characterization. Biochemistry 1972;11:4882–4891.

27. DiScipio RG, Hermodson MA, Yates SG, Davie EW. A comparison of human prothrombin, factor IX (Christmas factor), factor X (Stuart factor), and protein S. Biochemistry 1977;16:698–706.

28. Østerud B, Rapaport SI. Synthesis of intrinsic factor X activator. Inhibition of the function of formed activator by antibodies to factor VIII and to factor IX. Biochemistry 1970;9:1854–1861.

29. Jesty J, Nemerson Y. The activation of bovine coagulation factor X. Methods Enzymol 1979;45:95–107.

30. Jenny RJ, Pittman DD, Toole JJ, et al. Complete cDNA and derived amino acid sequence of human factor V. Proc Natl Acad Sci USA 1987;84:4846–4850.

31. Cripe LD, Moore KD Kane WH. Structure of the gene for human coagulation factor V. Biochemistry 1992;31:3777–3785.

32. Kane WH, Ichinose A, Hagen FS, Davie EW. Cloning of cDNAs coding for the heavy chain region and connecting region of human factor V, a blood coagulation factor with four types of internal repeats. Biochemistry 1987;26:6508–6514.

33. Tracy PB, Eide LL, Mann, KG. Human prothrombinase complex assembly on isolated peripheral blood cell populations. J Biol Chem 1985;258:7264–7267.

34. Kane WH, Majerus PW. Purification and characterization of human coagulation factor V. J Biol Chem 1981;256:1002–1007.

35. Camire RM, Pollak ES, Kaushansky K, Tracy PB. Secretable human platelet-derived factor V originates from the plasma pool. Blood 1998;92:3035–3041.

36. Degen SJ, MacGillivray RTA, Davie EW. Characterization of the complementary deoxyribonucleic acid and gene coding for human prothrombin. Biochemistry 1983;22:2087–2097.

37. Degen SJ, Davie EW. Nucleotide sequence of the gene for human prothrombin. Biochemistry 1987;26:6165–6177.

38. MacGillivray RTA, Davie EW. Characterization of bovine prothrombin mRNA and its translation product. Biochemistry 1984;23:1626–1634.

39. Lundblad RL, Kingdon HS, Mann KG. Thrombin. In: Lorand L, ed. Methods in Enzymology, Proteolytic Enzymes, Part B. Academic, New York, 1976, pp. 156–176.

40. Kisiel W, Hanahan DJ. Purification and characterization of human factor II. Biochem Biophys Acta 1973; 304:103-113.
41. Poort SR, Rosendal FR, Reitsma PH, Bertina RM. A common genetic variation in the 3'-untranslated region of the prothrombin gene is associated with elevated plasma prothrombin levels and an increase in venous thrombosis. Blood 1996;88:3698–3703.
42. Heldebrant CM, Butkowski RJ, Bajaj SP, Mann KG. The activation of prothrombin. II: partial reactions, physical and chemical characterization of the intermediates of activation. J Biol Chem 1973;248:7149–7163.
43. Nesheim ME, Mann KG. The kinetics and cofactor dependence of the two cleavages involved in prothrombin activation. J Biol Chem 1983;258:5386–5391.
44. Krishnaswamy S, Church WR, Nesheim ME, Mann KG. Activation of human prothrombin by human prothrombinase: influence of factor Va on the reaction mechanism. J Biol Chem 1987;262:3291–3299.
45. Bruffato N, Nesheim ME. Analysis of the kinetics of prothrombin activation and evidence that two equilibrating forms of prothjrombinase are involved in the process. J Biol Chem 2003;278:6755–6764.
46. Tracy PB, Peterson JM, Nesheim ME, McDuffie FC, Mann KG. Interaction of coagulation factor V and factor Va with platelets. J Biol Chem 1979;254:10354–10361.
47. Krishnaswamy S, Mann KG. The binding of factor Va to phospholipid vesicles. J Biol Chem 1988;263:5714–5723.
48. Tracy PB, Nesheim ME, Mann KG. Coordinate binding of factor Va and factor Xa to the unstimulated platelet. J Biol Chem 1981;253:743–751.
49. Tracy PB. Regulation of thrombin generation at cell surfaces. Semin Hemost Thromb 1988;14:227–233
50. Miletich JP, Kane WH, Hofmann SL, Stanford N, Majerus PW. Deficiency of factor Xa-factor Va binding sites on the platelets of a patient with a rare bleeding disorder. Blood 1979;54:1015–1022.
51. Miletich JP, Majerus DW, Majerus PW. Patients with congenital factor V deficiency have decreased factor Xa binding sites on their platelets. J Clin Invest 1978;62:824–831.
52. Miletich JP, Jackson CM, Majerus PW. Properties of the factor Xa binding site on human platelets. J Biol Chem 1978;253:6908–6916.
53. Altieri DC. Molecular cloning of effector cell protease receptor-1, a novel surface receptor for the protease factor Xa. J Biol Chem 1994;269:3139–3142.
54. Bouchard BA, Catcher CS, Thrash BR, Adida C, Tracy PB. Effector cell protease receptor-1, a platelet activation-dependent membrane protein, regulates prothrombinase-catalyzed thrombin generation. J Biol Chem 1997;272:9244–9251.
55. Zaman GJR, Conway EM. The elusive factor Xa receptor: failure to detect transcripts that correspond to the published sequence of EPR-1. Blood 2000;96:145–148.
56. Briede JJ, Heemskerk JW, van't Veer C, Hemker HC, Lindhout T. Contribution of platelet-derived factor Va to thrombin generation on immobilized collagen- and fibrinogen-adherent platelets. Thromb Haemost 2001;85:509–513.
57. Tulinsky A, Park CH, Rydel TJ. The structure of prothrombin fragment 1 at 3.5 Å resolution. J Biol Chem 1985;260:10771–10778.
58. Tulinsky A, Park CH, Skrzypczak-Jankun E. Structure of prothrombin fragment 1 refined at 2.8 Å resolution. Biochemistry 1988;28:6805–6810.
59. Soriano-Garcia M, Park CH, Tulinsky A, Ravichandran KG, Skrzypczak-Jankun E. Structure of Ca^{2+} prothrombin fragment 1 including the conformation of the Gla domain. Biochemistry 1989;28:6805–6810.
60. Soriano-Garcia M, Padmanabhan K, de Vos AM, Tulinsky A. The Ca^{2+} ion and membrane binding structure of the Gla domain of Ca-prothrombin fragment 1. Biochemistry 1992;31:2554–2566.

61. Weiss HJ, Vivic WJ, Lages BA, Rogers J. Isolated deficiency of platelet procoagulant activity. Am J Med 1979;67:206–213.
62. Weiss HJ. Scott syndrome: A disorder of platelet coagulant activity. Semin Hematol 1994;31:312–319.
63. Toti F, Satta N, Fressinaud E, Meyer D, Freyssinet JM. Scott syndrome, characterized by impaired transmembrane migration of procoagulant phosphatidylserine and hemorrhagic complications, is an inherited disorder. Blood 1996;87:1409–1415.
64. Wilson MJ, Richterlowney K, Daleke DL. Hyperglycemia induces a loss of phospholipid asymmetry in human erythrocytes. Biochemistry 1993;32:11302–11310.
65. Zhou Q, Sims PJ, Wiedmer T. Expression of proteins controlling transbilayer movement of plasma membrane phospholipids in the B lymphocytes from a patient with Scott syndrome. Blood 1998;92:1707–1712.
66. Munnix IC, Harmsma M, Giddings JC, et al. Store-mediated calcium entry in the regulation of phosphatidylserine exposure in blood cells from Scott patients. Thromb Haemost 2003;89:687–695.
67. Bevers EM, Wiedmer T, Comfurius P, Shattil SJ, Weiss HJ, Zwaal RFA, Sims PJ. Defective Ca^{2+}-induced microvesiculation and deficient expression of procoagulant activity in erythrocytes from a patient with a bleeding disorder: a study of the red blood cells of Scott syndrome. Blood 1992;79:380–388.
68. Bennett MR, Gibson DF, Schwartz SM, Tait JF. Binding and phagocytosis of apoptotic vascular smooth muscle cells is mediated in part by exposure of phosphatidylserine. Circ Res 1995;77:1136–1142.
69. Bombeli T, Karsan A, Tait JF, Harlan JM. Apoptotic vascular endothelial cells become procoagulant. Blood 1997;89:2429–2442.
70. Hynes RO. Integrins: A family of cell surface receptors. Cell 1987;48:549–550.
71. Hynes RO. Integrins: bidirectional, allosteric signaling machines. Cell 2002;110:673–687.
72. Quinn MJ, Byzova TV, Qin J, Topol EJ, Plow EF. Integrin $\alpha_{IIb}\beta_3$ and its antagonism. Arterioscler Thromb Vasc Biol 2003;23:945–952.
73. Wagner CL, Mascelli MA, Neblock DS, Weisman HF, Coller BS, Jordan RE. Analysis of GPIIb/IIIa receptor number by quanitification of 7E3 binding to human platelets. Blood 1996;88:907–914.
74. Coller BS, Cheresh DA, Asch E, Seligsohn U. Platelet vitronectin receptor expression differentiates Iraqi-Jewish from Arab patients with Glanzmann thrombasthenia in Israel. Blood 1991;77:75–83.
75. Suehiro K, Smith JW, Plow EF. The ligand recognition specificity of β_3 integrins. J Biol Chem 1996;271:10365–10371.
76. Plow EF, Haas TA, Zhang L, Loftus J, Smith JW. Ligand binding to integrins. J Biol Chem 2000;275:21785–21788.
77. Ruoslahti E. RGD and other recognition sequences for integrins. Annu Rev Cell Biol. 1996;12:697–715.
78. Bennett JS. Structural biology of glycoprotein IIb-IIIa. Trends Cardiovasc Med 1996;6:31–36.
79. Hato T, Ginsberg MH, Shattil SJ. Integrin αIIbβ3. In: Michelson AD, ed. Platelets. Academic, San Diego, 2002, pp. 105–116.
80. Hardisty RM, Dormandy KM, Hutton RA. Thrombasthenia. Studies on three cases. Br J Haematol 1964;10:371–387.
81. Zucker MB, Pert JH, Hilgartner MW. Platelet function in a patient with thrombasthenia. Blood 1966;28:524–534.
82. Weiss HJ, Kochwa S. Studies of platelet function and proteins in 3 patients with Glanzmann's thrombasthenia. J Lab Clin Med 1968;71:153–165.

83. Weiss HJ, Lages B. Platelet prothrombinase activity and intracellular calcium responses in patients with storage pool deficiency, glycoprotein IIb-IIIa deficiency, or impaired platelet coagulant activity—a comparison with Scott syndrome. Blood 1997;89:1599–1611.

84. Reverter JC, Beguin S, Kessels H, Kumar R, Hemker HC, Coller BS. Inhibition of platelet-mediated, tissue factor-induced thrombin generation by the mouse/human chimeric 7E3 antibody: potential implications for the effect of c7E3 Fab treatment on acute thrombosis and "clinical restenosis." J Clin Invest 1996;98:863–874.

85. Bar-Shavit R, Sabbah V, Lampugnani MG, et al. An arg-gly-asp sequence within thrombin promotes endothelial cell adhesion. J Cell Biol 1991;112:335–344.

86. Bar-Shavit R, Eskohjido Y, Fenton JW, II, Esko JD, Vlodavsky I. Thrombin adhesive properties: induction by plasmin and heparan sulfate. J Cell Biol 1993;123:1279–1287.

87. Byzova TV, Plow EF. Networking in the hemostatic system. Integrin $\alpha_{IIb}\beta_3$ binds prothrombin and influences its activation. J Biol Chem 1997;272:27183–27188.

88. Plow EF, Byzova T. Prothrombin as a ligand for $\alpha_{IIb}\beta_3$ and $\alpha_V\beta_3$ defines new paradigms in the recognition specificity of β_3 integrins. In: Anonymous. New Frontiers in Vascular Biology: Thrombosis and Hemostasis. Proceedings of Symposium on Thrombosis and Hemostasis, Osaka, Japan, 2000, pp. 65–73.

89. Smyth SS, Tsakiris DA, Scudder LE, Coller BS. Structure and function of murine $\alpha_{IIb}\beta_3$ (GPIIb/IIIa): studies using monoclonal antibodies and β_3-null mice. Thromb Haemost 2000;84:1103–1108.

90. Stubbs MT, Bode W. A player of many parts: the spotlight falls on thrombin structure. Thromb Res 1993;69:1–58.

91. Vijayalakshmi J, Padmanabhan KP, Mann KG, Tulinsky A. The isomorphous structures of prethrombin2, hirugen-, and PPACK-thrombin: changes accompanying activation and exosite binding to thrombin. Protein Sci 1994;3:2254–2271.

92. Coughlin SR. Sol Sherry lecture in thrombosis: how thrombin 'talks' to cells: molecular mechanisms and roles in vivo. Arterioscler Thromb Vasc Biol 1998;18:514–518.

93. Jamieson GA, Okumura T. Reduced thrombin binding and aggregation in Bernard-Soulier platelets. J Clin Invest 1978;61:861–864.

94. Dörmann D, Clemetson KJ, Kehrel BE. The GPIb thrombin-binding site is essential for thrombin-induced platelet procoagulant activity. Blood 2000;96:2469–2478.

95. Lefkovits J, Plow EF, Topol EJ. Platelet glycoprotein IIb/IIIa receptors in cardiovascular medicine. N Engl J Med 1995;332:1553–1559.

96. Coller BS. GPIIb-IIIa antagonists: pathophysiologic and therapeutic insights from studies of c7E3 Fab. Thromb Haemost 1997;78:730–735.

97. Agah R, Plow EF, Topol EJ. GPIIb-IIIa antagonists. In: Michelson AD, ed. Platelets. Academic, San Diego, 2002, pp. 769–785.

98. Moliterno DJ, Califf RM, Aguirre FV, et al. Effect of platelet glycoprotein IIb/IIIa integrin blockade on activated clotting time during percutaneous transluminal coronary angioplasty or directional atherectomy (the EPIC trial). Am J Cardiol 1995;75:559–562.

99. Ammar T, Scudder LE, Coller BS. In vitro effects of the platelet glycoprotein IIb/IIIa receptor antagonist c7E3 Fab on the activated clotting time. Circulation 1997;95:614–617.

100. Dangas G, Badimon JJ, Coller BS, et al. Administration of abciximab during percutaneous coronary intervention reduces both ex vivo platelet thrombus formation and fibrin deposition: implications for a potential anticoagulant effect of abciximab. Arterioscler Thromb Vasc Biol 1998;18:1342–1349.

101. Pedicord DL, Thomas BE, Mousa SA, Dicker IB. Glycoprotein IIb/IIIa receptor antagonist inhibit the developmetn of platelet procoagulant activity. Thromb Res 1998;90:247–258.

102. Furman MI, Krueger LA, Frelinger AL III, et al. GPIIb-IIIa antagonist-induced reduction in platelet surface factor V/Va binding and phosphatidylserine expression in whole blood. Thromb Haemost 2000;84:492–498.

103. Peter K, Schwarz M, Ylanne J, et al. Induction of fibrinogen binding and platelet aggregation as a potential intrinsic property of various glycoprotein IIb/IIIa ($\alpha_{IIb}\beta_3$) inhibitors. Blood 1998;92:3240–3249.

104. Frelinger AL, III, Furman MI, Krueger LA, Barnard MR, Michelson AD. Dissociation of glycoprotein IIb/IIIa antagonists from platelets does not result in fibrinogen binding or platelet aggregation. Circulation 2001;104:1374–1379.

105. Byzova TV, Plow EF. Activation of $\alpha_v\beta_3$ on vascular cells controls recognition of prothrombin. J Cell Biol 1998;143:2081–2092.

106. Khaspekova SG, Vlasik TN, Byzova TV, Vinogradov DV, Berndt MC, Mazurov AV. Detection of an epitope specific for the dissociated form of glycoprotein IIIa of platelet membrane glycoprotein IIb-IIIa complex and its expression on the surface of adherent platelets. Br J Haematol 1993;85:332–340.

107. Byzova TV, Goldman CK, Pampori N, et al. A mechanism for modulation of cellular responses to VEGF: activation of the integrins. Mol Cell 2000;6:851–860.

108. Smith EB, Staples EM. Haemostatic factors in human aortic intima. Lancet 1981;1:1171–1174.

109. McBane RD, II, Miller RS, Hassinger NL, Chesebro JH, Nemerson Y, Owen WG. Tissue prothrombin. Universal distribution in smooth muscle. Arterioscler Thromb Vasc Biol 1997;17:2430–2436.

110. Hatton MWC, Southward SMR, Serebrin SD, Kulczycky M, Blajchman MA. Catabolism of rabbit prothrombin in rabbits: uptake of prothrombin by the aorta wall before and after a de-endothelializing injury in vivo. J Lab Clin Med 1995;126:521–529.

13 Markers of Platelet Activation and Granule Secretion

Alan D. Michelson, MD, and Mark I. Furman, MD

INTRODUCTION

Platelet activation results in a complex series of changes including a physical redistribution of receptors, changes in the molecular conformation of receptors, secretion of granule contents, development of a procoagulant surface, generation of platelet-derived microparticles, and formation of leukocyte-platelet aggregates. Each of these changes can potentially be used as a marker of platelet activation. Whole blood flow cytometry *(1)* is the method of choice for the measurement of all these changes, except the secretion of soluble molecules, which are usually measured by enzyme-linked immunosorbent assay (ELISA). Whole blood flow cytometry has many advantages, including: only minuscule volumes (~5 µL) of blood are required; platelets are directly analyzed in their physiological milieu of whole blood; the minimal manipulation of samples prevents artifactual in vitro activation and potential loss of platelet subpopulations; both the activation state of circulating platelets and the reactivity of circulating platelets can be determined; and a spectrum of different activation-dependent changes can be determined. The spe-

From: *Contemporary Cardiology:*
Platelet Function: Assessment, Diagnosis, and Treatment
Edited by: M. Quinn and D. Fitzgerald © Humana Press Inc., Totowa, NJ

cific methodological details of the use of flow cytometry to measure platelet activation are described elsewhere *(1–3)*.

MARKERS OF PLATELET ACTIVATION

Activation-Dependent Monoclonal Antibodies

Activation-dependent monoclonal antibodies, i.e., antibodies that bind to activated but not resting platelets, can be used to detect conformational changes in integrin $\alpha_{IIb}\beta_3$ (the glycoprotein [GP]IIb-IIIa complex, CD41/CD61), plasma membrane expression of granule membrane proteins, platelet surface binding of secreted platelet proteins, and development of a procoagulant surface (Table 1). The two most widely studied types of activation-dependent monoclonal antibodies are those directed against conformational changes in $\alpha_{IIb}\beta_3$ and those directed against granule membrane proteins.

Integrin $\alpha_{IIb}\beta_3$ is a receptor for fibrinogen and von Willebrand factor that is essential for platelet aggregation *(4)*. Whereas most monoclonal antibodies directed against $\alpha_{IIb}\beta_3$ bind to resting platelets, the monoclonal antibody PAC-1 is directed against the fibrinogen binding site exposed by a conformational change in $\alpha_{IIb}\beta_3$ of activated platelets (Table 1) *(5)*. Thus, PAC-1 only binds to activated platelets, not to resting platelets. Other $\alpha_{IIb}\beta_3$-specific activation-dependent monoclonal antibodies are directed against either ligand-induced conformational changes in $\alpha_{IIb}\beta_3$ (ligand-induced binding sites [LIBS]) *(6)* or receptor-induced conformational changes in the bound ligand (fibrinogen; receptor-induced binding sites [RIBS]) *(7)* (Table 1). Rather than $\alpha_{IIb}\beta_3$-specific monoclonal antibodies, fluorescein-conjugated fibrinogen can also be used in flow cytometric assays to detect the activated form of platelet surface $\alpha_{IIb}\beta_3$ *(8,9)*, but the concentration of unlabeled plasma fibrinogen and unlabeled fibrinogen released from platelet α granules must also be considered in these assays.

The most widely studied type of activation-dependent monoclonal antibodies directed against granule membrane proteins are P-selectin (CD62P)-specific. P-selectin is a component of the α-granule membrane of resting platelets that is only expressed on the platelet surface membrane after α-granule secretion *(10)*. Therefore a P-selectin-specific monoclonal antibody only binds to degranulated platelets, not to resting platelets. The activation-dependent increase in platelet surface P-selectin is not reversible over time in vitro *(11,12)*. However, in vivo circulating degranulated platelets rapidly lose their surface P-selectin but continue to circulate and function *(13,14)*. Platelet surface P-selectin is therefore not an ideal marker for the detection of circulating degranulated platelets, unless (1) the blood sample is drawn immedi-

Table 1
Activation-Dependent Monoclonal Antibodies:
Antibodies That Bind to Activated But Not Resting Platelets

Activation-dependent platelet surface change	Prototypic antibodies	References
Conformational changes in integrin $a_{IIb}\beta_3$		
Activation-induced conformational change in $\alpha_{IIb}\beta_3$ resulting in exposure of the fibrinogen binding site	PAC-1	5
Ligand-induced conformational change in $\alpha_{IIb}\beta_3$	PM 1.1, LIBS-1, LIBS-6	6, 79, 80
Receptor-induced conformational change in bound ligand (fibrinogen)	2G5, 9F9, F26	7, 52, 81
Plasma membrane expression of granule membrane proteins		
P-selectin (α-granules)	S12, AC1.2, 1E3	82–84
CD63 (lysosomes)	CLB-gran/12	85
LAMP-1 (lysosomes)	H5G11	86
LAMP-2 (lysosomes)	H4B4	87
CD40L	TRAP-1	88
Lectin-like oxidized LDL receptor-1 (LOX-1)	JTX-68	89
Platelet surface binding of secreted platelet proteins		
Thrombospondin	P8, TSP-1	90, 91
Multimerin	JS-1	92, 93
Development of a procoagulant surface[a]		
Factor V/Va binding	V237	18
Factor X/Xa binding	5224	94
Factor VIII binding	1B3	19

[a]Development of a procoagulant platelet surface can also be detected by the binding of annexin V to phosphatidylserine (20). Reproduced with permission from ref. 1, with permission from Elsevier.

Abbreviations: LAMP, lysosome-associated membrane protein; LDL, low-density lipoprotein; LIBS, ligand-induced binding site; TSP-1, thrombospondin-1.

ately distal to the site of platelet activation, (2) the blood sample is drawn within 5 min of the activating stimulus, or (3) there is continuous activation of platelets. The length of time that other activation-dependent surface markers remain expressed on the platelet surface in vivo has not yet been definitively determined.

Leukocyte-Platelet Aggregates

P-selectin mediates the initial adhesion of activated platelets to monocytes and neutrophils via the P-selectin glycoprotein ligand-1 (PSGL-1) counterreceptor on the leukocyte surface *(10)*. Monocyte-platelet and neutrophil-platelet aggregates are readily identified by whole blood flow cytometry *(15)*.

Tracking of autologous infused biotinylated platelets in baboons by three-color whole blood flow cytometry *(15)* enabled us to demonstrate directly in vivo that: (1) platelets degranulated by thrombin very rapidly (within 1 min) form circulating aggregates with monocytes and neutrophils (Fig. 1A); (2) the percent of monocytes with adherent infused platelets is greater than the percent of neutrophils with adherent infused platelets (Fig. 1A); and (3) the in vivo half-life of detectable circulating monocyte-platelet aggregates (approx 30 min) is longer than both the in vivo half-life of neutrophil-platelet aggregates (approx 5 min) and the previously reported *(13)* rapid loss of surface P-selectin from nonaggregated infused platelets (Fig. 1A).

All these findings suggested that measurement of circulating monocyte-platelet aggregates may be a more sensitive indicator of in vivo platelet activation than either circulating neutrophil-platelet aggregates or circulating P-selectin-positive nonaggregated platelets. We therefore performed two clinical studies in patients with acute coronary syndromes *(15)*. First, after percutaneous coronary intervention (PCI), there was an increased number of circulating monocyte-platelet (and, to a lesser extent, neutrophil-platelet) aggregates, but not P-selectin-positive platelets, in peripheral blood. Second, of patients presenting to an Emergency Department with chest pain, patients with acute myocardial infarction had more circulating monocyte-platelet aggregates than patients without acute myocardial infarction and normal controls. However, circulating P-selectin-positive platelets were not increased in chest pain patients with or without acute myocardial infarction *(15)*.

In summary, we have demonstrated by five independent means (in vivo tracking of activated platelets in baboons; Fig. 1A) *(15)*, human PCI *(15)*, human acute myocardial infarction *(15)*, human stable coronary artery disease (*16*; discussed in the Acute Coronary Syndromes section below), and human chronic venous insufficiency (*17*; discussed in the Peripheral Vascular Disease section below) that circulating monocyte-platelet aggregates are a more sensitive marker of in vivo platelet activation than platelet surface P-selectin.

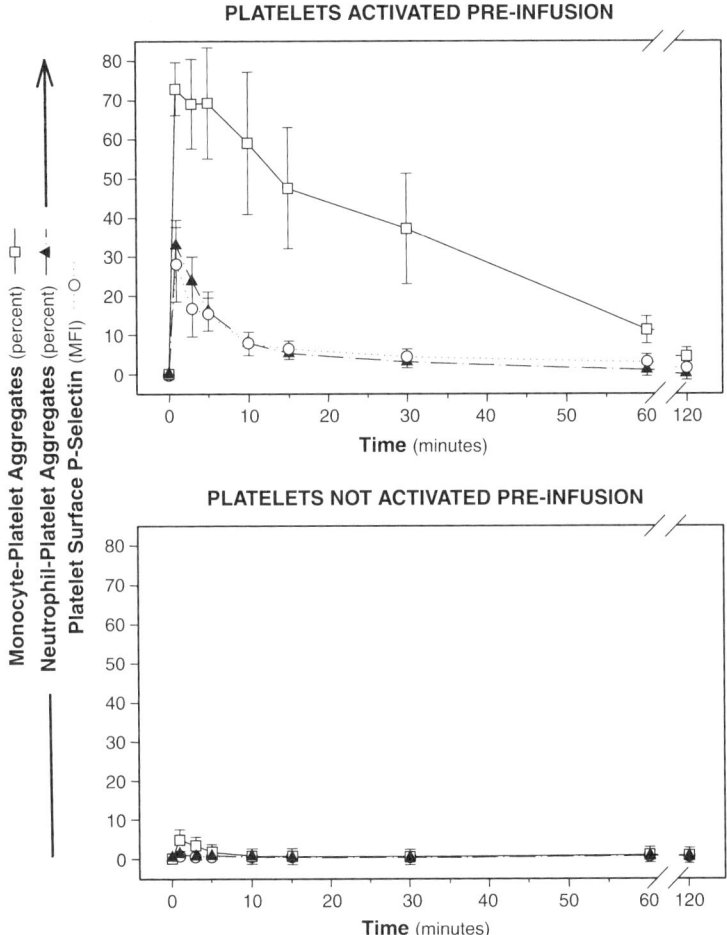

Fig. 1. In vivo tracking of platelets. Baboons were infused with autologous, biotinylated platelets that were **(upper)** or were not **(lower)** thrombin-activated pre-infusion. Surface P-selectin on the infused platelets and participation of the infused platelets in circulating monocyte-platelet and neutrophil-platelet aggregates were determined by three-color whole blood flow cytometric analysis of peripheral blood samples drawn at the indicated time points. The "0" time point refers to blood samples taken immediately pre-infusion. Platelet surface P-selectin (open circles) is expressed as mean fluorescence intensity (MFI), as a percentage of the fluorescence of a preinfusion maximally activated (10 U/mL) thrombin control sample. Monocyte-platelet (open squares) and neutrophil-platelet (closed triangles) aggregates are expressed as the percent of all monocytes and neutrophils with adherent infused platelets. Data are mean ± SEM. (From ref. *15*. Copyright 2001; with permission from Elsevier.)

Platelet-Derived Microparticles

As determined by flow cytometry, in vitro activation of platelets by some agonists (e.g., C5b-9, collagen/thrombin, and the calcium ionophore A23187) in the presence of extracellular calcium ions results in platelet-derived microparticles (defined by low forward-angle light scatter and binding of a platelet-specific monoclonal antibody) that are procoagulant (determined by binding of monoclonal antibodies to activated factors V or VIII or by annexin V) *(18–20)*. These findings suggest that procoagulant platelet-derived microparticles may play an important role in the assembly of the "tenase" and "prothrombinase" components of the coagulation system in vivo. A flow cytometric method for the direct detection of procoagulant platelet-derived microparticles in whole blood has been developed *(21)*.

Platelet-Derived Plasma Markers

Platelet secretion results in the release into plasma of numerous soluble molecules present in intracellular granules. Of these molecules, the most commonly measured as markers of platelet activation are the α-granule constituents soluble P-selectin *(22)*, β-thromboglobulin (β-TG) *(23,24)*, and platelet factor-4 (PF-4) *(23,24)*. However, as a result of the obligatory plasma separation procedures, these assays are particularly vulnerable to artifactual in vitro platelet activation *(23,24)*. Furthermore, soluble P-selectin in plasma may be of endothelial cell origin *(22)*. Lumiaggregometry can be used to measure the ex vivo release of ATP from dense granules in response to an exogenous agonist *(25)*.

A more useful plasma marker of in vivo platelet activation may be soluble CD40 ligand (sCD40L, CD154), because (1) release of sCD40L by activated platelets is the predominant source of plasma sCD40L *(26)*, and (2) the mechanism of sCD40L release is not platelet granule secretion but proteolysis of platelet surface CD40L *(26,27)*. sCD40L is prothrombotic via stabilization of arterial thrombi by a β_3-integrin-dependent mechanism *(28)* and proinflammatory via induction of leukocyte chemokine production *(29)* and endothelial cell adhesive proteins *(30)* (although not all studies agree on this latter point; *see* ref. 26). An important practical point is that in many published patient studies of sCD40L levels, the assay was performed in serum. However, blood clotting in a serum tube results in platelet activation and the ex vivo release of large amounts of sCD40L into the serum. Therefore, accurate measurement of in vivo circulating sCD40L requires assay in plasma rather than serum.

PLATELET ACTIVATION IN CLINICAL DISORDERS
Acute Coronary Syndromes

Whole blood flow cytometric studies have demonstrated circulating activated platelets, as determined by activation-dependent monoclonal antibodies, in patients with stable angina, unstable angina, and acute myocardial infarction *(16,31–34)*. In addition, as determined by activation-dependent monoclonal antibodies, coronary angioplasty results in platelet activation in coronary sinus blood *(35,36)*.

Flow cytometric analysis of platelet activation-dependent markers can be used to determine optimal antiplatelet therapy in clinical settings, e.g., in acute coronary syndromes *(37,38)* and after coronary stenting *(39,40)*. Flow cytometric analysis of platelet activation markers before angioplasty can predict an increased risk of acute and subacute ischemic events after angioplasty *(41–43)*. Flow cytometrically detected exposure of LIBS is strongly associated with the development and progression of heart transplant vasculopathy *(44)*.

Circulating leukocyte-platelet aggregates are increased in stable coronary artery disease *(16)*, unstable angina *(31)*, acute myocardial infarction *(45,46)*, and cardiopulmonary bypass *(47)*. Circulating leukocyte-platelet aggregates also increase after coronary angioplasty, with a greater magnitude in patients experiencing late clinical events *(48)*. As discussed in the Leukocyte-Platelet Aggregates section above, circulating monocyte-platelet aggregates (but not neutrophil-platelet aggregates) are a more sensitive marker of in vivo platelet activation than platelet surface P-selectin in the clinical settings of stable coronary artery disease *(16)*, PCI *(15)*, and acute myocardial infarction *(15)*. Furthermore, circulating monocyte-platelet aggregates are an early marker of acute myocardial infarction *(49)*.

Platelet-derived microparticles are increased in acute coronary syndromes *(50)* and cardiopulmonary bypass *(51,52)*.

Elevated plasma levels of sCD40L have been demonstrated in unstable angina *(53)*, PCI *(53)*, and cardiopulmonary bypass *(54)*. GPIIb-IIIa antagonists inhibit the release of sCD40L from platelets both in vitro *(27,55)* and in vivo *(56)*. A recent preliminary report suggests that measurement of sCD40L in the first 12 h after the onset of ischemic symptoms in patients with unstable angina identifies a subgroup of patients that has a much greater clinical benefit from abciximab treatment *(57)*. High plasma concentrations of sCD40L may be associated with increased cardiovascular risk in apparently healthy women *(58)*.

Cerebrovascular Ischemia

Increased circulating P-selectin-positive, CD63-positive, and activated $\alpha_{IIb}\beta_3$-positive platelets have been reported in acute cerebrovascular ischemia *(59–62)*. This platelet activation is evident 3 mo after the acute event, suggesting the possibility of an underlying prothrombotic state *(61)*. Furthermore, increased expression of surface P-selectin on platelets is a risk factor for silent cerebral infarction in patients with atrial fibrillation *(63)*.

Platelet-derived microparticles have been reported to be increased in transient ischemic attacks *(52,64)*. Increased platelet-derived microparticles and procoagulant activity occur in symptomatic patients with prosthetic heart valves and provide a potential pathophysiological explanation of cerebrovascular events in this patient group *(65)*.

Peripheral Vascular Disease

Circulating activated platelets and platelet hyperreactivity (as determined by P-selectin expression, platelet aggregates, and platelet-derived microparticle formation) were demonstrated in 50 patients with peripheral arterial occlusive disease compared with 50 healthy volunteers *(66)*. In addition, elevated plasma levels of sCD40L have been demonstrated in peripheral arterial occlusive disease *(67)*.

With regard to peripheral venous disease, Peyton et al. *(17)* demonstrated an increased number of circulating monocyte-platelet aggregates in patients with chronic venous stasis ulceration, compared with control individuals without venous disease. Interestingly, these changes were present not only in blood drawn from the lower extremity veins of affected individuals, but also in blood drawn from their arm veins, suggesting that the changes are systemic rather than localized to the lower extremities *(17)*. Powell et al. *(68)* further characterized these findings as being related to the presence of chronic venous disease rather than the presence of venous ulceration, since increased numbers of monocyte-platelet aggregates were noted in patients with all classes of venous disease, not just in patients with deep venous valvular insufficiency. Furthermore, increased levels of monocyte-platelet aggregates were noted even in patients with only superficial venous stasis disease manifested by the presence of varicose veins. Even more intriguing is the fact that the number of monocyte-platelet aggregates remains elevated 6 wk after total correction of the venous insufficiency by stripping of the abnormal veins, leaving normal venous physiology as documented by postoperative duplex scanning *(69)*. This finding suggests an underlying predisposition to the development of chronic venous disease in these patients, perhaps mediated by monocyte-platelet interactions.

Other Clinical Disorders Associated With Platelet Hyperreactivity and/or Circulating Activated Platelets

Other conditions in which whole blood flow cytometric measurement of platelet hyperreactivity, circulating activated platelets, and/or circulating leukocyte-platelet aggregates may prove to have a clinical role include diabetes mellitus *(70)*, preeclampsia *(71,72)*, hemodialysis *(73)*, sickle cell disease *(74)*, systemic inflammatory response syndrome *(75)*, septic multiple organ dysfunction syndrome *(76)*, myeloproliferative disorders *(77)*, and Alzheimer's disease *(78)*.

REFERENCES

1. Michelson AD, Barnard MR, Krueger LA, Frelinger AL III, Furman MI. Flow cytometry. In: Michelson AD, ed. Platelets. Academic/Elsevier Science, New York, 2002, pp. 297–315.
2. Krueger LA, Barnard MR, Frelinger III AL, Furman MI, Michelson AD. Immunophenotypic analysis of platelets. In: Robinson JP, Darzynkiewicz Z, Dean PN, et al., eds. Current Protocols in Cytometry. John Wiley, New York, 2002, pp. 6.10.1–6.10.17.
3. Barnard MR, Krueger LA, Frelinger III AL, Furman MI, Michelson AD. Whole blood analysis of leukocyte-platelet aggregates. In: Robinson JP, Darzynkiewicz Z, Dean PN, et al., eds. Current Protocols in Cytometry. John Wiley, New York, 2003, pp, 16.15.1–16.15.8.
4. Hato T, Ginsberg MH, Shattil SJ. Integrin alphaIIb-beta3. In: Michelson AD, ed. Platelets. Academic/Elsevier Science, New York, 2002, pp. 105–116.
5. Shattil SJ, Hoxie JA, Cunningham M, Brass LF. Changes in the platelet membrane glycoprotein IIb-IIIa complex during platelet activation. J Biol Chem 1985;260:11107–11114.
6. Frelinger AL, Lam SC, Plow EF, et al. Occupancy of an adhesive glycoprotein receptor modulates expression of an antigenic site involved in cell adhesion. J Biol Chem 1988;263:12397–12402.
7. Zamarron C, Ginsberg MH, Plow EF. Monoclonal antibodies specific for a conformationally altered state of fibrinogen. Thromb Haemost 1990;64:41–46.
8. Faraday N, Goldschmidt-Clermont P, Dise K, Bray PF. Quantitation of soluble fibrinogen binding to platelets by fluorescence-activated flow cytometry. J Lab Clin Med 1994;123:728–740.
9. Heilmann E, Hynes LA, Burstein SA, George JN, Dale GL. Fluorescein derivatization of fibrinogen for flow cytometric analysis of fibrinogen binding to platelets. Cytometry 1994;17:287–293.
10. McEver RP. P-selectin/PSGL-1 and other interactions between platelets, leukocytes, and endothelium. In: Michelson AD, ed. Platelets. Academic/Elsevier Science, New York, 2002, pp. 139–155.
11. Michelson AD, Benoit SE, Kroll MH, et al. The activation-induced decrease in the platelet surface expression of the glycoprotein Ib-IX complex is reversible. Blood 1994;83:3562–3573.
12. Ruf A, Patscheke H. Flow cytometric detection of activated platelets: comparison of determining shape change, fibrinogen binding, and P-selectin expression. Semin Thromb Hemost 1995;21:146–151.

13. Michelson AD, Barnard MR, Hechtman HB, et al. In vivo tracking of platelets: circulating degranulated platelets rapidly lose surface P-selectin but continue to circulate and function. Proc Natl Acad Sci USA 1996;93:11877–11882.

14. Berger G, Hartwell DW, Wagner DD. P-Selectin and platelet clearance. Blood 1998;92:4446–4452.

15. Michelson AD, Barnard MR, Krueger LA, Valeri CR, Furman MI. Circulating monocyte-platelet aggregates are a more sensitive marker of in vivo platelet activation than platelet surface P-selectin: studies in baboons, human coronary intervention, and human acute myocardial infarction. Circulation 2001;104:1533–1537.

16. Furman MI, Benoit SE, Barnard MR, et al. Increased platelet reactivity and circulating monocyte-platelet aggregates in patients with stable coronary artery disease. J Am Coll Cardiol 1998;31:352–358.

17. Peyton BD, Rohrer MJ, Furman MI, et al. Patients with venous stasis ulceration have increased monocyte-platelet aggregation. J Vasc Surg 1998;27:1109–1115.

18. Sims PJ, Faioni EM, Wiedmer T, Shattil SJ. Complement proteins C5b-9 cause release of membrane vesicles from the platelet surface that are enriched in the membrane receptor for coagulation factor Va and express prothrombinase activity. J Biol Chem 1988;263:18205–18212.

19. Gilbert GE, Sims PJ, Wiedmer T, et al. Platelet-derived microparticles express high affinity receptors for factor VIII. J Biol Chem 1991;266:17261–17268.

20. Furman MI, Krueger LA, Frelinger AL III, et al. GPIIb-IIIa antagonist-induced reduction in platelet surface factor V/Va binding and phosphatidylserine expression in whole blood. Thromb Haemost 2000;84:492–498.

21. Michelson AD, Rajasekhar D, Bednarek FJ, Barnard MR. Platelet and platelet-derived microparticle surface factor V/Va binding in whole blood: differences between neonates and adults. Thromb Haemost 2000;84:689–694.

22. Chong BH, Murray B, Berndt MC, et al. Plasma P-selectin is increased in thrombotic consumptive platelet disorders. Blood 1994;83:1535–1541.

23. Kaplan KL, Owen J. Radioimmunoassays of platelet alpha-granule proteins. In: Harker LA, Zimmerman TS, eds. Measurements of Platelet Function. Churchill Livingston, Edinburgh, 1983, pp. 115–125.

24. Levine SP. Secreted platelet proteins as markers for pathological disorders. In: Phillips DR, Shuman MA, eds. Biochemistry of Platelets. Academic, Orlando, FL, 1986, pp. 378–415.

25. Feinman RD, Lubowsky J, Charo I, Zabinski MP. The lumi-aggregometer: a new instrument for simultaneous measurement of secretion and aggregation by platelets. J Lab Clin Med 1977;90:125–129.

26. Henn V, Steinbach S, Buchner K, Presek P, Kroczek RA. The inflammatory action of CD40 ligand (CD154) expressed on activated human platelets is temporally limited by coexpressed CD40. Blood 2001;98:1047–1054.

27. Furman MI, Krueger LA, Barnard MR, Frelinger III AL, Michelson AD. Release of soluble CD40L from platelets is regulated by fibrinogen binding to GPIIb-IIIa and actin polymerization. J Am Coll Cardiol 2004;43:2319–2325.

28. Andre P, Prasad KS, Denis CV, et al. CD40L stabilizes arterial thrombi by a beta3 integrin-dependent mechanism. Nat Med 2002;8:247–252.

29. Kiener PA, Moran-Davis P, Rankin BM, et al. Stimulation of CD40 with purified soluble gp39 induces proinflammatory responses in human monocytes. J Immunol 1995;155:4917–4925.

30. Hollenbaugh D, Mischel-Petty N, Edwards CP, et al. Expression of functional CD40 by vascular endothelial cells. J Expl Med 1995;182:33–40.

31. Ott I, Neumann FJ, Gawaz M, Schmitt M, Schomig A. Increased neutrophil-platelet adhesion in patients with unstable angina. Circulation 1996;94:1239–1246.

32. Becker RC, Tracy RP, Bovill EG, Mann KG, Ault K. The clinical use of flow cytometry for assessing platelet activation in acute coronary syndromes. TIMI-III Thrombosis and Anticoagulation Group. Coron Artery Dis 1994;5:339–345.

33. Coulter SA, Cannon CP, Ault KA, et al. High levels of platelet inhibition with abciximab despite heightened platelet activation and aggregation during thrombolysis for acute myocardial infarction: results from TIMI (Thrombolysis in Myocardial Infarction) 14. Circulation 2000;101:2690–2695.

34. Schultheiss HP, Tschoepe D, Esser J, et al. Large platelets continue to circulate in an activated state after myocardial infarction. Eur J Clin Invest 1994;24:243–247.

35. Scharf RE, Tomer A, Marzec UM, et al. Activation of platelets in blood perfusing angioplasty-damaged coronary arteries. Flow cytometric detection. Arterioscler Thromb 1992;12:1475–1487.

36. Langford EJ, Brown AS, Wainwright RJ, et al. Inhibition of platelet activity by S-nitrosoglutathione during coronary angioplasty. Lancet 1994;344:1458–1460.

37. Langford EJ, Wainwright RJ, Martin JF. Platelet activation in acute myocardial infarction and unstable angina is inhibited by nitric oxide donors. Arterioscler Thromb Vasc Biol 1996;16:51–55.

38. Ault KA, Cannon CP, Mitchell J, et al. Platelet activation in patients after an acute coronary syndrome: results from the TIMI-12 trial. Thrombolysis in Myocardial Infarction. J Am Coll Cardiol 1999;33:634–639.

39. Gawaz M, Neumann FJ, Ott I, May A, Schomig A. Platelet activation and coronary stent implantation. Effect of antithrombotic therapy. Circulation 1996;94:279–285.

40. Neumann FJ, Gawaz M, Dickfeld T, et al. Antiplatelet effect of ticlopidine after coronary stenting. J Am Coll Cardiol 1997;29:1515–1519.

41. Tschoepe D, Schultheiss HP, Kolarov P, et al. Platelet membrane activation markers are predictive for increased risk of acute ischemic events after PTCA. Circulation 1993;88:37–42.

42. Gawaz M, Neumann FJ, Ott I, et al. Role of activation-dependent platelet membrane glycoproteins in development of subacute occlusive coronary stent thrombosis. Coron Artery Dis 1997;8:121–128.

43. Kabbani SS, Watkins MW, Ashikaga T, et al. Platelet reactivity characterized prospectively: a determinant of outcome 90 days after percutaneous coronary intervention. Circulation 2001;104:181–186.

44. Fateh-Moghadam S, Bocksch W, Ruf A, et al. Changes in surface expression of platelet membrane glycoproteins and progression of heart transplant vasculopathy. Circulation 2000;102:890–897.

45. Gawaz M, Reininger A, Neumann FJ. Platelet function and platelet-leukocyte adhesion in symptomatic coronary heart disease. Effects of intravenous magnesium. Thromb Res 1996;83:341–349.

46. Neumann FJ, Marx N, Gawaz M, et al. Induction of cytokine expression in leukocytes by binding of thrombin-stimulated platelets. Circulation 1997;95:2387–2394.

47. Rinder CS, Bonan JL, Rinder HM, et al. Cardiopulmonary bypass induces leukocyte-platelet adhesion. Blood 1992;79:1201–1205.

48. Mickelson JK, Lakkis NM, Villarreal-Levy G, Hughes BJ, Smith CW. Leukocyte activation with platelet adhesion after coronary angioplasty: a mechanism for recurrent disease? J Am Coll Cardiol 1996;28:345–353.

49. Furman MI, Barnard MR, Krueger LA, et al. Circulating monocyte-platelet aggregates are an early marker of acute myocardial infarction. J Am Coll Cardiol 2001;38:1002–1006.

50. Katopodis JN, Kolodny L, Jy W, et al. Platelet microparticles and calcium homeo-stasis in acute coronary ischemias. Am J Hematol 1997;54:95–101.
51. George JN, Pickett EB, Saucerman S, et al. Platelet surface glycoproteins. Studies on resting and activated platelets and platelet membrane microparticles in normal subjects, and observations in patients during adult respiratory distress syndrome and cardiac surgery. J Clin Invest 1986;78:340–348.
52. Abrams CS, Ellison N, Budzynski AZ, Shattil SJ. Direct detection of activated platelets and platelet-derived microparticles in humans. Blood 1990;75:128–138.
53. Aukrust P, Muller F, Ueland T, et al. Enhanced levels of soluble and membrane-bound CD40 ligand in patients with unstable angina. Possible reflection of T lym-phocyte and platelet involvement in the pathogenesis of acute coronary syndromes. Circulation 1999;100:614–620.
54. Nannizzi-Alaimo L, Rubenstein MH, Alves VL, et al. Cardiopulmonary bypass induces release of soluble CD40 ligand. Circulation 2002;105:2849–2854.
55. Nannizzi-Alaimo L, Alves VL, Phillips DR. Inhibitory effects of glycoprotein IIb/IIIa antagonists and aspirin on the release of soluble CD40 ligand during platelet stimulation. Circulation 2003;107:1123–1128.
56. Michelson AD, Krueger LA, Barnard MR, et al. GPIIb-IIIa antagonists reduce thromboinflammatory processes in patients with acute coronary syndromes under-going percutaneous coronary intervention [abstract]. J Thromb Haemost 2003.
57. Heeschen C, Hamm CW, van den Brand MJ, et al. CD40 ligand serum levels inde-pendently predicts outcome and effect of anti-platelet therapy in patients with un-stable angina [abstract]. Circulation 2002;106:II-402.
58. Schonbeck U, Varo N, Libby P, Buring J, Ridker PM. Soluble CD40L and cardio-vascular risk in women. Circulation 2001;104:2266–2268.
59. Grau AJ, Ruf A, Vogt A, et al. Increased fraction of circulating activated platelets in acute and previous cerebrovascular ischemia. Thromb Haemost 1998;80:298–301.
60. Zeller JA, Tschoepe D, Kessler C. Circulating platelets show increased activation in patients with acute cerebral ischemia. Thromb Haemost 1999;81:373–377.
61. Meiklejohn DJ, Vickers MA, Morrison ER, et al. In vivo platelet activation in atherothrombotic stroke is not determined by polymorphisms of human platelet glycoprotein IIIa or Ib. Br J Haematol 2001;112:621–631.
62. Yamazaki M, Uchiyama S, Iwata M. Measurement of platelet fibrinogen binding and P-selectin expression by flow cytometry in patients with cerebral infarction. Thromb Res 2001;104:197–205.
63. Minamino T, Kitakaze M, Sanada S, et al. Increased expression of P-selectin on platelets is a risk factor for silent cerebral infarction in patients with atrial fibrilla-tion: role of nitric oxide. Circulation 1998;98:1721–1727.
64. Lee YJ, Jy W, Horstman LL, et al. Elevated platelet microparticles in transient ischemic attacks, lacunar infarcts, and multiinfarct dementias. Thromb Res 1994;72:295–304.
65. Geiser T, Sturzenegger M, Genewein U, Haeberli A, Beer JH. Mechanisms of cerebrovascular events as assessed by procoagulant activity, cerebral microemboli, and platelet microparticles in patients with prosthetic heart valves. Stroke 1998;29:1770–1777.
66. Zeiger F, Stephan S, Hoheisel G, et al. P-Selectin expression, platelet aggregates, and platelet-derived microparticle formation are increased in peripheral arterial disease. Blood Coagul Fibrinol 2000;11:723–728.
67. Tsakiris DA, Tschopl M, Wolf F, et al. Platelets and cytokines in concert with endothelial activation in patients with peripheral arterial occlusive disease. Blood Coagul Fibrinol 2000;11:165–173.

68. Powell CC, Rohrer MJ, Barnard MR, et al. Chronic venous insufficiency is associated with increased platelet and monocyte activation and aggregation. J Vasc Surg 1999;30:844–851.

69. Rohrer MJ, Claytor RB, Garnette CSC, et al. Platelet-monocyte aggregates in patients with chronic venous insufficiency remain elevated following correction of reflux. Cardiovasc Surg 2002;10:464–469.

70. Tschoepe D, Roesen P, Esser J, et al. Large platelets circulate in an activated state in diabetes mellitus. Semin Thromb Hemost 1991;17:433–438.

71. Janes SL, Goodall AH. Flow cytometric detection of circulating activated platelets and platelet hyper-responsiveness in pre-eclampsia and pregnancy. Clin Sci 1994;86:731–739.

72. Konijnenberg A, van der Post JA, Mol BW, et al. Can flow cytometric detection of platelet activation early in pregnancy predict the occurrence of preeclampsia? A prospective study. Am J Obstet Gynecol 1997;177:434–442.

73. Gawaz MP, Mujais SK, Schmidt B, Blumenstein M, Gurland HJ. Platelet-leukocyte aggregates during hemodialysis: effect of membrane type. Artif Organs 1999;23:29–36.

74. Wun T, Cordoba M, Rangaswami A, Cheung AW, Paglieroni T. Activated monocytes and platelet-monocyte aggregates in patients with sickle cell disease. Clin Lab Haematol 2002;24:81–88.

75. Ogura H, Kawasaki T, Tanaka H, et al. Activated platelets enhance microparticle formation and platelet-leukocyte interaction in severe trauma and sepsis. J Trauma Injury Infect Crit Care 2001;50:801–809.

76. Gawaz M, Dickfeld T, Bogner C, Fateh-Moghadam S, Neumann FJ. Platelet function in septic multiple organ dysfunction syndrome. Intensive Care Med 1997;23:379–385.

77. Jensen MK, de Nully BP, Lund BV, Nielsen OJ, Hasselbalch HC. Increased circulating platelet-leukocyte aggregates in myeloproliferative disorders is correlated to previous thrombosis, platelet activation and platelet count. Eur J Haematol 2001;66:143–151.

78. Sevush S, Jy W, Horstman LL, et al. Platelet activation in Alzheimer disease. Arch Neurol 1998;55:530–536.

79. Ginsberg MH, Frelinger AL, Lam SC, et al. Analysis of platelet aggregation disorders based on flow cytometric analysis of membrane glycoprotein IIb-IIIa with conformation-specific monoclonal antibodies. Blood 1990;76:2017–2023.

80. Frelinger AL, Cohen I, Plow EF, et al. Selective inhibition of integrin function by antibodies specific for ligand-occupied receptor conformers. J Biol Chem 1990;265:6346–6352.

81. Gralnick HR, Williams SB, McKeown L, et al. Endogenous platelet fibrinogen: its modulation after surface expression is related to size-selective access to and conformational changes in the bound fibrinogen. Br J Haematol 1992;80:347–357.

82. Stenberg PE, McEver RP, Shuman MA, Jacques YV, Bainton DF. A platelet alpha-granule membrane protein (GMP-140) is expressed on the plasma membrane after activation. J Cell Biol 1985;101:880–886.

83. Carmody MW, Ault KA, Mitchell JG, Rote NS, Ng AK. Production of monoclonal antibodies specific for platelet activation antigens and their use in evaluating platelet function. Hybridoma 1990;9:631–641.

84. Larsen E, Celi A, Gilbert GE, et al. PADGEM protein: a receptor that mediates the interaction of activated platelets with neutrophils and monocytes. Cell 1989; 59:305–312.

85. Nieuwenhuis HK, van Oosterhout JJ, Rozemuller E, van Iwaarden F, Sixma JJ. Studies with a monoclonal antibody against activated platelets: evidence that a secreted 53,000-molecular weight lysosome-like granule protein is exposed on the surface of activated platelets in the circulation. Blood 1987;70:838–845.

86. Febbraio M, Silverstein RL. Identification and characterization of LAMP-1 as an activation-dependent platelet surface glycoprotein. J Biol Chem 1990; 265:18531–18537.

87. Silverstein RL, Febbraio M. Identification of lysosome-associated membrane protein-2 as an activation-dependent platelet surface glycoprotein. Blood 1992;80:1470–1475.

88. Henn V, Slupsky JR, Grafe M, et al. CD40 ligand on activated platelets triggers an inflammatory reaction of endothelial cells. Nature 1998;391:591–594.

89. Chen M, Kakutani M, Naruko T, et al. Activation-dependent surface expression of LOX-1 in human platelets. Biochem Biophys Res Commun 2001;282:153–158.

90. Boukerche H, McGregor JL. Characterization of an anti-thrombospondin monoclonal antibody (P8) that inhibits human blood platelet functions. Normal binding of P8 to thrombin-activated Glanzmann thrombasthenic platelets. Eur J Biochem 1988;171:383–392.

91. Aiken ML, Ginsberg MH, Plow EF. Mechanisms for expression of thrombospondin on the platelet cell surface. Semin Thromb Hemost 1987;13:307–316.

92. Hayward CP, Smith JW, Horsewood P, Warkentin TE, Kelton JG. p-155, a multimeric platelet protein that is expressed on activated platelets. J Biol Chem 1991;266:7114–7120.

93. Hayward CP, Bainton DF, Smith JW, et al. Multimerin is found in the alpha-granules of resting platelets and is synthesized by a megakaryocytic cell line. J Clin Invest 1993;91:2630–2639.

94. Holme PA, Brosstad F, Solum NO. Platelet-derived microvesicles and activated platelets express factor Xa activity. Blood Coagul Fibrinol 1995;6:302–310.

14 Genomic and Proteomic Analysis of Platelets

Clinical Applications

Andrew Maree, MD,
and James McRedmond, PhD

INTRODUCTION

The platelet is a circulating anucleate cell particle created from the cytoplasm of megakaryocytes in the bone marrow from whence it derives much of its cytoplasmic content. Deposited at sites of vascular injury, its role in the processes of thrombosis and haemostasis is well defined. Many important insights into the platelets haemostatic role were gained through genetic studies of rare inherited bleeding disorders such as Glanzmann's thrombesthenia and Bernard-Soulier disease [1,2]. It is now clear, however, that its physiological role extends beyond that of thrombosis to include regulation of inflammation, tissue repair, and the immune response, and one could argue that these are its predominant functions [3].

The contribution of platelets to certain pathological processes has also been extensively explored. Previously perceived as a passive component in atherothrombosis, the advent of newer molecular biology tech-

From: *Contemporary Cardiology:*
Platelet Function: Assessment, Diagnosis, and Treatment
Edited by: M. Quinn and D. Fitzgerald © Humana Press Inc., Totowa, NJ

niques to assess platelet function has revealed that platelets are involved in the earliest stages of vascular inflammation and have a complex interaction with both vascular cells and circulating blood cells. P-selectin (CD62P) release from α-granules is now understood to act as a receptor for monocytes and neutrophils in thrombin-activated platelets *(4)*. It has also been shown that activated platelets trigger an inflammatory response and procoagulant activity in endothelial cells and monocytes via a CD40/CD40L-dependent pathway *(5,6)*. Moreover, platelets incorporated into vascular plaque release platelet-derived growth factor, transforming growth factor, and chemokines, which modulate vessel wall adhesiveness, muscle cell proliferation, and inflammatory cell migration and thus may mediate coronary artery disease progression *(7)*.

As it becomes clear that platelet signaling and the resultant cell-cell interaction exceeds the perceived traditional thrombotic role, newer functional genomic techniques are being combined with complementary proteomic methods to advance our understanding of platelet biology. Such studies using a combined genomic–proteomic approach have demonstrated that platelet-secreted proteins such as RANTES and secretogranin III, thought to participate in vascular inflammation and cell proliferation, are present in human atherosclerotic plaque *(8,9)*. Integration of genomic and proteomic datasets using bioinformatics has also been used to study the platelet transcriptome *(10,11)*.

Definitions

Genetics is the study of patterns of inheritance of genetic information in organisms. This encompasses the study of genetic composition, heredity, variation and how that information is expressed.

Genomics is the study of the sequence, structure, and function of the genome. This involves the study of large numbers of genes and analysis of the relationship between gene activity and cell function and aims ultimately to assign useful biological information to all genes.

Proteomics is a complementary analysis to genomics in which the structure and function of proteins encoded by the genome are studied and catalogued. The ultimate aim is to understand entire protein systems, define component proteins, how they interact, and what kind of metabolic and signaling networks they form. Comparison of protein expression patterns in different environments helps to explain physiological and pathological roles.

The term *transcriptome* describes the cellular complement of all mRNA under a variety of cellular conditions. This is weighted by the expression level of molecules and incorporates results of alternative splicing. These products are continually changing in response to internal and external stimuli.

PLATELET RNA: ORIGIN, SIGNIFICANCE, AND CHALLENGES

Being anucleate and thus lacking transcriptional machinery, platelets are unable to transcribe nuclear genes or regulate gene expression at a transcriptional level. Therefore most regulation of function is effected at a posttranslational level. Platelets are, however, rich in mitochondria and contain approx 16 kb of genomic DNA, which encodes 13 genes and is thus likely to be actively transcribed in circulating platelets *(10)*. They also contain small amounts of mRNA derived from megakaryocytes, their nucleate precursor. The presence of rough endoplasmic reticulum and ribosomes in addition to mRNA means that platelets contain all the requirements for protein synthesis, and indeed *de novo* platelet protein synthesis has been confirmed *(12)* (Fig. 1).

Analysis of platelet mRNA provides information about platelet production, function, and the gene products present within. In contrast to this relatively static platelet profile, a more dynamic prospective is gained by studying the platelet proteome, which provides further insight into regulation of platelet function in both normal and pathological conditions. Although levels of translation in resting platelets are low, thrombin activation of platelets results in much higher levels of synthesis of several proteins. Thus, correlation of the platelet transcriptome with the proteome yields additional information about platelet physiology and its role in atherothrombotic pathology and may identify and validate novel therapeutic targets suitable for intervention.

The absence of nuclear DNA means that platelets do not lend themselves to analysis by traditional methods. Historically, platelet studies have employed techniques such as reverse transcriptase-polymerase chain reaction (RT-PCR), Northern blot hybridization, and, more recently, cDNA library construction. Although these studies confirmed the presence of various mRNA messages within the platelet, newer techniques such as microarray analysis and platelet proteomic analysis made it possible to characterize the platelet transcriptome and determine its contribution to platelet signaling and general function.

RNA isolation for transcriptional analysis using these newer techniques provides several challenges. Platelet isolates require an exceptionally high degree of purity. A single leukocyte contains 12,500 times the amount of RNA found in a platelet; thus minimal contamination makes the analysis redundant *(13)*. In addition, constant decay of mRNA in the absence of nuclear transcription and overrepresentation of more stable transcripts may obscure the presence of low-copy transcripts. Thus platelet RNA studies have significant limitations.

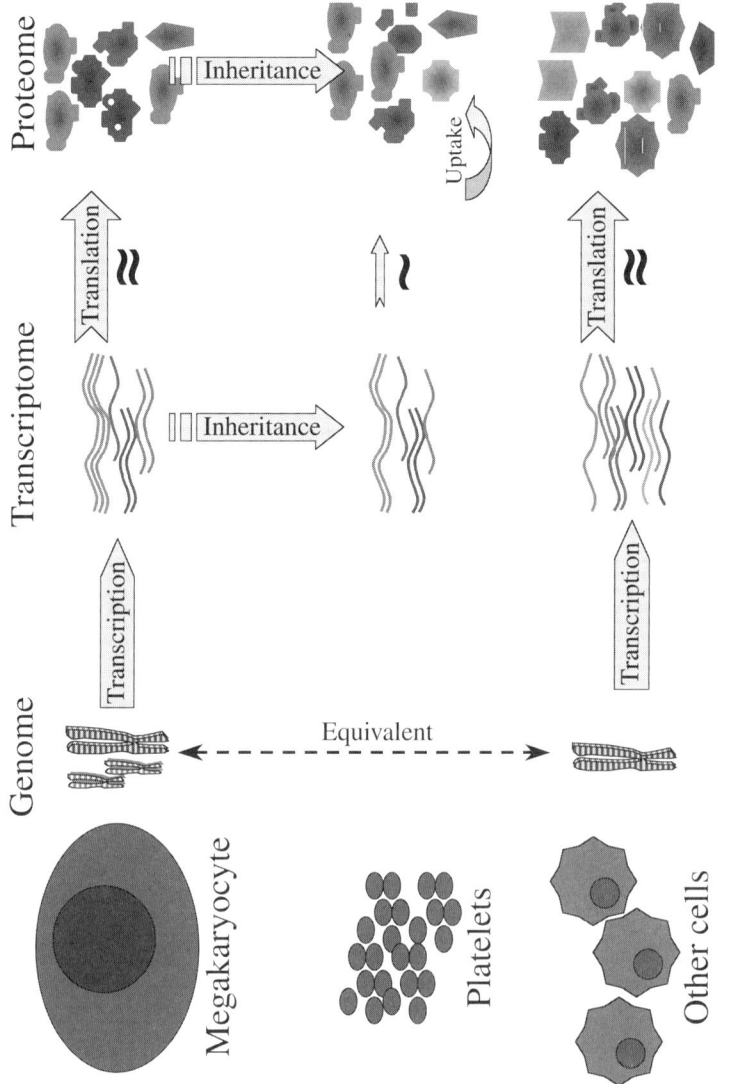

Proteome

Inheritance

Uptake

Translation

Translation

Inheritance

Genome

Equivalent

Megakaryocyte

Platelets

Other cells

THE COMPLEMENTARY NATURE OF GENOMICS AND PROTEOMICS

Most regulation of platelet function occurs at a posttranslational level. Indeed, more than a hundred posttranslational modifications have been described that alter enzyme activity, binding, and the length of time proteins remain active *(14)*. This becomes even more complex when one considers the often underestimated rate of splice variation that gives rise to a proteome and that significantly exceeds the number of genes *(15)*. Also noteworthy is the fact that gene-protein dynamics are nonlinear, and therefore correlation between gene activity and level of protein expression is unreliable *(16)*.

As with RNA analysis, current protein assays also have significant limitations. Unlike studies with DNA and RNA, protein analysis allows no amplification step, which therefore results in high-abundance proteins muffling low-abundance protein signals. This problem affects many regulatory proteins such as kinases and phosphatases, which exist in low copy numbers. Thus, limited and variable sample material in the absence of a reliable recombinant source to generate large amounts of protein is a considerable hurdle to be negotiated.

Despite early difficulties, platelet analysis using a combined genomic and proteomic approach is already starting to provide a macroscopic view of cell function and at the same time yield a comprehensive database of platelet gene function *(10,11)*. Initial studies have already advanced our understanding of the platelet's role in both physiological and

---

Fig. 1. *(opposite page)* Genomics and proteomics of platelets. Platelets largely inherit their transcriptome and proteome from megakaryocytes. Transcription of appropriate genes into mRNA and translation into protein results in a large degree of concordance between the identities of species in the transcriptome and proteome.

Platelets inherit their RNA and protein from megakaryocytes. Apparent attrition of RNA, failure to inherit all megakaryocyte proteins, and uptake of proteins from plasma by circulating platelets result in discrepancies between the RNA and protein content in platelets. Nevertheless, the transcriptome and proteome remain in reasonable agreement. Some translation of RNA into protein occurs in the platelet, at a basal level, and of specific transcripts in response to agonists.

The more direct routes of transcription and translation suggest that other cell types have a greater correspondence between the transcriptome and proteome, as well as a more diverse transcriptome than platelets. Nevertheless, the platelet transcriptome is complex, functional, and regulated. Many messages are relatively or absolutely platelet/megakaryocyte specific.

Megakaryocytes are polyploid but otherwise genetically identical to other cells. Genetic defects affecting platelet function are detectable in the DNA of any cell type.

pathological processes and should ultimately make early detection of patients at high risk of atherothrombotic disease attainable and thus facilitate primary and secondary disease prevention. Such analysis will also reveal novel targets for antiplatelet therapeutics and at the same time provide a means for their validation. Platelet pharmacogenomic studies that analyze platelet transcripts, their gene products, and drug response will make it possible to maximize treatment benefit, minimize side effects, and thus make "personalized medicine" more attainable. Ultimately the integration of platelet genomic and proteomic datasets thorough bioinformatics aims to provide a comprehensive database of platelet gene function.

METHODOLOGIES

A wide variety of molecular biological techniques in genomics and proteomics can be applied to the study of platelets. The following is not an exhaustive list but gives some of the more interesting methods, as well as precautions that must be taken owing to the peculiarities of platelets.

Mutation Detection

Mutation of protein coding sequences anywhere in the genome can give rise to defective proteins, and those in noncoding regions can alter patterns of protein expression. Platelet proteins are equally susceptible to such alterations; however, a comprehensive treatment of this topic is beyond the scope of this chapter.

Single-Nucleotide Polymorphisms

Single-nucleotide polymorphisms (SNPs; pronounced "snips"), the commonest form of polymorphism, are often benign and are used as markers of genetic similarity between individuals or populations. Defining a polymorphism as a difference occurring in more than 1% of the population, the reported incidence of 1 in approx 1300 bases implies that a "typical" genomic protein coding region of 27 kb *(17)* would be expected to contain approx 20 SNPs with the potential to alter protein expression. In fact, genes are less SNP dense than the rest of the genome, but the overall SNP frequency is higher. In keeping with this observation, a survey of 4000 genes found approx 16 SNPs per gene *(18)*.

Genes of interest can be scanned for SNPs, populations screened for their presence *(19)*, and an association sought between a particular allele and a phenotypic effect. Indeed, this has been done for certain genes expressed on platelets. In most cases, however, a strong association between SNP and disease is not provable.

One form of the most intensively investigated platelet SNP, the Pl (A)2 allele of glycoprotein (GP)IIIa, has been reported to be associated with cardiovascular disease in young men *(20)* and multivessel disease *(21)*, whereas other studies have failed to find any association with coronary artery disease *(22,23)*.

Pharmacogenomics is the study of how patient response to drugs varies depending on their genotype. Many pharmacogenomic effects found to date can be ascribed to differences in drug-metabolizing enzymes *(24)*; however, differences owing to genetic variation in the drug target are also evident. Patient responses to the antiplatelet drug orbofiban may vary depending on their Pl (A) genotype *(25)*. The phenomenon of aspirin resistance, which may be influenced by pharmacogenetic factors *(26)*, could also be caused by pharmacokinetic factors in many cases (Maree and Fitzgerald, unpublished data).

Platelet Genetic Diseases

Many heritable platelet disorders *(27)* are caused by genetic defects. Clinical symptoms may suggest a candidate gene, which is then scanned to pinpoint the molecular cause of the disease. This is usually performed using genomic DNA, which platelets lack. In some cases, however, extraction of the protein's mRNA from platelets can facilitate identification of the defect or provide further insight. Glanzmann's thrombasthenia is caused by a lack of or functional defect in the platelet integrin GPIIb-IIIa *(28)*. Owing to the myriad causative mutations *(29)*, as well as the complex genomic arrangement of the IIb and IIIa genes *(30,31)*, RT-PCR and sequencing of the IIb and IIIa cDNAs has been used to screen the coding region for the site of premature stop codons *(32,33)*; to determine which of two defective alleles is expressed *(34)*; to quantify the message level in response to a mutation-altering splicing; and to demonstrate the unexpected presence of extant mRNA owing to the use of a cryptic splice site *(35)*.

Platelet Isolation

Defensible genomic and proteomic analysis of platelets requires extremely pure cellular populations. As mentioned above, since the mass of RNA in a platelet is so low, even a small number of contaminating leukocytes could generate spurious transcriptional data *(13)*. Several protocols for the isolation of platelets have been developed that are more stringent than those used in platelet function analyses. These include filtration steps *(36)*, filtration and negative immunoselection *(10)*, and sequential differential centrifugation *(11)*. These methods often result in considerable attrition of platelets. The scarcity of RNA in platelets, together with the sample requirements for transcriptional (i.e., microarray) analysis, has led to development of various techniques to obtain sufficient sample, including pooling of multiple donor samples *(11)*, platelet apheresis *(10)*, and PCR-based amplification of the entire transcriptome *(37)*.

RT-PCR

RNA was previously considered irrelevant to platelet function. Reticulated platelets, in which RNA is detected through staining, are presumed to be "younger" and are thus used as an index of platelet turnover *(38)*. However, much of the reticulocyte staining can be ascribed to their greater size and granule contents, thus arguing against the notion that platelets inevitably lose RNA over time *(39)*. However, early reports noted that the major platelet proteins were synthesized in reticulated platelets isolated from patients with immune thrombocytopenia post splenectomy *(40)*.

Human platelet RNA has been used to synthesize a cDNA library, which was then screened for platelet messages *(41)*. The presence of many individual transcripts have since been confirmed in platelet RNA. These include chemokines *(42)*, kinases *(43)*, and receptors *(44)*. Recent work by Weyrich and co-workers *(45–48)* demonstrated the presence of transcripts that did not fit the established paradigm for platelet RNA, as well as the regulated translation of mRNA into protein in platelets.

Microarrays

The diversity of transcripts being found in platelets suggested that more comprehensive studies of the platelet mRNA population would be fruitful. The emergent technology of microarrays is facilitating such an approach.

DNA microarrays (chips) allow simultaneous detection and quantification of tens of thousands of mRNA species in complex biological samples. DNA strands corresponding to genes of interest (rather confusingly known as the *probe*) are arrayed on a solid support to which labeled sample (the *target*—cDNA or RNA) is hybridized, before being washed and scanned. (That which is referred to as "probe" and "target" is occasionally reversed). Hybridized sequences are detected by their label (usually fluorescent), and level of expression in the sample is determined. Many commercial and in-house arrays are available with a variety of probe formats, number of genes per chip, and detection systems.

Microarrays provide a snapshot of the transcriptional state of a tissue (its *transcriptome*; therefore comparison of microarray results obtained under different conditions allows changes in expression level of multiple messages in response to stimuli to be determined. They have been put to many uses, which include the classification of cancers *(49)*, toxicology *(50)*, infectious diseases *(51)*, and a myriad of other diseases, as well as for research purposes.

Message levels in platelets are minimally dynamic. With only mitochondrial DNA present, no new mRNA can be produced from the nuclear genome. It is proposed that megakaryocyte gene expression could change over time in response to environmental factors, such as drugs, hypertension, smoking, and so on and that these changes may manifest in the platelet transcriptome. To date, however, most microarray platelet studies have used the technology to catalog the platelet transcriptome and thus as a window into platelet function.

AFFYMETRIX

Arrays from Affymetrix consist of collections of short DNA oligonucleotides (*probesets*) for each arrayed gene. Half of these correspond exactly to sequences from the gene; the rest differ by a single base and are used to determine the specificity of sample binding. So-called copy RNA (cRNA) is generated from the sample of interest and is complementary in sequence to the mRNA. cRNA rather than cDNA is favored because of the slightly tighter binding of RNA to the DNA probesets. The cRNA is labeled with biotin, from which an amplified fluorescent signal is generated during the posthybridization steps.

Two studies of platelet RNA using Affymetrix chips have been published *(10,11)*. Both used the U95Av2 array of 12,625 probesets, which correspond to 9573 distinct, well-characterized genes. Subsequently released arrays cover the entire human genome, with 54,000 probesets on a single chip, but have not yet been applied to the study of platelets. These studies demonstrated the complexity of the platelet transcriptome and were in remarkable agreement with regard to the more abundant platelet transcripts. Gnatenko et al. *(10)* found 2147 out of 12,625 probesets present in platelet mRNA prepared from healthy volunteers by apheresis (~17%), a lower proportion of detectable messages than seen in other tissues. The authors note that whereas 11% of these are annotated as being involved in metabolism and a further 11% in signaling, 25% are miscellaneous, and 32% have no known function. The platelet transcriptome is very different from that of the leukocyte, with cytoskeletal machinery highly represented in the most abundant messages. McRedmond et al. *(11)* pooled RNA isolated from platelets of small whole blood samples and found broadly similar results. A more involved bioinformatics analysis allowed them to extend the number of probesets deemed "present" in platelets to 4000, some of which were confirmed by RT-PCR. Comparison with similar studies from other tissues allowed identification of relatively platelet-specific genes and gene categories, which included signaling proteins and immune/inflammatory response genes.

MWG

Microarrays from MWG Biotech consist of 50 base oligonucleotides that are sufficiently long that a single one can be used to detect each message specifically in the sample. Kluter and co-workers *(36)* investigated the platelet transcriptome using MWG arrays. Results from different array platforms are notoriously difficult to compare *(52)*, but this study confirmed the overall tenor of the platelet transcriptome seen in other studies. Platelets are enriched in messages for glycoproteins, chemokines, and receptors.

cDNA

Longer array probe sequences have been used historically and allow more stringent hybridization, which should allow greater confidence in transcript identification. A large array of 56,000 transcripts was hybridized with RNA from platelets *(2)*. The most notable finding was that the most abundant transcripts corresponded to genes encoded by mitochondria, a finding borne out by Serial Analysis of Gene Expression (SAGE) results *(see* section following). Mitochondrial messages are absent from most commercial arrays. Their preponderance in the platelet transcriptome has been invoked to explain the faint overall signal seen when platelet RNA is hybridized to Affymetrix arrays *(10,11)*.

SMART PCR

Since platelets contain little RNA, some amplification of the transcriptome is required if the transcriptomes of different individuals' platelets are to be compared. Switch Mechanism At the 5' end of Reverse Transcription (SMART) PCR is one such method, whereby known sequences are affixed to the ends of every transcript, allowing their amplification by the PCR method. Care must be taken that some transcripts are not selectively amplified in the exponential phase of the PCR *(53)*. A proof-of-principle applying this method to platelets has been performed *(37)*, opening the way to analysis of variations in the platelet transcriptome in disease states or in response to drugs.

Serial Analysis of Gene Expression

Microarrays can only detect messages for which probes are present on the array. For an unbiased snapshot of the transcriptional state of a tissue, other techniques are required, one of which is SAGE *(54,55)*. Gnatenko et al.'s *(10)* analysis of the platelet transcriptome included a SAGE component, which served to show that a small number of mitochondrial transcripts dominate the platelet transcriptome. Nonmitochondrial messages identified in platelets by SAGE agreed well with the most abundant mRNAs seen by microarray but also added several uncharacterized genes not present on the array *(10)*. Comprehensive SAGE analysis requires considerable investment of sequencing resources and is unlikely to be applied to mainstream gene expression studies, as both in silico gene identification and microarray technologies improve.

Relating Genomics and Proteomics

Proteomicists suggest that proteins are the "business end" of biology because analysis of proteins tells us how cells behave, whereas transcripts are only the message—messenger RNA, in fact. However, despite advances in proteomics, the messages in RNA remain easier to detect and decode. Even so, the proteomicists are right: ultimately, for the messages to be meaningful, they ought to have some correspondence with the presence and level of the proteins that they encode.

The delay between gene transcription to RNA (in the megakaryocyte) and RNA translation into protein (mostly in the megakaryocyte, some in "younger" platelets) and the detection of platelet messages and proteins (sampled from circulating platelets of various age) complicates the correlation of messages and proteins when one is studying platelets.

BIOINFORMATICS

Protein and message sequence data are stored in various databases and in a variety of formats, depending on how they were acquired and curated. These are best compared by matching both to a single, comprehensive data source, such as Unigene *(11)*. Transcriptional data are quantitative, and thus the "level" of message present is reported. Absolute levels cannot be compared between investigations, however, without rigorous standardization of technique. Nevertheless, relative abundance of platelet messages was found to be remarkably consistent between analyses using a common platform (Affymetrix) but performed on different continents, with different preparation, purification, and analysis techniques *(10,11)*. Forty five of the 50 most abundant platelet messages were common in these two studies.

Platelet proteomic data are mostly quantitative, and in many cases a protein is reported as detected, or not. With multiple proteomic studies, a very arbitrary quantification is possible, by counting the number of observations of a protein by independent groups *(11)*. Quantitative proteomic methodologies exist *(56)*, but these have not yet been applied to platelet studies. Thus comparison of platelet proteomics and genomics compares "detection" by two methodologies.

Differences in the technologies involved will affect how they can be compared. Like SAGE, proteomics is not limited by a prechosen set of detectable items, whereas arrays are. However, proteomic studies tend to report tens or hundreds of identified proteins, whereas transcriptional technologies allow the identification of thousands of messages at a time. If there is reasonable correlation, we would expect to find messages for most proteins detected, and many messages for which no protein is found.

THE COMPARISON

A comparison of platelet genomic and proteomic data found a re-markable correspondence between the two *(11)*. Three protein datasets were compared with a single transcriptional analysis; 70% of proteins in each dataset had a corresponding message detected in platelet RNA, much higher than might be expected by chance. Platelet proteins were more likely to have a transcript found in platelets than in other tissues (McRedmond and Fitzgerald, unpublished data).

By pooling several proteomic datasets, corresponding proteins were found for 4.6% of platelet messages. Although this figure may increase as further platelet proteomic studies are performed, some messages are unlikely to have their corresponding protein found in platelets. Histone messages are abundant in platelets, but, with no nuclear DNA, platelets are a highly unlikely location for histone proteins. This illustrates that platelet messages may reflect the transcriptional requirements of the megakaryocyte—the polyploidy of megakaryocytes most likely requires many times the normal cellular complement of histones, resulting in the ready detection of these rarely seen messages in the platelet. The persis-tence of useless histone messages also illustrates the stability or RNA in platelets.

The more usual correspondence of message and protein in platelets illustrates the utility of transcriptional analysis as a means of identifying novel platelet mediators. Novel platelet proteins, first identified at the message level, and subsequently as proteins secreted by activated plate-lets, have been detected in human atherosclerotic plaque, where they may contribute to disease progression *(8)*.

CLINICAL APPLICATION, THERAPEUTICS, AND THE FUTURE
Clinical Applications

Heritable factors determine platelet reactivity to a greater extent than environmental factors *(57)*. Studies of rare genetic disorders have resulted in important insights into human biological processes and led to the development of therapy for more common disease phenotypes. Indeed, when a single gene mutation results in a disease phenotype this may represent a key drug target in a disease pathway. Exploration and understanding Glanzmann's thrombasthenia, a rare recessive disorder with a clinical phenotype of bleeding and impaired platelet aggregation, led to the development of inhibitors of the protein complex GPIIb-IIIa that are now used routinely as an adjunct to coronary stent procedures *(58)*.

Genotype profiling of patients allows us to identify those at high risk for specific diseases and provides the opportunity for early institution of primary or secondary prevention measures and possibly gene therapy. Since completion of the human genome project, more studies have taken this approach, notably in the fields of vascular disease and oncology *(59–61)*. Common atherothrombotic disorders, however, result from complex pathology, which therefore makes genetic analysis less efficient. A combined genomic and proteomic approach will increase our understanding of platelet signaling in both the presence and the absence of normal physiology. Investigational techniques, which are still evolving, already provide the means to screen healthy and diseased populations for genetic variants and proteins associated with pathological processes. In the future, profiling of DNA, proteins, peptides, and antibodies in bodily fluids such as serum or cerebrospinal fluid may not only assist in the diagnosis and treatment of atherothrombosis but also facilitate development of novel therapeutic agents (www.bloodomics.de).

Therapeutics

Studies of the human platelet antigen A1/A2 variant in the platelet glycoprotein receptor GPIIIa demonstrate that genotype can determine response to antiplatelet pharmacotherapy *(25)*. Pharmacogenomics explores the possibility that common gene variants may predict drug response and therefore offers the opportunity to tailor drug therapy for maximum benefit and minimum side effects. The ability to predict those who will responds well, adversely, or even not at all owing to a defect in the drug target could impact immediately on patient care.

Therapeutics today, however, is based on relatively few drugs directed at between 300 and 400 drug targets *(14)*. Since completion of the human genome project, subsequent large-scale genomic and proteomic strategies have led to the discovery of many new gene products and significantly advanced the potential for drug discovery. Newer techniques are being used to identify novel target molecules, evaluate drug efficacy and safety, and refine target populations based on genetic profile. Initial studies have focused on enzyme families such as protein kinases and phosphatases, proteases, and G protein-coupled receptors.

The current challenge is to development high-throughput assays to identify further gene products, assign biological function, and evaluate their potential for as drug targets.

Ultimately integration of platelet genomic and proteomic datasets should provide a comprehensive database of gene function containing information about each platelet gene and resultant products, their sequence, domain structure, subcellular localization, posttranslational modification, variants, homologies to other proteins, and interacting partners *(14)*. This resource could be organized into an easily accessible database and linked to clinical information such as involvement in cellular mechanisms and disease.

REFERENCES

1. Nurden AT, Caen JP. An abnormal platelet glycoprotein pattern in three cases of Glanzmann's thrombasthenia. Br J Haematol 1974;28:253–260.
2. Hillman A. The platelet surface receptor glycoprotein (GP) Ib-V-IX: variants, structure, mutations and pleiotropy. Clinical Pharmacology. Royal College of Surgeons in Ireland, Dublin, 2002.
3. Maree A, Fitzgerald D. Glycoprotein IIb/IIIa antagonists in acute coronary syndromes: where are we now? Semin Vasc Med 2003;03:385–390.
4. Nurden A. Human platelet glycoproteins. In: Bloom AF, ed. Haemostasis and Thrombosis. Churchill Livingstone, New York, 1994, pp. 115–165.
5. Henn V, Slupsky JR, Grafe M, et al. CD40 ligand on activated platelets triggers an inflammatory reaction of endothelial cells. Nature 1998;391:591–594.
6. Lindmark E, Tenno T, Siegbahn A. Role of platelet P-selectin and CD40 ligand in the induction of monocytic tissue factor expression. Arterioscler Thromb Vasc Biol 2000;20:2322–2328.
7. Libby P, Ridker PM, Maseri A. Inflammation and atherosclerosis. Circulation 2002;105:1135–1143.
8. Coppinger JA, Cagney G, Toomey S, et al. Characterization of the proteins released from activated platelets leads to localization of novel platelet proteins in human atherosclerotic lesions. Blood 2004;103:2096–20104.
9. von Hundelshausen P, Weber KS, Huo Y, et al. RANTES deposition by platelets triggers monocyte arrest on inflamed and atherosclerotic endothelium. Circulation 2001;103:1772–1777.
10. Gnatenko DV, Dunn JJ, McCorkle SR, Weissmann D, Perrotta PL, Bahou WF. Transcript profiling of human platelets using microarray and serial analysis of gene expression. Blood 2003;101:2285–2293.
11. McRedmond JP, Park SD, Reilly DF, et al. Integration of proteomics and genomics in platelets: a profile of platelet proteins and platelet-specific genes. Mol Cell Proteomics 2004;3:133–144.
12. Booyse FM, Rafelson ME Jr. Studies on human platelets. I. synthesis of platelet protein in a cell-free system. Biochim Biophys Acta 1968;166:689–697.
13. Fink L, Holschermann H, Kwapiszewska G, et al. Characterization of platelet-specific mRNA by real-time PCR after laser-assisted microdissection. Thromb Haemost 2003;90:749–756.
14. Cahill DJ. Protein and antibody arrays and their medical applications. J Immunol Methods 2001;250:81–91.

15. Harrison PM, Kumar A, Lang N, Snyder M, Gerstein M. A question of size: the eukaryotic proteome and the problems in defining it. Nucleic Acids Res 2002;30:1083–1090.

16. Anderson L, Seilhamer J. A comparison of selected mRNA and protein abundances in human liver. Electrophoresis 1997;18:533–537.

17. Lander ES, Linton LM, Birren B, et al. Initial sequencing and analysis of the human genome. Nature 2001;409:860–921.

18. Salisbury BA, Pungliya M, Choi JY, Jiang R, Sun XJ, Stephens JC. SNP and haplotype variation in the human genome. Mutat Res 2003;526:53–61.

19. Chen X, Sullivan PF. Single nucleotide polymorphism genotyping: biochemistry, protocol, cost and throughput. Pharmacogenomics J 2003;3:77–96.

20. Bojesen SE, Juul K, Schnohr P, Tybjaerg-Hansen A, Nordestgaard BG. Platelet glycoprotein IIb/IIIa Pl(A2)/Pl(A2) homozygosity associated with risk of ischemic cardiovascular disease and myocardial infarction in young men: the Copenhagen City Heart Study. J Am Coll Cardiol 2003;42:661–667.

21. Gruchala M, Ciecwierz D, Ochman K, et al. Association between the Pl(A) platelet glycoprotein GPIIIa polymorphism and extent of coronary artery disease. Int J Cardiol 2003;88:229–237.

22. Bottiger C, Kastrati A, Koch W, et al. HPA-1 and HPA-3 polymorphisms of the platelet fibrinogen receptor and coronary artery disease and myocardial infarction. Thromb Haemost 2000;83:559–562.

23. Grove EL, Orntoft TF, Lassen JF, Jensen HK, Kristensen SD. The platelet polymorphism PlA2 is a genetic risk factor for myocardial infarction. J Intern Med 2004;255:637–644.

24. Evans WE. Pharmacogenomics: marshalling the human genome to individualise drug therapy. Gut 2003;52(Suppl 2):ii10–ii18.

25. O'Connor FF, Shields DC, Fitzgerald A, Cannon CP, Braunwald E, Fitzgerald DJ. Genetic variation in glycoprotein IIb/IIIa (GPIIb/IIIa) as a determinant of the responses to an oral GPIIb/IIIa antagonist in patients with unstable coronary syndromes. Blood 2001;98:3256–3260.

26. Halushka MK, Walker LP, Halushka PV. Genetic variation in cyclooxygenase 1: effects on response to aspirin. Clin Pharmacol Ther 2003;73:122–130.

27. Cattaneo M. Inherited platelet-based bleeding disorders. J Thromb Haemost 2003;1:1628–1636.

28. Nair S, Ghosh K, Kulkarni B, Shetty S, Mohanty D. Glanzmann's thrombasthenia: updated. Platelets 2002;13:387–393.

29. D'Andrea G, Colaizzo D, Vecchione G, Grandone E, Di Minno G, Margaglione M. Glanzmann's thrombasthenia: identification of 19 new mutations in 30 patients. Thromb Haemost 2002;87:1034–1042.

30. Heidenreich R, Eisman R, Surrey S, et al. Organization of the gene for platelet glycoprotein IIb. Biochemistry 1990;29:1232–1244.

31. Zimrin AB, Gidwitz S, Lord S, et al. The genomic organization of platelet glycoprotein IIIa. J Biol Chem 1990;265:8590–8595.

32. Schlegel N, Gayet O, Morel-Kopp MC, et al. The molecular genetic basis of Glanzmann's thrombasthenia in a gypsy population in France: identification of a new mutation on the alpha IIb gene. Blood 1995;86:977–982.

33. Simsek S, Heyboer H, de Bruijne-Admiraal LG, Goldschmeding R, Cuijpers HT, von dem Borne AE. Glanzmann's thrombasthenia caused by homozygosity for a splice defect that leads to deletion of the first coding exon of the glycoprotein IIIa mRNA. Blood 1993;81:2044–2049.

34. Peretz H, Rosenberg N, Usher S, et al. Glanzmann's thrombasthenia associated with deletion-insertion and alternative splicing in the glycoprotein IIb gene. Blood 1995;85:414–420.

35. Burk CD, Newman PJ, Lyman S, Gill J, Coller BS, Poncz M. A deletion in the gene for glycoprotein IIb associated with Glanzmann's thrombasthenia. J Clin Invest 1991;87:270–276.

36. Bugert P, Dugrillon A, Gunaydin A, Eichler H, Kluter H. Messenger RNA profiling of human platelets by microarray hybridization. Thromb Haemost 2003;90:738–7348.

37. Rox JM, Bugert P, Müller J, et al. Gene expression analysis in single donor platelets: evaluation of a PCR-based amplification technique. Clin Chem 2004;50:2271–2278.

38. Ault KA, Rinder HM, Mitchell J, Carmody MB, Vary CP, Hillman RS. The significance of platelets with increased RNA content (reticulated platelets). A measure of the rate of thrombopoiesis. Am J Clin Pathol 1992;98:637–646.

39. Balduini CL, Noris P, Spedini P, Belletti S, Zambelli A, Da Prada GA. Relationship between size and thiazole orange fluorescence of platelets in patients undergoing high-dose chemotherapy. Br J Haematol 1999;106:202–207.

40. Kieffer N, Guichard J, Farcet JP, Vainchenker W, Breton-Gorius J. Biosynthesis of major platelet proteins in human blood platelets. Eur J Biochem 1987;164:189–195.

41. Wicki AN, Walz A, Gerber-Huber SN, Wenger RH, Vornhagen R, Clemetson KJ. Isolation and characterization of human blood platelet mRNA and construction of a cDNA library in lambda gt11. Confirmation of the platelet derivation by identification of GPIb coding mRNA and cloning of a GPIb coding cDNA insert. Thromb Haemost 1989;61:448–453.

42. Power CA, Clemetson JM, Clemetson KJ, Wells TN. Chemokine and chemokine receptor mRNA expression in human platelets. Cytokine 1995;7:479–482.

43. Chang JD, Xu Y, Raychowdhury MK, Ware JA. Molecular cloning and expression of a cDNA encoding a novel isoenzyme of protein kinase C (nPKC). A new member of the nPKC family expressed in skeletal muscle, megakaryoblastic cells, and platelets. J Biol Chem 1993;268:14208–14214.

44. Vial C, Hechler B, Leon C, Cazenave JP, Gachet C. Presence of P2X1 purinoceptors in human platelets and megakaryoblastic cell lines. Thromb Haemost 1997;78:1500–1504.

45. Weyrich AS, Dixon DA, Pabla R, et al. Signal-dependent translation of a regulatory protein, Bcl-3, in activated human platelets. Proc Natl Acad Sci USA 1998; 95:5556–5561.

46. Pabla R, Weyrich AS, Dixon DA, et al. Integrin-dependent control of translation: engagement of integrin $\alpha_{IIb}\beta_3$ regulates synthesis of proteins in activated human platelets. J Cell Biol 1999;144:175–184.

47. Lindemann S, Tolley ND, Dixon DA, et al. Activated platelets mediate inflammatory signaling by regulated interleukin 1beta synthesis. J Cell Biol 2001;154:485–490.

48. Lindemann S, Tolley ND, Eyre JR, Kraiss LW, Mahoney TM, Weyrich AS. Integrins regulate the intracellular distribution of eukaryotic initiation factor 4E in platelets. A checkpoint for translational control. J Biol Chem 2001;276:33947–33951.

49. Wajapeyee N, Somasundaram K. Pharmacogenomics in breast cancer: current trends and future directions. Curr Opin Mol Ther 2004;6:296–301.

50. Vrana KE, Freeman WM, Aschner M. Use of microarray technologies in toxicology research. Neurotoxicology 2003;24:321–332.

51. Bryant PA, Venter D, Robins-Browne R, Curtis N. Chips with everything: DNA microarrays in infectious diseases. Lancet Infect Dis 2004;4:100–111.

52. Kuo WP, Jenssen TK, Butte AJ, Ohno-Machado L, Kohane IS. Analysis of matched mRNA measurements from two different microarray technologies. Bioinformatics 2002;18:405–412.

53. Puskas LG, Zvara A, Hackler L Jr, Van Hummelen P. RNA amplification results in reproducible microarray data with slight ratio bias. Biotechniques 2002;32:1330–1334, 1336, 1338, 1340.

54. Yamamoto M, Wakatsuki T, Hada A, Ryo A. Use of serial analysis of gene expression (SAGE) technology. J Immunol Methods 2001;250:45–66.

55. Ye SQ, Lavoie T, Usher DC, Zhang LQ. Microarray, SAGE and their applications to cardiovascular diseases. Cell Res 2002;12:105–115.

56. Righetti PG, Campostrini N, Pascali J, Hamdan M, Astner H. Quantitative proteomics: a review of different methodologies. Eur J Mass Spectrom (Chichester, Eng) 2004;10:335–348.

57. O'Donnell CJ, Larson MG, Feng D, et al. Genetic and environmental contributions to platelet aggregation: the Framingham heart study. Circulation 2001;103:3051–3056.

58. United Kingdom Transient Ischaemic Attack (UK-TIA) aspirin trial: interim results. UK-TIA Study Group. Br Med J (Clin Res Ed) 1988;296:316–320.

59. Wang L, Fan C, Topol SE, Topol EJ, Wang Q. Mutation of MEF2A in an inherited disorder with features of coronary artery disease. Science 2003;302:1578–1581.

60. Cipollone F, Toniato E, Martinotti S, et al. A polymorphism in the cyclooxygenase 2 gene as an inherited protective factor against myocardial infarction and stroke. JAMA 2004;291:2221–2228.

61. Panguluri RC, Long LO, Chen W, et al. COX-2 gene promoter haplotypes and prostate cancer risk. Carcinogenesis 2004;25:961–966.

III CLINICAL APPLICATIONS

15 Antiplatelet Agents

Jacqueline Saw, MD, and David J. Moliterno, MD

INTRODUCTION

Antiplatelet therapy has become indispensable in modern-day cardiology practice. Over 200,000 patients have been studied in randomized controlled trials of antiplatelet agents for cardiovascular diseases, supporting diverse clinical indications including primary and secondary preventions of thromboembolic diseases. The 2002 updated Antithrombotic Trialist Collaboration meta-analysis of antiplatelet trials established the clinical benefit of antiplatelet agents in patients at high risk of vascular events (such as those with underlying coronary artery disease, prior history of stroke, peripheral artery disease, and atrial fibrillation) (1) (Fig. 1). A detailed discussion encompassing all clinical indications of antiplatelet therapy is beyond the scope of this chapter. We will focus on representatives of the three major classes of antiplatelet agents (aspirin,

From: *Contemporary Cardiology:*
Platelet Function: Assessment, Diagnosis, and Treatment
Edited by: M. Quinn and D. Fitzgerald © Humana Press Inc., Totowa, NJ

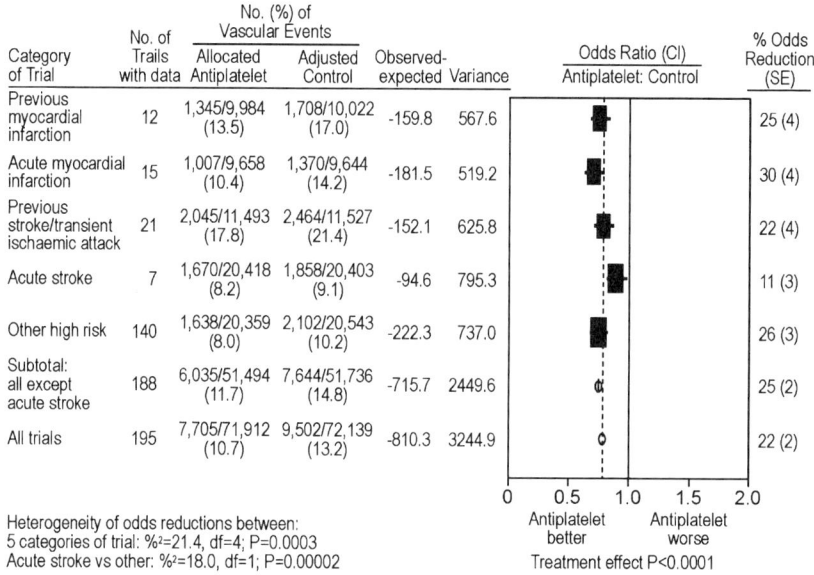

Category of Trial	No. of Trials with data	No. (%) of Vascular Events		Observed-expected	Variance	Odds Ratio (CI) Antiplatelet: Control	% Odds Reduction (SE)
		Allocated Antiplatelet	Adjusted Control				
Previous myocardial infarction	12	1,345/9,984 (13.5)	1,708/10,022 (17.0)	-159.8	567.6		25 (4)
Acute myocardial infarction	15	1,007/9,658 (10.4)	1,370/9,644 (14.2)	-181.5	519.2		30 (4)
Previous stroke/transient ischaemic attack	21	2,045/11,493 (17.8)	2,464/11,527 (21.4)	-152.1	625.8		22 (4)
Acute stroke	7	1,670/20,418 (8.2)	1,858/20,403 (9.1)	-94.6	795.3		11 (3)
Other high risk	140	1,638/20,359 (8.0)	2,102/20,543 (10.2)	-222.3	737.0		26 (3)
Subtotal: all except acute stroke	188	6,035/51,494 (11.7)	7,644/51,736 (14.8)	-715.7	2449.6		25 (2)
All trials	195	7,705/71,912 (10.7)	9,502/72,139 (13.2)	-810.3	3244.9		22 (2)

Heterogeneity of odds reductions between:
5 categories of trial: $\%^2$=21.4, df=4; P=0.0003
Acute stroke vs other: $\%^2$=18.0, df=1; P=0.00002

Antiplatelet better   Antiplatelet worse
Treatment effect P<0.0001

Fig. 1. Effects of antiplatelet therapy in high-risk patients from the Antithrombotic Trialists Collaboration metaanalysis of 195 trials. (From ref. *1* with permission from the BMJ Publishing Group).

thienopyridines, glycoprotein (GP)IIb-IIIa receptor antagonists) highlighting sentinel clinical trial results of coronary disease and interventions, and discuss platelet function assessments.

PATHOBIOLOGY OF PLATELET AGGREGATION

Platelets play an integral role in primary hemostasis at locations of spontaneous or traumatic endothelial injury. The formation of platelet hemostatic plugs entails a complex process of platelet adhesion, activation, secretion, and aggregation. The exposure of subendothelial connective tissue matrix promotes release of cytokines, with ensuing expression of adhesion molecules on the endothelium, encouraging platelet and leukocyte binding. Platelet adhesion incites a cascade of platelet-activation events, initiating conformational changes that allow binding of fibrinogen and von Willebrand factor to glycoprotein (GP)IIb-IIIa receptors, culminating in platelet aggregation (Fig. 2). In the setting of percutaneous interventions, balloon angioplasty produces mechanical plaque rupture, exposing subendothelial matrix, with further amplification of platelet activation and deposition when stents are placed *(2,3)*. Numerous targets for inhibiting these platelet processes have been identified.

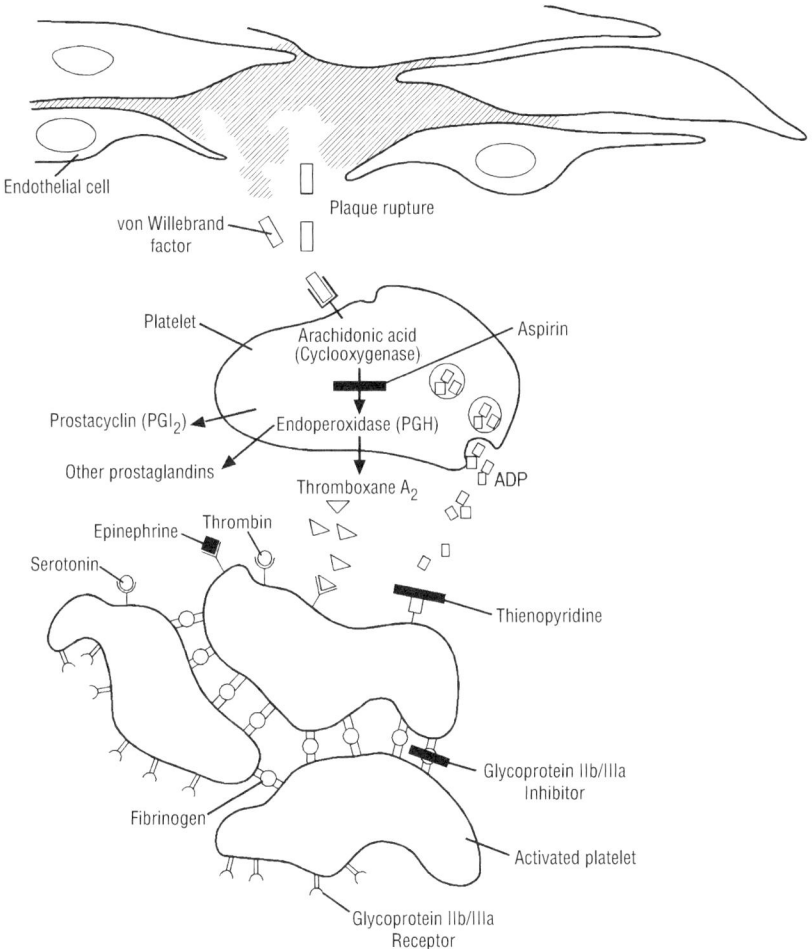

Fig. 2. Activated platelets, functionalized receptors, and mediators of thrombosis and inflammation associated with plaque rupture. Blocking the cascade of platelet aggregation can occur at several different levels. (Adapted from Sharis et al., Ann Intern Med 1998;129:394–405.)

ASPIRIN

Aspirin is by the far the most widely administered antiplatelet agent and constitutes the reference standard for comparison of novel agents. It is an irreversible inhibitor of cyclooxygenase (COX), being highly selective for COX-1 but it also inhibits COX-2 at higher doses *(4)*. COX-1 inhibition is dose dependent, causing reduction of thromboxane A_2 (TXA_2; a potent vasoconstrictor and stimulant of platelet aggregation) synthesis from arachidonic acid. A single dose of 160 mg produces almost complete inhibition of COX-1, whereas lower doses of 30–50 mg require 7–10 d to achieve maximum inhibition *(5)*. The Antithrombotic Trialists' Collaboration found no evidence that long-term administration of high-dose (500–1500 mg daily) aspirin is superior to lower doses (75–325 mg daily) *(1)*. Aspirin use is relatively safe but has been associated with nasal polyps and can cause major bleeding (such as gastrointestinal and intracranial bleed). Bleeding risk may be related to dose.

Overall, aspirin's antiplatelet effect is relatively weak, since it only inhibits one of a multitude of platelet activation pathways (Fig. 2). In addition, "aspirin resistance" has been clinically identified and loosely described as thrombotic complications or "excess" residual platelet activity via laboratory testing despite aspirin therapy. Proposed mechanisms of this resistance include inadequate aspirin dosage and increased platelet sensitivity to collagen *(6)*. Thus, aspirin monotherapy has inadequacies that may justify combination therapy with other antiplatelet agents in selected patient cohorts.

Clinical Trials of Aspirin for Cardiovascular Diseases

Aspirin is indicated for a variety of cardiovascular diseases, although mainly for primary and secondary prevention of ischemic vascular events *(1)*. The Physician's Health Study *(7)*, HOT (Hypertension Optimal Treatment) *(8)*, and the Primary Prevention Project *(9)* showed reduction in cardiovascular event rates with the use of aspirin for primary prevention of cardiovascular diseases in healthy patients or those with atherosclerotic risk factors. However, there was a small increase in the incidence of major bleeding in these trials *(7–9)*. The evidence for secondary prevention with aspirin is more robust and substantial, with an overall reduction of major cardiovascular event rates by 23% (in high-risk patients with acute myocardial infarction [MI], unstable angina, prior history of MI, stroke, transient ischemic attack [TIA]) *(1)*, which considerably outweighs the risks of major bleeding.

Aspirin also has a major role in preventing arterial thrombosis after percutaneous coronary interventions (PCIs). In a retrospective study by Barnathan et al. *(10)*, aspirin (with or without dipyridamole) given before angioplasty reduced total coronary occlusions by approx 85%. Administration of aspirin alone for PCI was never studied in a randomized placebo-controlled trial. However, aspirin in combination with dipyridamole given 24 h before angioplasty was superior to placebo in reducing periprocedural MI (1.6% vs 6.9%) *(11)*. A small randomized study subsequently revealed no benefit of adding dipyridamole to aspirin therapy *(12)*. The current PCI guidelines recommend that an empiric dose of 80–325 mg of aspirin be given at least 2 h prior to the procedure

(13). Long-term aspirin therapy probably does not importantly affect restenosis, but it is recommended for secondary prevention of cardiovascular events *(14)*.

THIENOPYRIDINES

Ticlopidine and clopidogrel are both thienopyridine derivatives that inhibit ADP-induced platelet aggregation and the resultant conformational change of GPIIb-IIIa receptors. They also inhibit thrombin, collagen, and shear-stress-induced platelet aggregation.

Ticlopidine

Ticlopidine is inactive in vitro and needs to be metabolized by the liver into its active forms. It has a plasma half-life of 12 h, and only 2% is excreted unchanged. Administration of 250 mg twice daily reaches maximal platelet inhibition in 3–5 d *(15)*. After stopping therapy, the platelet-inhibitory effects progressively dissipate over 4–10 d, correlating to platelet life span *(16)*. Unfortunately, ticlopidine has rare but serious side effects such as neutropenia (1–2.4%), thrombotic thrombocytopenic purpura (very rare, but associated with high mortality rate of ~33%), aplastic anemia, and pancytopenia. These life-threatening hematologic complications usually occur during the first few months of therapy (necessitating blood counts every 2 wk initially for about 3 mo) and may resolve with cessation of therapy. More often, ticlodipine causes rash (5%), nausea and vomiting (5%), or diarrhea (6%). For safety reasons, clopidogrel has largely replaced ticlopidine.

Clinical Trials of Ticlopidine for Cardiovascular Diseases

Ticlopidine was shown to be beneficial in reducing death, MI, and stroke in patients with acute coronary syndromes (ACS) *(17,18)*. In the setting of PCI, a randomized trial showed ticlopidine alone to be superior to placebo (2% vs 14%) in reducing ischemic complications after angioplasty, but it was equivalent to the combination of aspirin and dipyridamole (2% vs 5%) *(19)*. This supported the use of ticlopidine as an alternative to aspirin for patients who are aspirin intolerant. Subsequent studies showed that the combination of ticlopidine and aspirin reduced subacute thrombosis after stent placement and was superior to anticoagulant regimens (aspirin, warfarin, or both). These studies were the Intracoronary Stenting and Antithrombotic Regimen study (ISAR) *(20)*, the Full Anticoagulation versus Aspirin and Ticlopidine study (FANTASTIC) *(21)*, and the Stent Anticoagulation Restenosis Study (STARS) *(22)*.

Clopidogrel

Clopidogrel is an orally administered prodrug that requires liver metabolism by cytochrome P450 enzymes into an active metabolite *(23)*. Clopidogrel inhibits platelet aggregation via the irreversible binding and inactivation of $P2Y_{12}$ ADP receptors. This antagonizes ADP-induced adenyl cyclase inhibition, affecting intracellular signaling and protein phosphorylation *(24,25)*. A single loading dose of 375 mg produces maximal platelet aggregation inhibition (~80%) in 5 h *(26)*. Without a loading-dose, a 75-mg daily dose produces steady-state platelet inhibition in 3–7 d *(26)*. Unlike ticlopidine, the safety profile of clopidogrel is excellent, with a very low risk of thrombocytopenic thrombotic purpura and no association with neutropenia *(27)*. The CAPRIE (Clopidogrel versus Aspirin in Patients at Risk of Ischemic Events) study showed a lower incidence of gastrointestinal hemorrhage with clopidogrel compared with aspirin, but there were more occurrences of diarrhea and rash *(27)*. In addition to inhibiting the thrombotic activities of platelets, clopidogrel may also have an important role in reducing inflammation by decreasing platelet expression of CD40 ligand *(28)*.

CLINICAL TRIALS OF CLOPIDOGREL FOR CARDIOVASCULAR DISEASES

Large randomized trials support the use of clopidogrel for atherosclerotic diseases, including both stable and unstable plaques. The CAPRIE study demonstrated marginal superiority of clopidogrel compared with aspirin in reducing a composite of secondary ischemic events (stroke, MI, or vascular death—relative reduction of 8.7%) in more than 19,000 patients *(27)*. The CURE (Clopidogrel in Unstable angina to prevent Recurrent Events) trial showed that combining clopidogrel with aspirin reduced the composite end points of cardiovascular death, nonfatal MI, and stroke by 20% in more than 12,000 patients with non-ST elevation ACS, compared with aspirin alone *(29)*.

In the setting of PCI, early observational registries and randomized trials showed equivalent clinical efficacy of a clopidogrel-aspirin combination compared with ticlopidine and aspirin, with the added advantage of lower adverse events with clopidogrel *(30–33)*. A routine practice is to administer clopidogrel either before PCI or soon after stent placement, with a loading dose (usually 300 mg) followed by 75 mg daily, although data now show that advance pretreatment is superior. The post-PCI duration of clopidogrel treatment was generally 2–4 wk, until recent publications (CREDO [Clopidogrel for the Reduction of Events During Observation] and PCI-CURE trials) *(34,35)* supported longer term therapy.

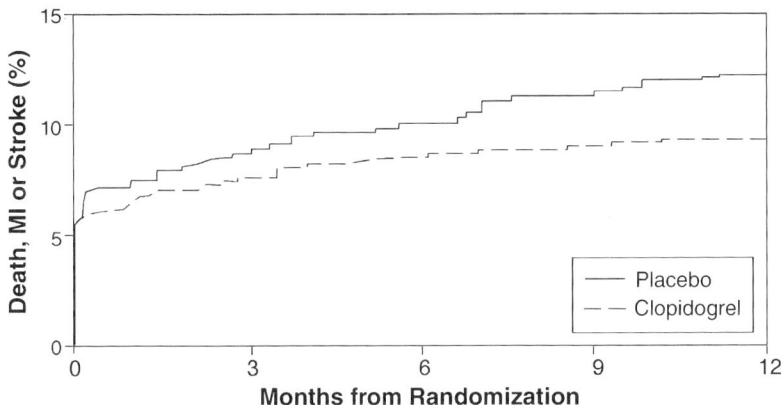

Fig. 3. One-year incidence of the composite of death, MI, or stroke in the CREDO study. (Reproduced with permission from ref. *34*. Copyright 2002 American Medical Association.)

PCI-CURE was a prespecified subgroup analysis of the CURE trial, comprising 2658 patients with non-ST elevation MI who underwent PCI. Pretreatment (median 10 d prior to PCI) and long-term (mean 8 mo) therapy with clopidogrel was compared with placebo, with open-label clopidogrel administration for 4 wk post-PCI to all patients. Clopidogrel pretreatment reduced the primary composite end point of cardiovascular death, MI, or urgent target vessel revascularization (TVR) by 30% within 30 d of PCI. Pre- and long-term clopidogrel treatment following PCI also reduced cardiovascular death and MI by 25% at long-term follow-up (mean 8 mo) *(35)*.

The CREDO study was a double-blind, randomized, placebo-controlled trial comparing short-term (4 wk) with long-term (1 yr) clopidogrel therapy post-PCI. Additionally, the long-term group received a 300 mg clopidogrel loading dose 3–24 h before PCI, vs preprocedural placebo given to the short-term group. The primary composite of death, MI, or stroke at 1 yr was reduced by 27% in the pretreatment/long-term clopidogrel arm (8.5% vs 11.5%, $p = 0.02$) (Fig. 3). In a prespecified subgroup analysis, those who received clopidogrel 6 h or more before PCI had a 39% reduction in the primary end point, whereas those given clopidogrel less than 6 h before PCI had no end point reduction. However, the design of this study hampered the ability to differentiate clearly pretreatment from long-term treatment effect with clopidogrel *(34)*. Overall, both the PCI-CURE and CREDO studies support pretreatment and long-term therapy with clopidogrel for PCI.

Clopidogrel is now an established crucial adjunct to aspirin therapy before and after PCI, and for patients presenting with non-ST elevation ACS. It is also the substitute of choice for those who are unable to tolerate aspirin for cardiovascular disease prevention. An important ongoing trial is CHARISMA (Clopidogrel for High Atherothrombotic Risk and Ischemic Stabilization Management and Avoidance), which is enrolling patients aged 55 yr or older at risk for atherothrombotic events to evaluate the combination of clopidogrel with aspirin for more than 1 yr. This study, which anticipates more than 15,000 patient enrollments, will further address the question of the benefit of long-term combination clopidogrel and aspirin therapy.

PLATELET GLYCOPROTEIN IIb-IIIa RECEPTOR ANTAGONISTS

Activated GPIIb-IIIa receptors mediate the final common pathway of platelet aggregation via the binding of fibrinogen and von Willebrand factor, leading to crosslinking of adjacent platelets (Fig. 2). GPIIb-IIIa receptors ($\alpha_{IIb}\beta_3$ integrin) are part of the integrin family of heterodimeric adhesion receptors implicated in cell-matrix and cell-cell interactions. Selective antagonism of $\alpha_{IIb}\beta_3$ can powerfully inhibit platelet aggregation and thrombus formation, translating to unequivocal clinical benefits when administered during PCI. Of the numerous agents developed, only three parenteral forms are currently approved by the Food and Drug Administration (FDA) in the United States currently: abciximab (Reopro®, Centocor), eptifibatide (Integrilin®, Millennium-COR Therapeutics), and tirofiban (Aggrastat®, Merck). We will limit our discussions to these intravenous agents, since the oral formulations are not efficacious. The use of intravenous GPIIb-IIIa agents during PCI necessitates heparin coadministration to achieve an activated clotting time (ACT) of around 250 s. Low-molecular-weight heparins also appear to be safe and efficacious when coadministered with GPIIb-IIIa inhibitors, as observed in the National Investigators Collaborating on Enoxaparin (NICE) 3 and 4 trials (36). A more recent small head-to-head study comparing enoxaparin with unfractionated heparins (both in combination with eptifibatide) during PCI showed no difference in bleeding or clinical ischemic events between the heparins (37).

Abciximab

Abciximab is a human chimeric antibody fragment that binds to both active and inactive $\alpha_{IIb}\beta_3$ integrin with high affinity. It is relatively nonselective, also adhering to other integrins: vitronectin ($\alpha_V\beta_3$) receptors on smooth muscle cells and Mac-1 receptors on leukocytes (38). An intravenous loading dose of 0.25 mg/kg followed by a 12-h infusion of 0.125 µg/kg/min achieves more than 80% GPIIb-IIIa receptor blockade in most patients within 3 min *(39,40)*. After binding $\alpha_{IIb}\beta_3$, abciximab slowly dissociates from $\alpha_{IIb}\beta_3$ and can redistribute to other platelets *(39)*, consequently having a longer biologic half-life than other small-molecule or nonantibody antagonists. Platelet function gradually returns to baseline level over approx 48 h after cessation of infusion. However, small fractions of abciximab can still be bound to platelets 2 wk after stopping therapy *(39)*. Abciximab is not cleared renally; the exact excretion mechanism is not entirely known but probably involves reticuloendothelial destruction. Unlike eptifibatide or tirofiban, platelet infusion can be successfully used for bleeding complications since abciximab redistribution to other platelets will reduce the number of blocked receptors per platelet *(41)*.

Eptifibatide

Eptifibatide is a synthetic cyclic heptapeptide that contains the Lys-Gly-Asp sequence. It is more selective than abciximab for inhibiting $\alpha_{IIb}\beta_3$ but also binds $\alpha_V\beta_3$ integrin *(42)*. The recommended PCI dosage is two boluses of 180 µg/kg 10 min apart, followed by 18–24-h infusion of 2 µg/kg/min, which will achieve more than 90% platelet inhibition at steady state *(41)*. Its predominant renal excretion is accompanied by a short 2.5-h plasma half-life, with platelet function returning to normal within 4 h after drug cessation *(41)*.

Tirobifan

Tirofiban is a nonpeptide tyrosine-derived mimetic of the Arg-Gly-Asp sequence that is highly selective for $\alpha_{IIb}\beta_3$ without crossreacting with other integrins. The recommended dosage for ACS is 0.4 µg/kg/min for 30 min (which achieves >90% platelet inhibition after 30 min), followed by an infusion of 0.1 µg/kg/min for 12–24 h *(42)*. It is excreted renally and has a short plasma half-life of 2 h; platelet function returns to normal 4–8 h after stopping infusion *(41)*. Although not approved solely for PCI, a bolus of 10 µg/kg with an infusion of 15 µg/kg/min has been used in clinical trials.

The main but infrequent complications associated with the use of GPIIb-IIIa receptor antagonists are bleeding and thrombocytopenia. The incidence of major and minor bleeding with these agents is dependent on the heparin dosage used and the ACT obtained during PCI (Fig. 4). As shown in the EPILOG (Evaluation in PTCA to Improve Long-term Outcome with abciximab GPIIb-IIIa blockade) study *(43)*, the use of lower dose heparin (70 U/kg) with abciximab reduced major bleeding

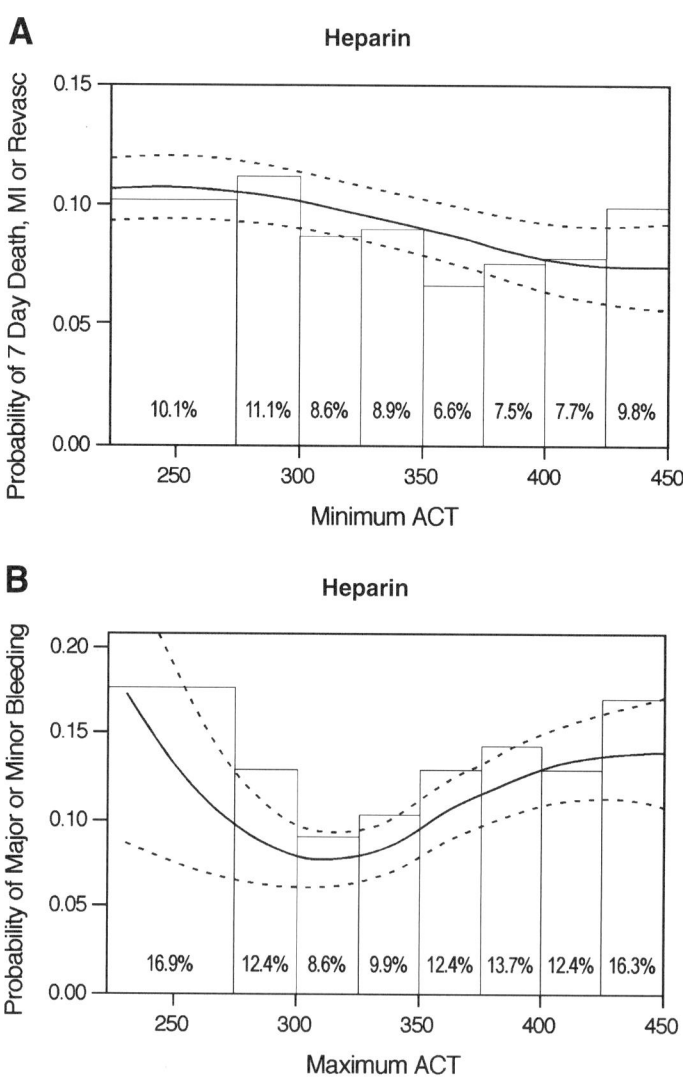

Fig. 4. (A) Relationship between minimum activated clotting time (ACT) and 7-d ischemic events (death, myocardial infarction [MI] or revascularization). **(B)** Relationship between maximum ACT and 7-d major or minor bleeding events. (Reproduced from ref. *45.*)

complications compared with the higher dose heparin (100 U/kg) used in EPIC (Evaluation of c7E3 Fab in the Prevention of Ischemic Complications) *(44)* (2% compared with 14%). Chew et al. *(45)* showed increasing risk of bleeding complications with an ACT greater than 250 s without incremental benefit of ischemic end point reduction (with ACT between

250 and 350 s) when patients received concomitant intravenous heparin and GPIIb-IIIa blockade *(45)*. In addition, stopping heparin immediately post-PCI with early removal of the arterial sheath (2–6 h post-PCI) when the ACT is less than 175 s also reduces access site bleeding complications. In patients who require coronary artery bypass surgery after a diagnostic catheterization, abciximab should be discontinued immediately and eptifibatide and tirofiban stopped at least 4 h before surgery.

Thrombocytopenia (platelets < 100,000/cm^3) occurs not infrequently with the use of GPIIb-IIIa antagonists, in 1–5% of patients overall. Acute profound thrombocytopenia (platelets < 20,000/cm^3) occurs in only 0.2–0.7% of cases *(46)* and is more frequent with abciximab than the small-molecule agents. It tends to occur within 1–4 h after starting therapy, with recovery of platelet count within a few days of stopping the drug. Early readministration (within 2 wk of first administration) of abciximab may increase the risk of severe thrombocytopenia (platelets < 50,000/cm^3) (12% in those readministered within 2 wk vs 2% with readministration >2 wk, p = 0.046) *(47)* and may result in a more profound platelet count nadir. The etiology of thrombocytopenia is not entirely clear, but it is most likely immune mediated. Treatment strategy depends on the severity of thrombocytopenia: (1) consider stopping GPIIb-IIIa antagonists for platelet counts of 50,000–100,000/cm^3, (2) stop GPIIb-IIIa antagonists for counts more than 50,000, (3) stop all antiplatelet agents (including aspirin and thienopyridines) for counts more than 20,000, or (4) platelet transfusions for bleeding or generalized petechiae and purpura *(48)*.

Clinical Trials for PCI

To date, clinical trials collectively involving more than 20,000 patients have indisputably confirmed the benefit of GPIIb-IIIa antagonists in reducing ischemic events during PCI. These agents benefited almost all subgroups, particularly those with ACS and positive troponin levels. These randomized trials included patients undergoing high- and low-risk procedures and those who had undergone primary angioplasty for acute MI (Fig. 5). The most extensive and definitive data were derived from abciximab used adjunctively during PCI, supporting its reputation as the reference agent. Moreover, abciximab is the only GPIIb-IIIa antagonist exhibiting long-term mortality reduction at multiyear follow-up (Fig. 6) *(49)*. As summarized in Table 1 *(43,44,50–62)*, abciximab reduced the composite end points of death, MI, and urgent revascularization at 30 d by 29–56%. Lesser degrees of benefit were achieved with eptifibatide and tirofiban, possibly explained by insufficient dose with inadequate platelet inhibition *(56,57)*. Benefits extend to 6 mo and 1 yr in most trials *(50,51,55,59)*. Abciximab is the only agent studied in

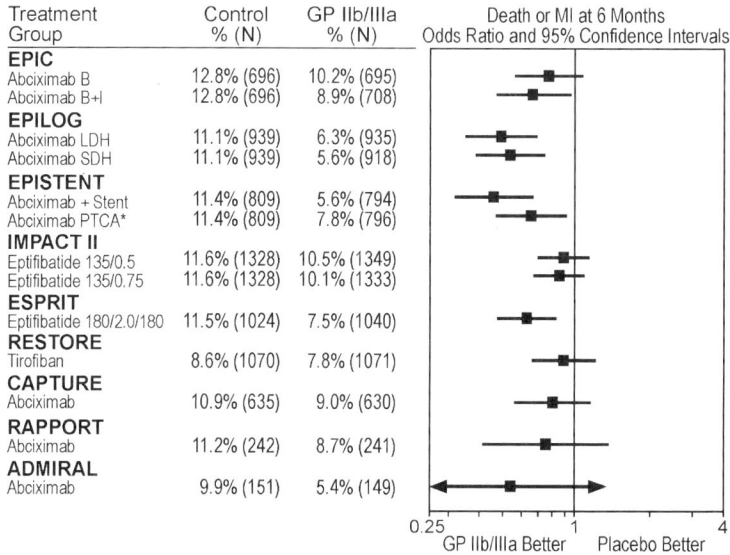

Fig. 5. Odds ratio of 6-mo death or MI event rates for randomized controlled trials of GPIIb-IIIa antagonists. (Reproduced with permission from Lincoff AM, ed. Platelet Glycoprotein IIb/IIIa Inhibitors in Cardiovascular Disease, 2nd ed. Humana, Totowa, NJ, 2003, p. 184.)

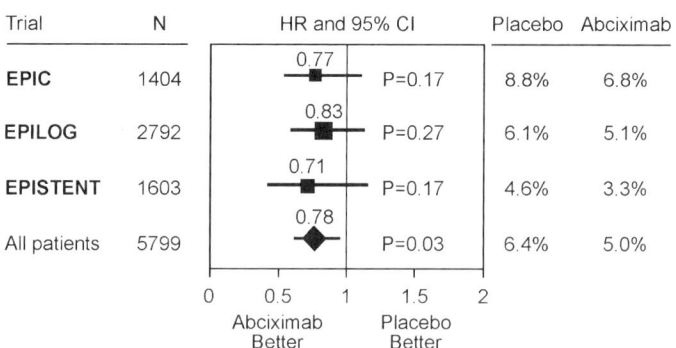

Fig. 6. Hazard ratios (HR) and 95% confidence intervals (CI) for long-term mortality reduction from abciximab in clinical trials of coronary intervention. (From ref. *49*. Copyright 2002, with permission from Excerpta Medica, Inc.)

sizeable primary PCI trials for acute MI, showing reduction in 30-d ischemic events, but less robust evidence for benefit at 6 mo *(60–62)*.

TARGET (Tirofiban And Reopro Give similar Efficacy outcomes Trial) was the only trial that directly compared two different GPIIb-IIIa antagonists, showing superiority of abciximab over tirofiban in the primary composite end point at 30 d (death, MI, urgent TVR) *(63)*. This difference was predominantly accounted for by periprocedural MI reduction with abciximab (5.4% vs 6.9% tirofiban, $p = 0.04$), with persistence of benefit at 6-mo follow-up (6.6% abciximab, 8.0% tirofiban, $p = 0.07$) (64). Potential explanations for more frequent periprocedural MI with tirofiban include insufficient bolus dose for adequate early platelet inhibition, or inadequate pretreatment duration to achieve steady-state concentration from the infusion.

GPIIb-IIIa antagonists have demonstrated superior clinical outcomes in nearly every subgroup. An exception is the use of such agents during percutaneous revascularization of coronary bypass grafts, although no randomized trial specifically addressed this indication. A pooled analysis of five major trials (EPIC, EPILOG, EPISTENT, IMPACT-II, and PURSUIT) assessed the efficacy of GPIIb-IIIa antagonists in graft interventions and found the composite end point of death, MI, or revascularization to be nonsignificantly increased by 24% at 30 d (16.5% with GPIIb-IIIa antagonists, 12.6% placebo, $p = 0.18$) (65).

Another consideration limiting the routine use of GPIIb-IIIa antagonists with PCI is when bivalirudin is used adjunctively with PCI. In the REPLACE-2 trial (Randomized Evaluation in PCI Linking Angiomax to Reduce Clinical Events) (66), bivalirudin with provisional GPIIb-IIIa blockade (given to 7.2% of patients) was shown to be noninferior to the combination of heparin and routine GPIIb-IIIa blockade during PCI (30-d secondary composite end point of death, MI, or urgent revascularization were 7.6% bivalirudin and 7.1% heparin + GPIIb-IIIa blockade). The incidence of major bleeding as defined by the REPLACE-2 study was lower with bivalirudin (2.4% vs 4.1%, $p < 0.001$). However, the incidence of major bleeding by Thrombolysis in Myocardial Infarction (TIMI) criteria was similar (0.6% bivalirudin, 0.9% heparin + GPIIb-IIIa blockade, $p = 0.3$). This study has prompted some interventional cardiologists to select bivalirudin for low-risk procedures or those adequately pretreated with clopidogrel, reserving heparin with GPIIb-IIIa antagonists for high-risk patients.

Ongoing key research focuses include GPIIb-IIIa blockade as part of facilitated PCI (combined GPIIb-IIIa antagonists with thrombolytic therapy) for acute ST-elevation MI. Studies such as FINESSE (Facilitated Intervention with Enhanced reperfusion Speed to Stop Events), ASSENT-4 (Fourth Assessment of the Safety and Efficacy of a New Thrombolytic), and ADVANCE-MI (Addressing the Value of facilitated Angioplasty after Combination treatment or Eptifibatide monotherapy in acute MI) trials are addressing whether this is a beneficial strategy for PCI in acute ST-elevation.

Table 1
Randomized Placebo-Controlled Trials of GPIIb-IIIa Antagonists in PCI

Trials	Agent used	Study cohort	No.	Drug dose and duration	Primary end points	Primary results	Long-term data and comments
EPIC (44,50)	Abciximab	High-risk PCI	2099	a. 0.25-mg/kg bolus, 0.125 µg/kg/min, 12 h b. Placebo	Death/MI/ TVR, 30 d	8.3% abciximab, 12.8% placebo $p = 0.008$	6 mo: a. 27% b. 35.1% $p = 0.001$ 3 yr: a. 41% b. 47.2% $p = 0.009$
EPILOG (43,51)	Abciximab	High- + low-risk PCI	2792	a. Abciximab (0.25-mg/kg bolus, 0.125 µg/kg/min, 12 h) + 100 U/kg hep b. Abciximab + 70 U/kg hep c. Placebo + 100 U/kg hep	Death/MI/ TVR, 30 d	a. 5.4% b. 5.2% c. 11.7% $p < 0.001$	1 yr: a. 9.5% b. 9.6% c. 16.1% $p < 0.001$
CAPTURE (52)	Abciximab	High-risk PCI	1265	a. 0.25-mg/kg bolus, 0.125 µg/kg/min, 18–24 h pre-procedure, continued 1 h post-procedure b. Placebo	Death/MI/ TVR, 30 d	11.3% abciximab, 15.9% placebo $p = 0.012$	Not significantly different at 6 mo; study stopped prematurely Thought due to short infusion duration post PCI
EPISTENT (53–55)	Abciximab	Elective or urgent PCI	2399	a. 0.25-mg/kg bolus, 0.125 µg/kg/min, 12 h b. Placebo	Death/MI/TVR, 30 d	Stent + a. 5.3% PTCA + a. 6.9% Stent + b. 10.8%	Death/MI at 6 mo: 5.6%, 7.8%, 11.4%, respectively

(continued)

Table 1 (*continued*)
Randomized Placebo-Controlled Trials of GPIIb-IIIa Antagonists in PCI

Trials	Agent used	Study cohort	No.	Drug dose and duration	Primary end points	Primary results	Long-term data and comments
RESTORE (56)	Tirofiban	Within 72 h	2139 ACS	a. 10 µg/kg bolus, 0.15 µg/kg/min 36 h b. Placebo	Death/MI/TVR, 30 d	10.3% tirofiban, 12.2% placebo $p = 0.16$	Drug started only after wire crossed lesion
IMPACT-II (57)	Eptifibatide	High- + low-risk PCI	4010	a. 135-µg/kg bolus, 0.5 µg/kg/min 20–24 h b. 135-µg/kg bolus, 0.75 µg/kg/min c. Placebo	Death/MI/TVR, 30 d	a. 9.2% b. 9.9% c. 11.4% $p = $ NS	Eptifibatide dose probably too low
ESPRIT (58,59)	Eptifibatide	Elective PCI	2064	a. 180-µg/kg bolus X2, 2 µg/kg/min, 18–24 h b. Placebo	Death/MI/TVR, 30 d	6.8% eptifibatide, 10.5% placebo $p = 0.0034$	1 yr: 17.5% eptifibatide, 12.4% placebo $p = 0.007$
Acute MI							
RAPPORT (60)	Abciximab	Acute MI Primary PTCA (stenting discouraged)	483	a. 0.25-mg/kg bolus, 0.125 µg/kg/min, 12 h b. Placebo	Death/MI/TVR, 6 mo	28.2% abciximab, 28.1% placebo $p = 0.97$	Lower composite end point with abciximab in treatment-received analysis
ADMIRAL (61)	Abciximab	Acute MI Primary stent	300	a. 0.25-mg/kg bolus, 0.125 µg/kg/min, 12 h b. Placebo	Death/MI/TVR, 30 d	6.0% abciximab, 14.6% placebo $p = 0.01$	6 mo: 7.4% abciximab, 15.9% placebo $p = 0.02$
CADILLAC (62)	Abciximab	Acute MI 2 × 2 factorial design	2665	a. 0.25-mg/kg bolus, 0.125 µg/kg/min, 12 h b. Placebo	Death/MI/TVR/ stroke 6 mo	PTCA + b. 20% PTCA + a. 16.5% Stent + b. 11.5% Stent + a. 10.2%	Addition of abciximab to stent group did not improve outcomes Lower risk patients

Abbreviations: ACS, acute coronary syndromes; hep, heparin; MI, myocardial infarction; PCI, percutaneous coronary intervention; PTCA, percutaneous transluminal coronary angioplasty; TVR, target vessel revascularization.

Clinical Trials for ACS

Several large randomized studies have assessed the use of intravenous GPIIb-IIIa antagonists for ACS, with or without early PCI *(67)*. Six main trials are summarized in Table 2: GUSTO-IV ACS (Global Use of Strategies to Open occluded arteries), PRISM (Platelet Receptro Inhibition in Ischemic Syndrome Management), PRISM-PLUS (PRISM in Patients Limited by Unstable Signs and Symptoms), PURSUIT (Platelet Glycoprotein IIb/IIIa in Unstable Angina Receptor Suppression Using Integrilin Therapy), and PARAGON- A and B (Platelet IIb/IIIa Antagonism for the Reduction of Acute Coronary Syndrome Events in a Global Organization Network) *(68–72)*. In a metaanalysis of these six trials by Boersma et al. *(73)*, a small reduction in death or MI was observed with a GPIIb-IIIa antagonist (11.8% compared with 10.8% with placebo, p = 0.015). The relative treatment benefit was similar irrespective of baseline characteristics, except for the female subgroup (Fig. 7). Data from GPIIb-IIIa antagonist PCI trials also showed similar results, with enhanced benefit in those presenting with ACS *(43,44,52,53,56,59)*. Pooled data from the EPIC, EPILOG, and EPISTENT trials similarly showed reduction in 1-yr death or MI rates in 3478 ACS patients with abciximab (6.7% compared with 13.3% for placebo) *(74)*.

In summary, based on the evidence of randomized clinical trials, the use of a GPIIb-IIIa antagonist should be strongly considered for ACS and PCI. Either eptifibatide or tirofiban could be administered upstream for ACS patients prior to PCI and continued up to 18–24 h post-PCI. For those ACS patients (including ST-elevation MI) undergoing PCI, who are not already receiving a GPIIb-IIIa antagonist when presenting to the catheterization laboratory, the agent of choice is abciximab.

OTHER ANTIPLATELET AGENTS

Dipyridamole

Dipyridamole is a reversible phosphodiesterase inhibitor that blocks the degradation of cyclic AMP and uptake of adenosine; its mechanism of antiplatelet effects is unknown. Dipyridamole is metabolized by the liver and has a relatively short half-life of 10 h. Early small trials in the 1980s showed no benefit of adding dipyridamole to aspirin for stroke prevention among patients with cerebrovascular diseases *(75–77)*. However, the much larger ESPS-2 (European Stroke Prevention Study 2) secondary prevention trial involving 6602 patients demonstrated that the combination of very-low-dose aspirin (50 mg daily) with dipyridamole (400 mg extended-release daily) reduced the risk of stroke by 37%, compared with 16.3% for dipyridamole alone (p = 0.039) and 18.1% for

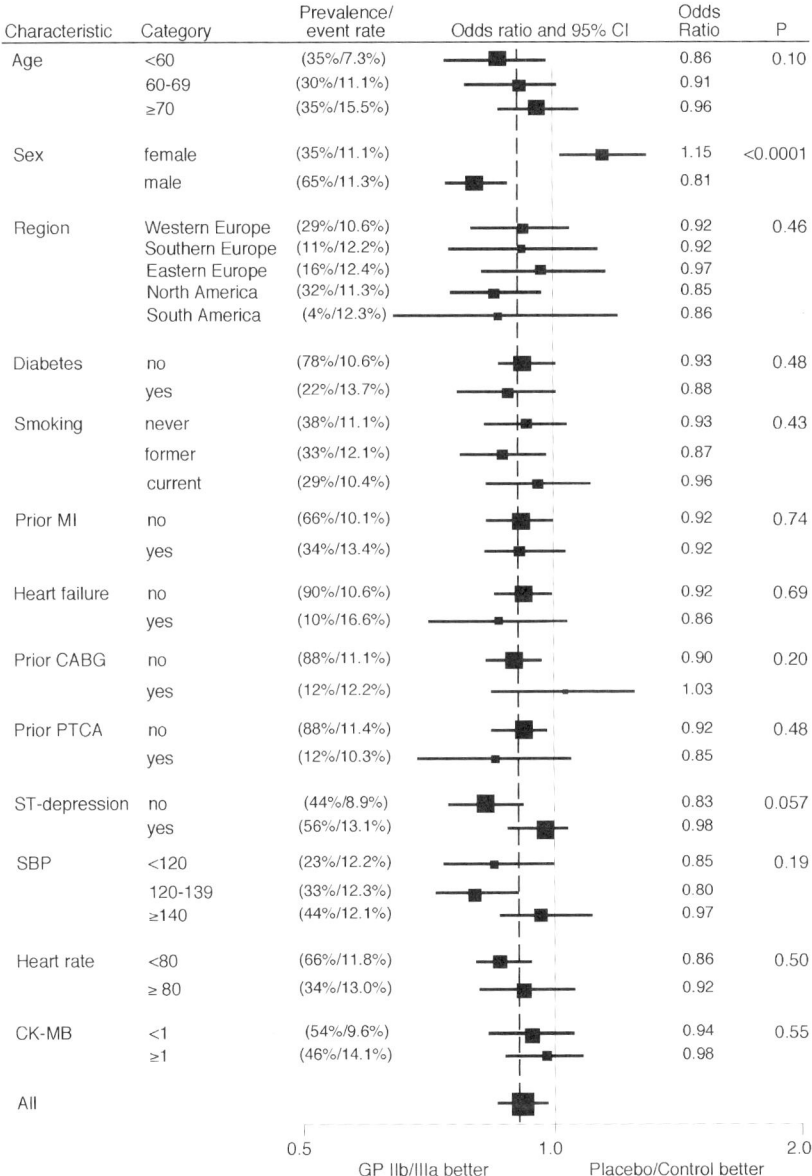

Characteristic	Category	Prevalence/ event rate	Odds ratio and 95% CI	Odds Ratio	P
Age	<60	(35%/7.3%)		0.86	0.10
	60-69	(30%/11.1%)		0.91	
	≥70	(35%/15.5%)		0.96	
Sex	female	(35%/11.1%)		1.15	<0.0001
	male	(65%/11.3%)		0.81	
Region	Western Europe	(29%/10.6%)		0.92	0.46
	Southern Europe	(11%/12.2%)		0.92	
	Eastern Europe	(16%/12.4%)		0.97	
	North America	(32%/11.3%)		0.85	
	South America	(4%/12.3%)		0.86	
Diabetes	no	(78%/10.6%)		0.93	0.48
	yes	(22%/13.7%)		0.88	
Smoking	never	(38%/11.1%)		0.93	0.43
	former	(33%/12.1%)		0.87	
	current	(29%/10.4%)		0.96	
Prior MI	no	(66%/10.1%)		0.92	0.74
	yes	(34%/13.4%)		0.92	
Heart failure	no	(90%/10.6%)		0.92	0.69
	yes	(10%/16.6%)		0.86	
Prior CABG	no	(88%/11.1%)		0.90	0.20
	yes	(12%/12.2%)		1.03	
Prior PTCA	no	(88%/11.4%)		0.92	0.48
	yes	(12%/10.3%)		0.85	
ST-depression	no	(44%/8.9%)		0.83	0.057
	yes	(56%/13.1%)		0.98	
SBP	<120	(23%/12.2%)		0.85	0.19
	120-139	(33%/12.3%)		0.80	
	≥140	(44%/12.1%)		0.97	
Heart rate	<80	(66%/11.8%)		0.86	0.50
	≥ 80	(34%/13.0%)		0.92	
CK-MB	<1	(54%/9.6%)		0.94	0.55
	≥1	(46%/14.1%)		0.98	
All					

0.5   1.0   2.0

GP IIb/IIIa better   Placebo/Control better

Fig. 7. Odds ratio of 30-d death or MI based on clinical baseline characteristics in a metaanalysis of six randomized controlled trials using GPIIb-IIIa blockade in acute coronary syndromes. CABG, coronary artery bypass graft; CK-MB, creatine kinase myocardial bound; PTCA, percutaneous transluminal coronary angioplasty; SBP, systolic blood pressure. (From ref. *73*, with permission from Elsevier.)

Table 2
Randomized Placebo-Controlled Trials of GP IIb-IIIa Antagonists for ACS

Trials	Agent used	Study cohort	No.	Drug dose and duration	Primary end points	Primary results	Long-term data and comments
PURSUIT (71)	Eptifibatide	Unstable angina or NQMI 89.8% received heparin	10948	a. 180-µg/kg bolus + 1.3 µg/kg/min b. 180 µg/kg bolus + c. Placebo 72-h infusion, 96 h if PCI done	30-d death or MI	Comparison between b. and c. groups: 14.2% eptifibatide vs 15.7% placebo p = 0.04	6-mo follow-up showed preservation of benefit with eptifibatide The low-dose group a. was discontinued after high-dose eptifibatide was shown to be safe
PRISM (69)	Tirofiban	ACS without ST elevation Only 2% PCI	3232	a. 0.6 µg/kg bolus + 0.15 µg/kg/min b. Placebo	48-h death, MI, or refractory ischemia	3.8% tirofiban vs 5.9% placebo p = 0.007	30-d events not significantly different (5.8% tirofiban vs 7.1% placebo)
PRISM-PLUS (70)	Tirofiban	Unstable angina or NQMI 30.5% had PCI	1915	a. 0.4-µg/kg bolus + 0.1 µg/kg/min + heparin b. 6-mg/kg bolus + 0.15 µg/kg/min + no heparin c. Heparin only	7-d death, MI, or refractory ischemia	a. 12.9% tirofiban/ heparin vs c. 17.9% heparin alone p = 0.004	Tirofiban alone arm b. was discontinued prematurely because of increased mortality (4.6%) compared with heparin alone (1.1%) Benefit of tirofiban/ heparin extended to 30 d

(Continued)

Table 2 (continued)

Randomized Placebo-Controlled Trials of GP IIb-IIIa Antagonists for ACS

Trials	Agent used	Study cohort	No.	Drug dose and duration	Primary end points	Primary results	Long-term data and comments
PARA-GON-A (72)	Lamifiban	ACS	2282	a. 300-μg bolus + 1 μg/min with or w/o heparin b. 500 μg + 5 μg/min with or w/o heparin c. Heparin only, infusion 72–120 h	30-d death, MI, or refractory ischemia	No difference in all lamifiban groups compared with placebo	6-mo death or MI was lower in the low-dose lamifiban a. group (13.7% vs 17.9% for placebo, $p = 0.03$), but no difference for the high-dose lamifiban b. group (16.4% vs 17.9%, $p = 0.45$)
PARA-GON-B (73)	Lamifiban	ACS All received heparin	5225	a. 500-μg bolus + 1–2 μg/min b. Heparin only	30-d death, MI, or refractory ischemia	No difference: 10.6% lamifiban vs 11.4% placebo	Troponin-positive patients had significant benefit with lamifiban However, commercial development did not proceed
GUSTO-IV ACS (68)	Abciximab	Unstable angina or NQMI All received heparin PCI in 1.6% of patients within 48 h	7800	a. 24-h 0.25-mg/kg bolus + 0.125 μg/kg/min b. 48-h 0.25 mg/kg bolus + 0.125μg/kg/min c. Heparin only	30-d death or MI	No difference between groups: a. 8.2%, b. 9.1%, c. 8.0%	Negative results may be explained by low-risk patients enrolled and low numbers of PCIs performed

Abbreviations: ACS, acute coronary syndromes; MI, myocardial infarction; NQMI, non-Q-wave MI; PCI, percutaneous coronary intervention.

aspirin alone ($p = 0.013$) *(78)*. Importantly, the meta-analysis of 10,404 patients in 25 trials of the Antithrombotic Trialists' Collaboration showed no difference in reduction of serious vascular events when comparing dipyridamole plus aspirin (11.8%) with aspirin alone (12.4%) *(1)*. Thus, the use of this agent in combination with aspirin for stroke prevention remains contentious. Based on the ESPS-2 trial, Aggrenox® (combination of aspirin [25 mg] and dipyridamole [extended-release 200 mg]) was recently FDA-approved for secondary prevention of stroke. In the setting of PCI, the combination of dipyridamole and aspirin was not superior to aspirin alone in a small randomized trial *(12)*.

Cilostazol

Cilostazol is a new antiplatelet agent that inhibits phosphodiesterase type III, thus increasing cyclic AMP and blocking platelet aggregation. It is also a vasodilator and has been increasingly used for symptomatic treatment of claudication. Another emerging indication is for PCI, as both an antiplatelet and potentially antirestenotic agent. Cilostazol plus aspirin has been compared with ticlopidine plus aspirin in a few small randomized PCI trials, showing no difference in major cardiac events including subacute stent thrombosis *(79–82)*. However, results were less consistent regarding restenosis, with most trials showing reduction with cilostazol *(81–84)*. In the Asian Paclitaxel-Eluting Clinical Trial (ASPECT) which randomized 180 PCI patients to either paclitaxel-eluting or bare-metal stents, the use of cilostazol plus aspirin was associated with higher major cardiac event rates (including four subacute stent thrombosis) compared with patients who received clopidogrel or ticlopidine plus aspirin (no subacute stent thrombosis) *(85)*.

ANTIPLATELET THERAPY
AND ANTIINFLAMMATORY EFFECTS

The additive benefit of combining antiplatelet agents was initially believed to be a consequence of enhanced antithrombotic potency. We have since realized that these agents also have antiinflammatory effects that may result from inhibition of platelet activation, inhibition of immune-active cells, or protection of endothelial function. Activated platelets can increase inflammation by mechanisms such as the release of CD40 ligand, synthesis of interleukin-1β, and expression of P-selectin *(86)*. This suggests that inhibition of platelet activation may curtail inflammation and the pathophysiologic link with thrombosis. However, the influence of antiplatelet therapy on inflammation is complex, as evidenced from the varying effects of GPIIb-IIIa blockade on inflammation (high GPIIb-IIIa receptor occupancy inhibits inflammation, whereas low receptor occupancy enhances inflammation) *(87).* Nevertheless, patients with the highest levels of inflammatory markers seem to derive the greatest benefit from antiplatelet therapy *(88).* Therefore, future research endeavoring to elucidate the effects of antiplatelet therapy on inflammation is imperative. This will help clarify the best strategy of antiplatelet combination for both PCI and systemic atherosclerosis.

PLATELET MONITORING

Platelet function testing can evaluate platelet adhesion, activation, aggregation, and secretion. This might be useful during invasive procedures to monitor the risk of thrombotic and hemorrhagic events and potentially optimize antiplatelet therapy during PCI. Presuming an ideal target of 80% receptor occupancy *(89),* current weight-adjusted GPIIb-IIIa antagonist dosing produces noteworthy interindividual variability. For example, with the current recommended abciximab dose of 0.25 mg/kg bolus and 0.125 µg/kg/min infusion, 13% of patients had less than 80% receptor blockade by 8 h during infusion, with greater variability immediately after cessation of the infusion (Fig. 8) *(90).*

Several studies have suggested the importance of adequate receptor blockade in patients undergoing PCI with adjunctive use of GPIIb-IIIa antagonists. The GOLD (AU-Assessing Ultegra) study prospectively enrolled 469 patients and correlated percent aggregation inhibition (measured with the Ultegra-RPFA device) to clinical events (death, MI, or urgent target revascularization) *(91).* The composite ischemic outcome was much lower in patients who achieved 95% or more of platelet inhibition, compared with patients with less than 95% inhibition (6.4% vs 14.4%, $p = 0.006$). In the study by Steinhubl et al. *(90),* 100 patients who received abciximab for PCI were prospectively evaluated, and platelet function inhibition was measured with the Ultegra-RPFA device. Although clinical outcome evaluation was not a predefined objective of this study, complete clinical follow-up data were available in 88 patients. Six of the 13 patients (46%) who had platelet inhibition of less than 80% at 8 h had an adverse cardiac event, compared with 5 of 75 patients (7%) who had 80% or more inhibition at 8 hours ($p < 0.001$). Both these studies indicate that specific levels of platelet inhibition should be achieved to prevent thromboembolic events associated with PCI. Kabbani et al. *(92)* performed ex vivo measurements of platelet function in ACS patients randomized to abciximab ($n = 8$) or tirofiban ($n = 10$) using light transmission aggregometry. The maximal platelet aggregation by 20 µM of ADP was inhibited to a greater extent with abciximab than tirofiban

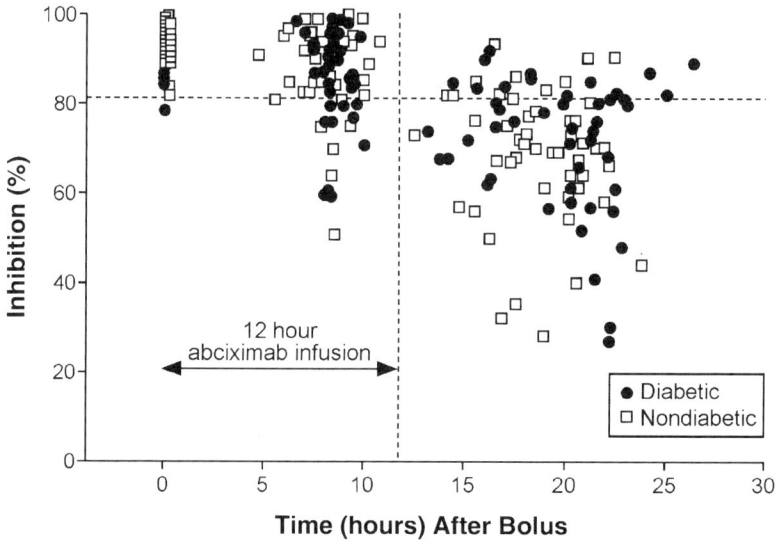

Fig. 8. Percent platelet function inhibition at various time points in patients undergoing PCI who received standard dose of abciximab. (Reproduced with permission from ref. *90.*)

treatment at 15–60 min after initiation of therapy (Fig. 9). This ex vivo finding may explain the initial 30-d composite outcome superiority of abciximab over tirofiban in the TARGET study.

Monitoring of platelet inhibition may also be valuable in patients with so-called aspirin resistance, and perhaps those on concomitant aspirin and nonsteroidal antiinflammatory drug (NSAID) therapies. A prospective study performed by Gum et al. *(93)* showed that aspirin resistance, as measured by optical platelet aggregometry, was associated with a higher risk of death, MI, or stroke at 2-yr follow-up (24% [4/17 patients] with aspirin resistant vs 10% [30/309 patients] aspirin sensitive, *p* = 0.03). Recent noncontrolled trials also suggest worse cardiovascular outcomes (including mortality) among those on both aspirin and ibuprofen *(94,95)*. Inadequate platelet inhibition in these scenarios may encourage substitution with thienopyridines or cessation of NSAIDs, respectively. Rapid platelet monitoring may also be beneficial when interchange of GPIIb-IIIa inhibitors is required, when combination antiplatelet therapy is needed, during bleeding complications to confirm excess inhibition, and prior to emergency surgery to confirm adequate restoration of aggregation.

Numerous tests evaluating a diversity of platelet functions are available, including measuring plasma drug levels, bleeding time, percent

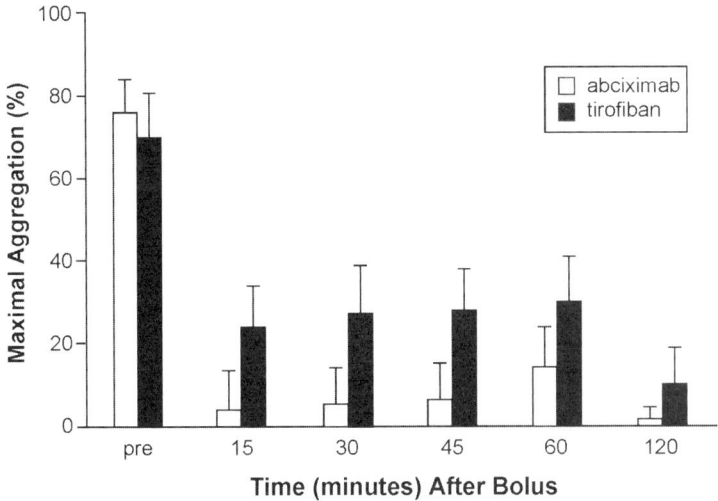

Fig. 9. Maximal platelet aggregation induced by 20 μ*M* ADP in patients randomized to abciximab or tirofiban. (From ref. *92*. Copyright 2002, with permission from Excerpta Medica, Inc.)

occupation of GPIIb-IIIa receptors, number of occupied GPIIb-IIIa receptors, extent of platelet aggregation inhibition, and clot strength. Such tests can be divided into central laboratory tests or point-of-care tests. Central laboratory tests are more accurate and precise; however, they are time consuming and cumbersome for rapid and routine clinical use. On the other hand, point-of-care tests, even though they produce more variable results, are practical and allow rapid bedside measurements. We will focus our discussion on current devices that are more commonly used, with emphasis on point-of-care tests. The different methods of assessing platelet function are discussed in more depth in Chapter 12.

Laboratory Platelet Aggregometry

PHOTO-OPTICAL PLATELET AGGREGOMETRY

Classical platelet aggregometry was invented in the 1960s *(96)*. Currently, several commercially available instruments employ this technique: Chrono-Log (Havertown, PA), Bio-Data (Hatboro, PA), Payton-Scientific (Buffalo, NY), and Helena Laboratories (Beaumont, TX). Platelet-rich plasma (PRP) is required to run this test, which is obtained from centrifugation of whole blood to sediment red cells and leukocytes, leaving platelets in the supernatant. This PRP is pipeted into cuvets and placed in the aggregometer between a light source and a photocell; then a platelet agonist (such as ADP, collagen, or epinephrine) is added and stirred at 37°C. As platelet aggregation occurs, turbidity decreases and light transmitted through the sample is increased. This change in light transmission is recorded with time and expressed as a percentage of aggregation. Disadvantages of this test include laborious sample preparation (PRP preparation is time consuming and may alter platelet behavior), the need for quality control, different standardizations between hospitals (precluding accurate comparison between different clinical sites), and unavailability for bedside testing.

IMPEDENCE AGGREGOMETRY

To circumvent the disadvantage of using PRP, impedence aggregometry was introduced as an alternative measurement of platelet aggregation utilizing whole blood by electrical impedence (97). A probe consisting of two platinum wire electrodes is inserted into cuvets containing whole blood diluted with normal saline. The resistance between the electrodes is measured at baseline and after addition of platelet agonist. Resistance increases as platelet aggregates accumulate between the electrodes and is reported as the change in impedence with time. This test also has a few disadvantages including higher variability than conventional aggregometry, necessary delicate care and cleaning of the electrodes, and expensive equipment. In addition, this method may not correlate well with conventional aggregometry when monitoring antiplatelet therapy.

LIGHT-SCATTERING PLATELET AGGREGOMETRY

A newer aggregometer was developed utilizing a combination of laser light scattering and aggregometry to monitor platelet microaggregate formation (98). It is more sensitive than conventional aggregometry, in which aggregates of less than 100 platelets cannot be detected. This improved instrument can detect microaggregates of two or three platelets, permitting identification of platelet hypersensitivity. It also requires much lower agonist concentration (<1000 times that of conventional aggregometry).

Point-of-Care Platelet Function Tests

ULTEGRA RAPID PLATELET FUNCTION ASSAY (RPFA)

The Ultegra RPFA (Accumetrics, San Diego, CA) is a simple and fast, automated point-of-care device that monitors GPIIb-IIIa inhibition. This test is based on platelet agglutination from interaction between unblocked GPIIb-IIIa receptors and fibrinogen-coated beads (99). A blood sample is collected into a citrate tube (except with eptifibatide and tirofiban, for which Phe-Pro-Arg chloromethyl ketone is used as the anticoagulant) and inserted into a disposible cartridge that contains TRAP (thrombin receptor-activating peptide) and fibrinogen-coated beads. TRAP activates platelets, exposing GPIIb-IIIa receptors to bind the fibrinogen-coated beads. Progressive increase in light transmission occurs as platelets agglutinate, which is impeded by GPIIb-IIIa inhibitors. The light absorbance is measured as a function of time, with agglutination rate quantified as platelet activation units (PAUs). Accumetrics also developed the Ultegra RPFA-ASA cartridge to measure aspirin resistance, but this has not been formally launched. The advantages of these automated tests are their simplicity of performance, the use of whole blood, and the fact that the data obtained correlate reasonably well with other tests of platelet function.

PLATELET-ACTIVATING CLOTTING TEST (PACT) ASSAY

The PACT assay, Hemostatus (Medtronic, Parker, CO), measures ACT without a platelet activator, comparing it with ACTs obtained with increasing concentrations of platelet-activating factor (PAF) *(100)*. The PAF-accelerated coagulation is measured in a multiwell cartridge containing a combination of kaolin and varied concentrations of PAF. The percent reduction of the ACT with PAF is related to the ability of the platelets to be activated and to shorten coagulation time. This rapid assay requires less than 3 min to perform, but the results obtained are highly variable. The instrument is also felt to be too large and cumbersome for routine use.

PFA-100 ANALYZER

The Dade Behring (Miami, FL) Platelet Function Analyzer (PFA-100) exposes platelets within citrated whole blood to high shear stress through a capillary tube, followed by an aperture in a membrane coated with collagen and either ADP or epinephrine *(101)*. The platelets adhere and aggregate until the aperture is occluded, and the time to this closure is recorded. This point-of-care assay is a quick and automatic way of evaluating primary hemostasis, with a normal closure time of 100 s. With GPIIb-IIIa inhibitors, the closure time is increased much beyond 300 s. This assay is highly dependent on von Willebrand factor but is coagulation independent. The collagen/epinephrine cartridge is sensitive to aspirin administration and may be useful for assessment of aspirin resistance. Among the advantages of this test are that it is an easy-to-use, rapid, automated, bedside test that uses whole blood. However, the results obtained are somewhat variable, and the relationship to PRP aggregometry and outcomes is uncertain.

PLATELETWORKS TEST

The Plateletworks (Helena Laboratories, Beaumont, TX) is a point-of-care test that uses a Coulter counter to measure platelet-count ratio, red blood cell count, hemoglobin, and hematocrit. Platelet count is measured in a control sample in which aggregation is prevented by EDTA and compared with the platelet count in an agonist-stimulated (ADP or collagen) sample *(102)*. The difference between these counts is expressed as a platelet-count ratio, which is reported as a percent platelet aggregation. This test is convenient and uses whole blood, and results are available within 5 min.

CLOT SIGNATURE ANALYZER

This instrument, from Xylum Corporation (Scarsdale, NY), measures several aspects of platelet function and clotting properties *(103)*. Non-anticoagulated blood is perfused through a collagen channel at a high shear rate, simulating blood flow in a thrombogenic subendothelial tissue. This activates platelets to aggregate and form thrombus. Simultaneously, a 0.15-mm needle is used to punch two fine holes in a channel without collagen, resulting in a high shear rate and promoting platelet adhesion, activation, and aggregation at the punch site. Growing fibrin clots then reduce blood flow, causing a fall in pressure, which is plotted against time for both channels to produce a clot signature. This test uses non-anticoagulated whole blood and can be performed at the bedside. The instrument is large, and interpretation of results is complex, precluding widespread use.

THROMBOELASTOGRAPHY

This device measures clot strength and gives a global assessment of hemostasis *(104)*. A clot is allowed to form between a cylindrical cup and a sensing device. The cup is then oscillated to and fro, and the transduction of the movement sensed by a torsion wire is represented graphically. This measurement relates directly to the physical properties of the clot, which is dependent on platelet function and its interaction with fibrin. Incremental strength of the clot formation translates to greater magnitude of output. This technique uses whole blood and has been utilized as point-of-care testing in surgical departments to detect hemostatic abnormalities. It is cumbersome and time consuming to perform, and some data suggest that it is insensitive to patients on aspirin.

In summary, platelet function testing is useful in many scenarios, especially during PCI with the use of antiplatelet agents. It has been shown that an adequate level of platelet inhibition is necessary for clinical efficacy and safety, particularly with the use of intravenous GPIIb-

IIIa antagonists. However, despite the wide variety of techniques available commercially, none of them are considered an ideal test. Many are simple to perform at the bedside during PCI, and results can be obtained promptly to facilitate clinical decisions. There is no clear winner at this juncture, and no study has been performed to demonstrate that measuring and adjusting extent of platelet inhibition improves outcomes.

CONCLUSIONS

Antiplatelet therapy is essential for numerous cardiovascular diseases including the prevention and treatment of thromboembolic processes. In many scenarios of increased platelet activity, combinations of antiplatelet agents are indicated (e.g., aspirin resistance, PCI, ACS). In most instances, monitoring of platelet activity is not necessary. However, when antiplatelet resistance is suspected or during PCI with intravenous GPIIb-IIIa antagonist use, the availability of prompt platelet monitoring will be valuable. Our understanding of antiplatelet therapy continues to expand in many dimensions, including the development of novel agents, exploitation of their antiinflammatory effects, and experimentation with concomitant fibrinolytic (i.e., facilitated PCI) and anticoagulant (low-molecular weight heparin) therapies. Further expansion of their clinical indications for cardiovascular diseases is anticipated.

REFERENCES

1. Antithrombotic Trialists' Collaboration. Collaborative metaanalysis of randomised trials of antiplatelet therapy for prevention of death, myocardial infarction, and stroke in high risk patients. BMJ 2002;324:71–86.
2. Gawaz M, Neumann F, Ott I, May A, Rudiger S, Schomig A. Changes in membrane glycoproteins of circulating platelets after coronary stent implantation. Heart 1996;76:166–172.
3. Parson H, Cwikiel W, Johansson K, Swartbol P, Norgren L. Deposition of platelets and neutrophils in porcine iliac arteries angioplasty and Wallstent placement compared with angioplasty alone. Cardiovasc Intervent Radiol 1994;17:190–196.
4. Higgs G, Salmon J, Henderson B, Vane J. Pharmacokinetics of aspirin and salicylate in relation to inhibition of arachidonate cyclooxygenase and anti-inflammatory activity. Proc Natl Acad Sci USA 1987;84:1417–1420.
5. Patrono C. Aspirin as an antiplatelet drug. N Engl J Med 1994;330:1287–1294.
6. Cambria-Kiely J, Gandhi P. Possible mechanisms of aspirin resistance. J Thromb Thrombol 2002;13:49–56.
7. Steering Committee of the Physicians' Health Study Research Group. Final report on the aspirin component of the ongoing physicians' health study. N Engl J Med 1989;321:129–135.
8. Hansson L, Zanchetti A, for the HOT Study Group. Effects of intensive blood pressure lowering and low dose aspirin in patients with hypertension: principal results of the hypertension optimal treatment (HOT) randomized trial. Lancet 1998;351:1755–1762.

9. Collaborative Group of the Primary Prevention Project (PPP). Low-dose aspirin and
    vitamin E in people at cardiovascular risk: a randomised trial in general practice.
    Lancet 2001;357:89–95.
10. Barnathan E, Schwartz J, Taylor L, et al. Aspirin and dipyridamole in the prevention
    of acute coronary thrombosis complicating coronary angioplasty. Circulation
    1987;76:125–134.
11. Schwartz L, Bourassa M, Lesperance J, et al. Aspirin and dipyridamole in the
    prevention of restenosis after percutaneous transluminal coronary angioplasty. N
    Engl J Med 1988;318:1714–1719.
12. Lembo N, Black A, Roubin G, et al. Effect of pretreatment with aspirin versus
    aspirin plus dipyridamole on frequency and type of acute complications of percu-
    taneous transluminal coronary angioplasty. Am J Cardiol 1990;65:422–426.
13. Smith S, Dove J, Kern M, et al. ACC/AHA guidelines for percutaneous coronary
    intervention (revision of the 1993 PTCA guidelines)—executive summary. J Am
    Coll Cardiol 2001;37:2215–2239.
14. Popma J, Ohman M, Weitz J, Lincoff M, Harrington R, Berger P. Antithrombotic
    therapy in patients undergoing percutaneous coronary intervention. Chest
    2001;119:321S–336S.
15. Desager J. Clinical pharmacokinetics of ticlopidine. Clin Pharmacokinet
    1994;26:347–355.
16. Defreyn G, Bernat A, Delebassee D, Maffrand J. Pharmacology of ticlopidine: a
    review. Semin Thromb Hemost 1989;15:159–166.
17. Haas W, Easton J, Adams H, et al. A randomized trial comparing ticlopidine hydro-
    chloride with aspirin for the prevention of stroke in high-risk patients. N Engl J Med
    1989;321:501–505.
18. Balsano F, Rizzon P, Violi F, et al. Antiplatelet treatment with ticlopidine in un-
    stable angina: a controlled multicenter device trial. Circulation 1990;82:17–22.
19. White C, Chaitman B, Lassar T, et al. Antiplatelet agents are effective in reducing
    the immediate complications of PTCA: results from the ticlopidine multicenter trial
    [abstract]. Circulation 1987;76:IV-400.
20. Schomig A, Neumann F, Kastrati A, et al. A randomized comparison of antiplatelet
    and anticoagulant therapy after the placement of coronary-artery stents. N Engl J
    Med 1996;334:1084–1089.
21. Bertrand M, Legrand V, Boland J, et al. Randomized multicenter comparison of
    conventional anticoagulation versus antiplatelet therapy in unplanned and elective
    coronary stenting: the full anticoagulation versus aspirin and ticlopidine (FANTAS-
    TIC) study. Circulation 1998;98:1597–1603.
22. Leon M, Baim D, Popma J, et al. A randomized trial comparing three drug regimens
    to prevent thrombosis following elective coronary stenting. N Engl J Med
    1998;339:1665–1671.
23. Savi P, Combalbert J, Gaich C, et al. The antiaggregating activity of clopidogrel is
    due to a metabolic activation by the hepatic cytochrome P450-1A. Thromb Haemost
    1994;72:313–317.
24. Savi P, Labouret C, Delesque N, Guette F, Lupker J, Herbert J. P2y(12), a new
    platelet ADP receptor, target of clopidogrel. Biochem Biophys Res Commun
    2001;283:379–383.
25. Geiger J, Brich J, Honig-Liedl P, et al. Specific impairment of human platelet P2Yac
    ADP receptor-mediated signaling by the antiplatelet drug clopidogrel. Arterioscler
    Thromb Vasc Biol 1999;19:2007–2011.

26. Savcic M, Hauert J, Bachmann F, Wyld P, Geudelin B, Cariou R. Clopidogrel loading dose regimens: kinetic profile of pharmacodynamic response in healthy subjects. Semin Thromb Haemost 1999;25:15–19.
27. CAPRIE Steering Committee. A randomized, blinded trial of clopidogrel versus aspirin in patients at risk of ischemic events (CAPRIE). Lancet 1996;348:1329–1339.
28. Hermann A, Rauch B, Braun M, Schror K, Weber A. Platelet CD40 ligand (CD40L)—subcellular localization, regulation of expression, and inhibition by clopidogrel. Platelets 2001;12:74–82.
29. Yusuf S, Zhao F, Mehta S, Chrolavicius S, Tognoni G, Fox K. Effects of clopidogrel in addition to aspirin in patients with acute coronary syndrome without ST-segment elevation. N Engl J Med 2001;345:494–502.
30. Muller C, Buttner H, Petersen J, Roskamm H. A randomized comparison of clopidogrel and aspirin versus ticlopidine and aspirin after the placement of coronary-artery stents. Circulation 2000;101:590–593.
31. Moussa I, Oetgen M, Roubin G, et al. Effectiveness of clopidogrel and aspirin versus ticlopidine and aspirin in preventing stent thrombosis after coronary stent implantation. Circulation 1999;99:2364–2366.
32. Berger P, Bell M, Rihal C, et al. Clopidogrel versus ticlopidine after intracoronary stent placement. J Am Coll Cardiol 1999;34:1892–1894.
33. Mishkel G, Aguirre F, Ligon R, Rocha-Singh K, Lucore C. Clopidogrel as adjunctive antiplatelet therapy during coronary stenting. J Am Coll Cardiol 1999;34:1884–1890.
34. Steinhubl S, Berger P, Mann J, et al. Early and sustained dual oral antiplatelet therapy following percutaneous coronary intervention. JAMA 2002;288:2411–2420.
35. Mehta S, Yusuf S, Peters R, et al. Effects of pretreatment with clopidogrel and aspirin followed by long-term therapy in patients undergoing percutaneous coronary intervention: the PCI-CURE study. Lancet 2001;358:527–533.
36. Kereiakes D, Grines C, Fry E, et al. Enoxaparin and abciximab adjunctive pharmacotherapy during percutaneous coronary intervention. J Invasive Cardiol 2001;13:272–278.
37. Bhatt D, Lee B, Casterella P, et al. Safety of concomitant therapy with eptifibatide and enoxaparin in patients undergoing percutaneous coronary intervention. Results of the Coronary Revascularization Using Integrilin and Single Bolus Enoxaparin Study. J Am Coll Cardiol 2003;41:20–25.
38. Coller B. Potential non-glycoprotein IIb/IIIa effects of abciximab. Am Heart J 1999;138:S1–S5.
39. Mascelli M, Lance E, Damaraju L, Wagner C, Weisman H, Jordan R. Pharmacodynamic profile of short-term abciximab treatment demonstrates prolonged platelet inhibition with gradual recovery from GP IIb/IIIa receptor blockade. Circulation 1998;97:1680–1688.
40. Quinn M, Murphy R, Dooley M, Foley J, Fitzgerald D. Occupancy of the internal and external pools of glycoprotein IIb/IIIa following abciximab bolus and infusion. J Pharmacol Exp Ther 2001;297:496–500.
41. Leclerc J. Platelet glycoprotein IIb/IIIa antagonists: lessons learned from clinical trials and future directions. Crit Care Med 2002;30:S332–S340.
42. Lele M, Sajid M, Wajih N, Stouffer G. Eptifibatide and 7E3, but not tirofiban, inhibit $\alpha v \beta 3$ integrin-mediated binding of smooth muscle cells to thrombospondin and prothrombin. Circulation 2001;104:582–587.
43. The EPILOG Investigators. Platelet glycoprotein IIb/IIIa receptor blockade and low dose heparin during percutaneous coronary revascularization. N Engl J Med 1997;336:1689–1696.

44. The EPIC Investigators. Use of a monoclonal antibody directed against the platelet glycoprotein IIb/IIIa receptor in high-risk coronary angioplasty. N Engl J Med 1994;330:956–961.

45. Chew D, Bhatt D, Lincoff A, et al. Defining the optimal activated clotting time during percutaneous coronary intervention. Aggregate results from 6 randomized, controlled trials. Circulation 2001;103:961–966.

46. Berkowitz S, Harrington R, Rund M, Tcheng J. Acute profound thrombocytopenia after c7E3 Fab (abciximab) therapy. Circulation 1997;330:956–961.

47. Madan M, Kereiakes D, Hermiller J, et al. Efficacy of abciximab readministration in coronary intervention. Am J Cardiol 2000;85:435–440.

48. Llevadot J, Coulter S, Giugliano R. A practical approach to the diagnosis and management of thrombocytopenia associated with glycoprotein IIb/IIIa receptor inhibitors. J Thromb Thrombol 2000;9:175–180.

49. Topol E, Lincoff A, Kereiakes D, et al. Multi-year follow-up of abciximab therapy in three randomized, placebo-controlled trials of percutaneous coronary revascularization. Am J Med 2002;113:1–6.

50. Topol E, Ferguson J, Weisman H, et al. Long-term protection from myocardial ischemic events in a randomized trial of brief integrin beta3 blockade with percutaneous coronary intervention. JAMA 1997;278:479–484.

51. Lincoff A, Tcheng J, Califf R, et al. Sustained suppression of ischemic complications of coronary intervention by platelet GP IIb/IIIa blockade with abciximab. One year outcome in the EPILOG Trial. Circulation 1999;99:1951–1958.

52. The CAPTURE Investigators. Randomized placebo-controlled trial of abciximab before and during coronary intervention in refractory unstable angina: the CAPTURE investigators. Lancet 1997;349:1429–1435.

53. The EPISTENT Investigators. Randomized placebo-controlled and balloon angioplasty controlled trial to assess safety of coronary stenting with use of platelet glycoprotein IIb/IIIa blockade. Lancet 1998;352:87–92.

54. Lincoff A, Califf R, Moliterno D, et al. Complementary clinical benefits of coronary-artery stenting and blockade of platelet glycoprotein IIb/IIIa receptors. N Engl J Med 1999;341:319–327.

55. Marso S, Lincoff A, Ellis S, et al. Optimizing the percutaneous interventional outcomes for patients with diabetes mellitus: results of the EPISTENT (Evaluation of Platelet IIb/IIIa Inhibitor for Stenting Trial) Diabetic Substudy. Circulation 1999;100:2488–2484.

56. The RESTORE Investigators. Effects of platelet glycoprotein IIb/IIIa blockade with tirofiban on adverse cardiac events in patients with unstable angina or acute myocardial infarction undergoing coronary angioplasty. Circulation 1997;96:1445–1453.

57. The IMPACT-II Investigators. Randomized, placebo-controlled trial of effect of eptifibatide on complications of percutaneous coronary intervention: IMPACT-II. Lancet 1997;349:1422–1428.

58. Blankenship J, Tasissa G, O'Shea J, et al. Effect of glycoprotein IIb/IIIa receptor inhibition on angiographic complications during percutaneous coronary intervention in the ESPRIT Trial. J Am Coll Cardiol 2001;38:653–658.

59. O'Shea J, Buller C, Cantor W, et al. Long-term efficacy of platelet glycoprotein IIb/IIIa integrin blockade with eptifibatide in coronary stent intervention. JAMA 2002;287:618–621.

60. Brener S, Barr L, Burchenal J, et al. Randomized, placebo-controlled trial of platelet glycoprotein IIb/IIIa blockade with primary angioplasty for acute myocardial infarction. Circulation 1998;98:734–741.

61. Montalescot G, Barragan P, Wittenberg O, et al. Platelet glycoprotein IIb/IIIa inhibition with coronary stenting for acute myocardial infarction. N Engl J Med 2001;1895–1903.

62. Stone G, Grines C, Cox D, et al. Comparison of angioplasty with stenting, with or without abciximab, in acute myocardial infarction. N Engl J Med 2002;346:958–966.

63. Topol E, Moliterno D, Herrmann H, et al. Comparison of two platelet glycoprotein IIb/IIIa inhibitors, tirofiban and abciximab, for the prevention of ischemic events with percutaneous coronary revascularization. N Engl J Med 2001;344:1888–1894.

64. Moliterno D, Yakubov S, DiBattiste P, et al. Outcomes at 6 months for the direct comparison of tirofiban and abciximab during percutaneous coronary revascularisation with stent placement: the TARGET follow-up study. Lancet 2002;360:355–360.

65. Roffi M, Mukherjee D, Chew D, et al. Lack of benefit from intravenous platelet glycoprotein IIb/IIIa receptor inhibition as adjunctive treatment for percutaneous interventions of aortocoronary bypass grafts. A pooled analysis of five randomized clinical trials. Circulation 2002;106:3063–307.

66. Lincoff A, Bittl J, Harrington R, et al. Bivalirudin and provisional glycoprotein IIb/IIIa blockade compared with heparin and planned glycoprotein IIb/IIIa blockade during percutaneous coronary intervention. JAMA 2003;289:853–863.

67. Bhatt D, Topol E. Current role of platelet glycoprotein IIb/IIIa inhibitors in acute coronary syndromes. JAMA 2000;284:1549–1558.

68. The GUSTO-IV ACS Investigators. Effect of glycoprotein IIb/IIIa receptor blocker abciximab on outcome in patients with acute coronary syndromes without early coronary revascularisation: the GUSTO IV-ACS randomised trial. Lancet 2001;357:1915–1924.

69. The PRISM Investigators. A comparison of aspirin plus tirofiban with aspirin plus heparin for unstable angina. N Engl J Med 1998;338:1498–1505.

70. The PRISM-PLUS Investigators. Inhibition of the platelet glycoprotein IIb/IIIa receptor with tirofiban in unstable angina and non-Q-wave myocardial infarction. N Engl J Med 1998;338:1488–1497.

71. The PURSUIT Investigators. Inhibition of platelet glycoprotein IIb/IIIa with eptifibitide in patients with acute coronary syndromes. N Engl J Med 1998; 339:436–443.

72. The PARAGON Investigators. International, randomized, controlled trial of lamifiban (a platelet glycoprotein IIb/IIIa inhibitor), heparin, or both in unstable angina. Circulation 1998;97:2386–2395.

73. Boersma E, Harrington R, Moliterno D, et al. Platelet glycoprotein IIb/IIIa inhibitors in acute coronary syndromes: a meta-analysis of all major randomised clinical trials. Lancet 2002;359:189–198.

74. Roe M, Gum P, Booth J, et al. Consistent and durable reduction in death and myocardial infarction with abciximab during coronary intervention in acute coronary syndromes and stable angina. Circulation 1999;100:I-187.

75. Guiraud-Chaumeil B, Rascol A, David J, Boneu B, Clanet M, Bierme R. Prevention des recidives des accidents vasculaires cérébraux ischemiques par les anti-agregants plaquettaires. Rev Neurol 1982;138:367–385.

76. Bousser M, Eschwege E, Haguenau M, et al. "AICLA" controlled trial of aspirin and dipyridamole in the secondary prevention of athero-thrombotic cerebral ischemia. Stroke 1983;14:5–14.

77. The American-Canadian Co-operative Study Group. Persantine aspirin trial in cerebral ischemia. Part II: Endpoint results. Stroke 1985;16:406–415.

78. Diener H, Cunha L, Forbes C, Sivenius J, Smets P, Lowenthal A. European Stroke Prevention Study 2: dipyridamole and acetylsalicylic acid in the secondary prevention of stroke. J Neurol Sci 1996;143:1–13.
79. Yoon Y, Shim W, Lee D, et al. Usefulness of cilostazol versus ticlopidine in coronary artery stenting. Am J Cardiol 1999;84:1375–1380.
80. Park S, Lee C, Kim H, et al. Comparison of cilostazol versus ticlopidine therapy after stent implantation. Am J Cardiol 1999;84:511–514.
81. Tanabe Y, Ito E, Nakagawa I, Suzuki K. Effect of cilostazol on restenosis after coronary angioplasty and stenting in comparison to conventional coronary artery stenting with ticlopidine. Int J Cardiol 2001;78:285–291.
82. Kamishirado H, Inoue T, Mizoguchi K, et al. Randomized comparison of cilostazol versus ticlopidine hydrochloride for antiplatelet therapy after coronary stent implantation for prevention of late restenosis. Am Heart J 2002;144:303–308.
83. Tsuchikane E, Fukuhara A, Kobayashi T, et al. Impact of cilostazol on restenosis after percutaneous coronary balloon angioplasty. Circulation 1999;100:21–26.
84. Park S, Lee C, Kim H, et al. Effects of cilostazol on angiographic restenosis after coronary stent placement. Am J Cardiol 2000;86:499–503.
85. Park S, Shim W, Ho D, et al. A paclitaxel-eluting stent for the prevention of coronary restenosis. N Engl J Med 2003;348:1537–1545.
86. Aukrust P, Waehre T, Damas J, Gullestad L, Solum N. Inflammatory role of platelets in acute coronary syndromes. Heart 2001;86:605–606.
87. Nannizzi-Alaimo N, Alves V, Prasad S, et al. GP IIb-IIIa antagonists demonstrate a dose-dependent inhibition and potentiation of soluble CD40L (CD154) release during platelet stimulation. Circulation 2001;104:II-318.
88. Chew D, Bhatt D, Robbins M, et al. Effect of clopidogrel added to aspirin before percutaneous coronary intervention on the risk associated with C-reactive protein. Am J Cardiol 2001;88:672–674.
89. Coller B, Peerschke E, Scudder L, Sullivan C. A murine monoclonal antibody that completely blocks the binding of fibrinogen to platelets produces a thrombasthenic-like state in normal platelets and binds to glycoproteins IIb and/or IIIa. J Clin Invest 1983;72:325–338.
90. Steinhubl S, Kottke-Marchant K, Moliterno D, et al. Attainment and maintenance of platelet inhibition through standard dosing of abciximab in diabetic and nondiabetic patients undergoing percutaneous coronary intervention. Circulation 1999;100:1977–1982.
91. Steinhubl S, Talley J, Braden G, et al. Point-of-care measured platelet inhibition correlates with a reduced risk of an adverse cardiac event after percutaneous coronary intervention. Results of the GOLD (AU-Assessing Ultegra) multicenter study. Circulation 2001;103:2572–2578.
92. Kabbani S, Aggarwal A, Terrien E, DiBattiste P, Sobel B, Schneider D. Suboptimal early inhibition of platelets by treatment with tirofiban and implications for coronary interventions. Am J Cardiol 2002;89:647–650.
93. Gum P, Kottke-Marchant K, Welsh P, White J, Topol E. A prospective, blinded determination of the natural history of aspirin resistance among stable patients with cardiovascular disease. J Am Coll Cardiol 2003;41:961–965.
94. MacDonald T, Wei L. Effect of ibuprofen on cardioprotective effect of aspirin. Lancet 2003;361:573–574.
95. Ray W, Stein C, Hall K, Daugherty J, Griffin M. Non-steroidal anti-inflammatory drugs and risk of serious coronary heart disease. Lancet 2002;359:118–123.
96. Born G. Aggregation of blood platelets by adenosine and its reversal. Nature 1962;194:927–929.

97. Cardinal D, Flower R. The electronic aggregometer: a novel device for assessing platelet behaviour. J Pharmacol Methods 1980;3:135–138.
98. Ozaki Y, Satoh K, Yatomi Y, Yamamoto T, Shirasawa Y, Kume S. Detection of platelet aggregates using light scattering. Anal Biochem 1994;218:284–294.
99. Coller B, Lang D, Scudder L. Rapid and simple platelet function assay to assess glycoprotein IIb/IIIa blockade. Circulation 1997;4:860–867.
100. Despotis G, Levine V, Filos K, et al. Evaluation of a new point of care test that measures PAF-mediated acceleration of coagulation in cardiac surgical patients. Anesthesiology 1996;85:1311–1323.
101. Kundu S, Heilmann E, Sio R, Garcia C, Davidson R, Ostgaard R. Description of an in vitro platelet function analyzer—PFA-100. Semin Thromb Haemost 1995;21:106–112.
102. Nicholson N, Panzer-Knodle S, Haas N, et al. Assessment of platelet function assays. Am Heart J 1998;135:S170–S178.
103. Li C, Hoffmann T, Hsieh P, Malik S, Watson W. Xylum CSA: automated system for assessing haemostasis in simulated vascular flow. Clin Chem 1997;43:1788–1790.
104. Mallet S, Cox D. Thromboelastography. Br J Anaesth 1992;69:307–313.

16 Assessing Platelet Function in Clinical Trials

Neal Kleiman, MD

INTRODUCTION: CLINICAL STATUS OF ANTIPLATELET AGENTS

Since the 1970s, the role of antiplatelet therapy in patients with coronary artery disease has become established. Aspirin was the first drug to be used as an antiaggregant. Although early trials of aspirin lacked adequate statistical power to detect clinical benefits, two metaanalyses by the antiplatelet trialist group established the place of aspirin in the management of coronary artery disease and provided significant insight into the lack of a documented dose-response effect (1,2). Although the administration of aspirin to suitable patients still lags behind desired targets, most surveys indicate that more than 90% of appropriate patients are treated with it at the time of hospital discharge.

Clinical research in more recent years has highlighted the thienopyridines ticlopidine and clopidogrel. A combination of these drugs, so-called "dual antiplatelet therapy" initially began in patients receiving intracoronary stents (3), and has more recently been shown to reduce a composite of ischemic sequelae in patients hospitalized with an acute coronary syndrome (4), and is now undergoing evaluation in a variety of chronic disease states. Antagonists of platelet (GP)IIb-IIIa provide more potent

From: *Contemporary Cardiology:*
Platelet Function: Assessment, Diagnosis, and Treatment
Edited by: M. Quinn and D. Fitzgerald © Humana Press Inc., Totowa, NJ

inhibition of platelet aggregation and are currently used in patients undergoing percutaneous coronary intervention (PCI) and in patients presenting with acute coronary syndromes. The evidence supporting the use
of these therapies is reviewed elsewhere in this text. The purpose of the
current chapter is to outline the role that tests of platelet function have
played in the evolution of the clinical trials in which these agents were
evaluated.

Purposes of Testing

Testing platelet function in preparation for clinical trials has generally
been directed at evaluation of individual drug therapies and has served
two general purposes. The first aim is to confirm that the selected
antiplatelet therapy is physiologically active within a clinical syndrome.
The second is to select appropriate drug doses for clinical testing in
patients with or at risk for atherosclerosis and its clinical manifestations.
In most cases, initial dose selection is derived from experimental studies
and is refined in volunteer subjects. However, there are several ways in
which patients with atherosclerosis are likely to differ from volunteer
subjects. In general, subjects with atherosclerosis are older and have
more comorbidities than volunteer subjects. As a result, drug absorption
and disposition may be different than seen in volunteer subjects and may
also be more variable. Disruption of an atherosclerotic plaque may also
increase the proportion of circulating platelets that are in an activated
state. Compared with quiescent platelets, activated platelets express
greater numbers of GPIIb-IIIa receptors, a greater proportion of GPIIb-
IIIa in a ligand binding-permissive state, and a number of surface proteins, such as P-selectin, which mediates adhesion to leukocytes and
possibly other platelets *(5,6)* and CD 40 ligand (CD-154).

The literature is replete with documentation of increased levels of
activated platelets *(7)*, platelet-leukocyte complexes *(8)*, increased generation of thrombin *(9)*, and increased levels of circulating markers of
thrombotic and inflammatory processes in patients with acute coronary
syndromes *(10)*. It has also been recognized for more than a decade that
platelet activation follows PCI almost immediately *(11)*. The activity of
the disease process itself may therefore enhance resistance to antiplatelet
drugs, thereby altering dose requirements. Finally, much attention has
been drawn to the fact that patient response to any of the antiplatelet
drugs in common use is heterogeneous rather than homogeneous. It is
this last observation that argues most strongly for the use of platelet
functional testing in clinical trials, so that relationships can be observed
between physiologic responses and clinical outcomes. In fact, as the
patient population under study shifts from the relatively homogeneous

groups studied in dose-ranging trials to the more heterogeneous groups studied in larger trials, which are more representative of the sorts of patients likely to be encountered in clinical practice, comorbidities increase in frequency, and the spectrum of drug response is also likely to increase.

Pitfalls of Platelet Function Testing

Unfortunately, assessment of platelet function for the purposes of clinical trials suffers from several important limitations. Primary among these is the fact that physiologic understanding of platelet function has advanced more rapidly than drug development. A primary requisite of any drug development program is the assumption that all pertinent mechanisms of action of any drug have been elucidated and that their relationship to the activity of the disease being treated have been established. Unfortunately, this has rarely turned out to be the case, as numerous "collateral" effects, some deleterious and some beneficial, of antiplatelet agents have been described since their inception.

It is important to recognize two other important pitfalls of platelet function assessment that are particularly applicable to GPIIb-IIIa antagonists. First, most assessments in the early phases of clinical development have been performed in patients who receive antithrombotic treatment with unfractionated heparin. Multiple studies have indicated increases in platelet aggregability following bolus doses of unfractionated heparin *(10,12–14)*. Although the mechanism is not clearly elucidated, the increase associated with heparin bolus dosing appears to be dose dependent and occurs within minutes of administration. These findings may have particular relevance in the early studies of GPIIb-IIIa antagonists, which were performed in patients undergoing percutaneous coronary interventions at a time when heparin doses were considerably higher than those used today. The more recent adoption of bivalirudin and possibly of unfractionated heparins, which appear to have little to no effect *(14,15)* on platelet aggregation, may mitigate these findings in the future.

A second, more recently recognized variable is the use of thienopyridines, particularly clopidogrel, prior to intracoronary stenting. Clopidogrel's activity occurs through blockade of the purinergic P2Y12 receptor *(16)*, which is responsible for platelet aggregation and secretion *(17)*. Blockade of this receptor inhibits adenosine diphosphate (ADP)-induced activation and aggregation of platelets and appears to have an effect on platelet responses to other antagonists, probably by limiting the secondary response to platelet secretion of ADP. When a thienopyridine is given in conjunction with a GPIIb-IIIa antagonist, the inhibition of platelet aggregation is usually overwhelmingly modulated by the GPIIb-IIIa antagonist, although when the dose of the GPIIb-IIIa antagonist is low, there may be a synergistic effect. Recent trends toward increasing the initial dose of clopidogrel to 600 mg may affect subsequent measurement of the platelet aggregation response to a GPIIb-IIIa antagonist, although unpublished data from our own laboratory do not suggest that this is likely to be the case. The situation may be further complicated by a recently recognized phenomenon of clopidogrel "resistance," which has been reported in nearly 25%–40% of patients given a clopidogrel dose prior to coronary stent placement (18).

CLINICAL ASSESSMENT OF PLATELET MEASUREMENT TECHNIQUES

Impact of Platelet Tests on Clinical Trials: GPIIb-IIIa Antagonists

The observation by Marguerie et al. (19,20) that platelet aggregation was mediated by expression of a constitutive surface glycoprotein led to the development of antibodies and eventually peptides and peptidomimetic compounds designed to prevent the ligation of this receptor (integrin $\alpha_{IIb}\beta_3$, or GPIIb-IIIa) (21). The subsequent model of platelet aggregation proposed that following platelet exposure to a variety of stressors (biochemical agonists as well as biophysical shear), quiescent GPIIb-IIIa receptors on the platelet surface assumed an active conformation and were able to ligate fibrinogen as well as a variety of other circulating macromolecules and form stable platelet aggregates. Signaling through this integrin was thus assumed to occur in an "inside-out" fashion.

Initial observations with the murine antibody m7E3 F(ab')2, a precursor of abciximab, in a canine thrombosis and thrombolysis model indicated that expression of the receptor appeared redundant. Occupancy of approx 80% of surface receptors was required to inhibit turbidimetric platelet aggregation in response to 20 μM ADP by approx 80% (22). This level of receptor occupancy appeared to be the threshold at which platelet participation in vascular occlusion following thrombolysis was prevented. This model has served as a paradigm for the development of GPIIb-IIIa antagonists. However, the existence of threshold levels for either receptor occupancy or inhibition of platelet aggregation in response to other lower binding affinity antagonists has not been established, nor has a threshold been established in less intensely prothrombotic settings.

The paradigm of a "final common pathway" for platelet aggregation is now understood to be considerably more complex than initially envisioned. It is now clear that the formation of firmly bonded aggregates on an injured surface continues to progress after ligation of GPIIb-IIIa has occurred. It is also appreciated that in addition to inside-out signaling, messages also appear to be transmitted to the platelet from GPIIb-IIIa in an "outside-in" fashion. Within this model, ligation of GPIIb-IIIa by macromolecules results in activation of the platelet and further participation in thrombotic as well as inflammatory processes. The implication for pharmacologic concentrations of GPIIb-IIIa antagonists is that when they ligate GPIIb-IIIa, they simultaneously activate the platelet, but suppress the ability of the activated platelet to form aggregates. The economy of these competing processes appears to be driven by the observation that low levels of GPIIb-IIIa ligation can initiate receptor signaling, whereas higher levels of receptor occupancy are required to inhibit aggregation.

Although less well established than the simple model that was originally conceived, this more complex paradigm would seem to explain several "paradoxical" phenomena that have been observed in clinical trials. Thus, when bolus doses of an antagonist are administered, platelet activation is inhibited effectively, but as drug levels and consequently receptor occupancy levels decline, either during a maintenance infusion or after it is terminated, the prothrombotic effects of platelet activation may predominate. Each of the three commercially available antagonists has been tested at doses selected almost entirely based on turbidimetric platelet aggregometry. Each has taught a valuable lesson concerning the assumptions one makes when selecting a drug dose based entirely on pharmacodynamic assumptions.

ABCIXIMAB

The currently indicated bolus dose of abciximab was selected based on inhibition of turbidimetric platelet aggregation in response to a $20 \mu M$ concentration of ADP. The initial studies were performed using larger antibody fragments that were eventually refined to develop the pharmacologic compound abciximab. Pilot studies by Tcheng et al. in the setting of PCI (23), Simoons et al. in the setting of acute coronary syndromes (24), and Kleiman et al. in the setting of acute myocardial infarction (25) indicated that this bolus dose would inhibit platelet aggregation by a median value of approx 80% in each of the patient populations investigated. The study by Tcheng et al. (23) also established that a bolus dose of 0.25 mg/kg followed by a continuous infusion of 10 μg/min could persistently suppress platelet aggregation for the duration of the infusion.

The sequence of events that led to dose selection is remarkable. Stoichiometric calculations were performed based on the number of receptors measured per platelet and the known dissociation constant for abciximab. Subsequently, a canine model was selected to derive dosing

data. Measurements of receptor occupancy using radioimmunoassay
(26) with ^{125}I-labeled abciximab and platelet aggregation using turbidimetric aggregrometry in response to a 20 μ*M* concentration of ADP were
readily translated into appropriate dose selection information for patients. Subsequent dosing studies were then designed primarily to test
gross safety of the selected doses. In the previously referenced study,
only four patients received the 0.25-mg/kg bolus and 0.1-mg/min infusion that was ultimately selected for the pivotal trial in humans *(23)*. This
dosing regimen was subsequently tested in a randomized trial of 2099
patients undergoing PCI in the Evaluation of Platelet Inhibition to Prevent Complications (EPIC) study. The bolus dose alone was ineffective
at preventing periprocedural ischemic events, whereas the bolus followed by the infusion successfully reduced the event rate.

These results showed that in the setting of the complex procedures
performed in clinical settings, along with higher doses of heparin (average approx 14,000 U of unfractionated heparin), a composite of ischemic
complications was reduced from 12.8 to 8.3%, but the risk of receiving
a blood transfusion was increased from 7 to 15% *(27)*. Beyond this
almost fortuitous dose selection process, clinical data indirectly supported data derived from the animal model. Pharmacokinetic studies
revealed that either 6 h after administering a bolus or 6 h after terminat-
ing an infusion of abciximab, platelet receptor occupancy returned to
about 80% of the baseline value *(23)*. In EPIC, the group receiving the
bolus dose alone began to experience ischemic events 6 h after the bolus
was administered, and the bolus and infusion group experienced a nomi-
nal but not significant increase in event rates at about the same point after
the infusion was terminated *(27)*. These findings lent support to the
observation made in the canine studies that occupancy of more than 80%
of platelet GPIIb-IIIa, or availability of less than 20% of the surface pool,
was required for arterial thrombosis to be inhibited.

A second trial, the Evaluation of Percutaneous Transluminal Coronary Angioplasty to Improve Long-Term Outcome with Abciximab
Glycoprotein IIb/IIIa Blockade (EPILOG), was performed in an attempt
to reduce hemorrhagic complications while maintaining antiischemic
efficacy. The bolus dose of abciximab was unchanged, but the infusion
dose was reduced from 0.10 mg/min to 0.125 μg/kg/min. This trial
revealed that when the original bolus dose (0.25 μg/kg) was coupled
with the weight-based infusion dose, along with a reduction in the dose
of heparin from 100 to 70 U/kg, the composite of death, myocardial
infarction, and urgent revascularization, compared with a placebo and
the standard (100 U/kg) heparin dose, fell from 10.6% to 5.5%; the risk
of major bleeding increased only from 3.15% to 3.5%, with a fall in the

rate of red blood cell transfusion from 3.9% to 3.3% *(28)*. A subsequent trial confirmed the applicability of these findings to patients receiving intracoronary stents and ticlopidine *(29)*.

The results of these trials are critically important for two reasons. First, these findings led to widespread use of GPIIb-IIIa antagonists as clinically useful drugs during percutaneous revascularization procedures. Equally, and perhaps more important, they cemented the concept that with effective inhibition of platelet aggregation, the accompanying dose of antithrombin therapy (unfractionated heparin in this case) could and should be reduced, with the result being a notable increase in the safety of antiplatelet therapy and maintenance of the antithrombotic effect of this treatment.

However, newer developments in the understanding of platelet physiology also raised new questions concerning abciximab dosing. In the clinical pilot studies, inhibition to less than 80% occurred in approx 20% of patients. In the study by Simoons et al. *(24)*, low levels of inhibition were most evident in two patients, both of whom had markedly elevated platelet counts (and hence more receptors available to ligate circulatory abciximab). However, the development of a bedside assay of platelet agglutination *(30)* led to investigation of the degree of inhibition that actually occurred when abciximab was used clinically. In the Assessing Ultegra (Au; GOLD) study of 500 patients treated with a GPIIb-IIIa antagonist (84% abciximab) during elective PCI, Steinhubl et al. *(31)* observed that the inhibitory response was variable and documented that the proportion of patients "escaping" from high-level platelet inhibition increased during the duration of the infusion. Ten minutes after initiating therapy, 4.5% of patients had less than 85% inhibition, 6% had inhibition of 85–89%, and 16% had inhibition between 90 and 94%. After 8 h, the proportions were 6.4% with inhibition less than 70%, 4.8% with inhibition of 70–79%, and 20% with inhibition of 80–90%. Major adverse cardiovascular events (MACE) occurred in 25% of patients whose platelets were inhibited less than 70% at the 8-h point compared with 8.1% in patients with more than 70% inhibition *(31)*.

Although the implication of these findings is that low levels of inhibition of platelet aggregation are associated with an increased risk of vascular thrombosis, the study did not test the utility of supplemental doses of abciximab to achieve a target antiplatelet effect, nor did it test whether a lower bolus dose of abciximab followed by supplemental boluses, given until a predetermined level of inhibition is obtained, would be an effective therapeutic regimen. Notably, the greatest association between events and the level of inhibition was observed at a point 8 h after beginning the abciximab infusion. It is also likely that most events had already occurred by the time the observation was made. Smaller studies using ^{125}I-labeled abciximab to detect receptor occupancy and turbidimetric platelet aggregation have also reported increasing variability of receptor occupancy and inhibition of aggregation during the last 6 h of a 12-h infusion of abciximab *(32)*. Similarly, Quinn et al. *(33)* observed in 15 patients subjected to a 36-h-long infusion of abciximab that after the end of the first hour of the infusion, mean receptor availability and platelet aggregation in response to ADP and a thrombin receptor agonist peptide (TRAP) progressively increased.

These observations have implications beyond the realm of percutaneous coronary intervention as well. In the Global Use of Streptokinase and Tissue Plasminogen Activator for Occluded Arteries (GUSTO)-IV study, patients with acute coronary syndromes were randomized to receive a placebo, an abciximab bolus followed by a 24-h-long infusion, or an abciximab bolus followed by a 48-h-long infusion. Unlike the observations made in previous trials of percutaneous coronary interventions, patients in GUSTO-IV who received abciximab had slightly higher rates of death and myocardial infarction than patients assigned to placebo. The group receiving the 48-h-long infusion of abciximab had slightly higher rates than did the group receiving the 24-h-long infusion *(34)*. One of the potential explanations for this observation is that as the duration of abciximab infusion increased, the level of platelet aggregation inhibition decreased and a substantial proportion of patients developed subthreshold levels of inhibition, possibly accompanied by paradoxical drug-induced platelet activation.

Eptifibatide

The clinical development of eptifibatide has also reflected advances in the understanding of assays of platelet function. Eptifibatide is a cyclic heptapeptide developed to provide highly specific ligation of GPIIb-IIIa *(35,36)*. The physiochemical properties of eptifibatide, specifically its high dissociation constant for GPIIb-IIIa *(37)*, have led to a very different development course than that for abciximab. Unlike what is seen as a result of high-affinity binding of abciximab to GPIIb-IIIa, direct measurement of GPIIb-IIIa receptor occupancy by eptifibatide is extremely difficult and relies on indirect expression of a neoepitope induced by eptifibatide binding to GPIIb-IIIa *(38)*. The second direct consequence of the considerably more rapid association and dissociation of eptifibatide from its receptor is that measurement of plasma levels of eptifibatide are directly related to the number of molecules bound to platelet GPIIb-IIIa and are therefore representative of its efficacy at preventing platelet aggregation *(39)*.

Initial dose-ranging studies involved what are by contemporary standards extremely low doses. Schulman et al. *(40)* studied a 45-µg/kg bolus followed by an 0.5-µg/kg/min infusion and a 90-µg/kg/ bolus dose followed by a 1.0-µg/kg/min infusion in patients with unstable angina. Subsequent dosing studies were performed in patients undergoing PCI, using the 90-µg/kg dose and an infusion rate of 1.0 µg/kg/min, for either 4 or 12 h *(41)*. In a subsequent trial of eptifibatide in the setting of PCI, doses were modified based on pharmacokinetic modeling. Bolus doses of 90 and 180 µg/kg were compared followed by infusion rates of 0.5 and 1.0 µg/kg/min, respectively, in six and four patients respectively. Groups of 16 and 28 patients were studied using doses of 135 µg/kg bolus and 0.5 and 0.75 µg/kg/min, respectively. In response to the latter two doses, the platelet aggregation response to 20 µM ADP was inhibited by more than 90% initially, but after 24 h of infusion had returned to 60 and 80% of baseline, respectively. Four hours after termination of the infusion, platelet aggregation had returned to the baseline value *(42)*.

These doses were selected for a larger trial of 4010 patients undergoing PCI. The two infusion rates were compared to test the concept that the gradual recovery of platelet aggregation observed with the lower infusion rate would be associated with fewer bleeding complications. However, reduction in clinical events at the 30-d end point did not occur in either eptifibatide-treated group, nor was there a significant increase in major bleeding associated with either dose of eptifibatide *(43)*.

Subsequent recognition that eptifibatide binding to GPIIb-IIIa was dependent on exogenous calcium concentration led to a reassessment of platelet aggregation determination and ultimately to revision of the doses of eptifibatide tested. By chelating calcium, the anticoagulant disodium citrate removes divalent cation binding sites on GPIIb-IIIa and simulataneously decreases the affinity of GPIIb-IIIa for fibrinogen while increasing its affinity for eptifibatide. Dose ranging had been performed using blood samples collected in disodium citrate, which reduced ambient calcium concentrations approx 25-fold and increased the inhibitory concentration of 50% (IC_{50}) of eptifibatide approx 3-fold *(44)*. This caused enhanced in vitro inhibition of platelet aggregation and consequently led to overestimation of the antiaggregant effect of each of the previously assessed doses of eptifibatide. Anticoagulation of blood samples in tubes containing either heparin or the direct thrombin antagonist D-phenylalanyl-L-propyl-L arginine cholomethylketone (PPACK) did not alter calcium concentration and lesser levels of inhibition were reported. In subsequent dosing studies, higher doses of eptifibatide were used, and blood samples were collected in PPACK-anticoagulated tubes. Pharmacokinetic modeling of plasma eptifibatide concentrations predicted that a 180-µg/kg bolus followed by a 2-μg/kg/min infusion would result in drug levels able to produce sustained inhibition of platelet aggregation. The combination of higher concentrations of eptifibatide and an anticoagulant is less likely to enhance the pharmacologic effect of eptifibatide as shown by higher levels of inhibition of platelet aggregation.

Tardiff et al. *(45)* demonstrated that in patients with acute coronary syndromes manifested by either elevated plasma biomarkers or ST segment deviation, platelet inhibition using this bolus/infusion regimen suppressed platelet aggregation by approx 80–90% in response to ADP 20 μ*M* and by 40–50% in response to a 6-mer TRAP. When the anticoagulants disodium citrate and PPACK were compared in samples drawn at the same time points, nearly all samples collected in citrated tubes had inhibition exceeding the 80% level compared with about three-fourths of samples collected in PPACK-anticoagulated tubes *(45)*. In fact, in the Platelet IIb/IIIa Underpinning the Receptor for Suppression of Unstable Ischemia Trial (PURSUIT) of more than 12,000 patients with an acute coronary syndrome, this dose of eptifibatide led to a 15% relative reduction in a composite clinical end point of death or myocardial infarction compared with a placebo *(46)*.

Both pharmacokinetic modeling and pharmacodynamic measurements in the latter study indicated that between the first and fourth hour after delivering the bolus, plasma levels of eptifibatide and inhibition of platelet aggregation declined transiently, only to reach steady state after approximately the fourth hour. Although such a strategy proved useful for preventing a composite of death and myocardial infarction in a large study of patients presenting with acute coronary syndromes, it posed a serious concern in patients undergoing PCI soon after hospital presentation, since coronary arterial manipulations were frequently performed during the time when antiplatelet activity was at or near a trough value. Further pharmacokinetic modeling suggested that a revised regimen consisting of two bolus doses of eptifibatide and the same 2-mg/kg/min infusion would eliminate this trough level and provide sustained inhibition of platelet aggregation during this critical period.

Using two boluses of 180 μg/kg separated by 10 min and a 2-μg/kg/min infusion, Tcheng et al. *(41)* demonstrated sustained inhibition of platelet aggregation over a 24-h period. A clinical trial performed using this dosing regimen documented a reduction in a composite of death, myocardial infarction, and urgent revascularization from 10.5 to 6.6%. It must be kept in mind, however, that, in contrast to the clinical trial performed at the lower dose, 96% of patients in the latter trial were treated with an intracoronary stent at the time of PCI and received subsequent therapy with a thienopyridine. Thus, in addition to the altered dose, the substrate treated was also altered. This dual bolus dose regimen is now undergoing clinical testing in a large trial of patients with evidence of an acute coronary syndrome and high risk features in whom early angiography is planned. Based on findings from a recently completed study of enoxaparin, also in patients with high-risk acute coronary syndromes (47), approx 50% of these patients can be expected to undergo PCI while they are being treated with the study regimen, 20% will undergo coronary bypass surgery, and the remainder will be managed medically.

TIROFIBAN

Tirofiban is a peptidomimetic antagonist of GPIIb-IIIa designed with high specificity and a rapid off-rate (i.e., high K_D). Clinical development of tirofiban paralleled the development of eptifibatide. As with the other two commercially available antagonists of GPIIb-IIIa, early dose ranging of tirofiban was performed in patients undergoing elective PCI. Samples were collected in citrated tubes. Although several investigators have reported that assessment of the platelet aggregation response in the presence of tirofiban is also subject to the same effects of calcium chelation as were observed with eptifibatide, the effect may be less profound (48).

A more pertinent and incompletely answered issue concerns the agonist used to provoke platelet aggregation in these studies. The dose-ranging trials by both Theroux et al. (49) in patients with acute coronary syndromes and Kereiakes et al. (50) in patients undergoing PCI studied the inhibitory effects of tirofiban on platelets stimulated with ADP 5 μM. This technique stands in contradistinction to the 20 μM concentration used to assess doses of abciximab and eptifibatide. In most patients, in our own laboratory, the aggregation response to ADP exhibits linear characteristics as the concentration of ADP is increased until a level somewhere between 6 and 10 μM is reached. After this point, further increases in the concentration of ADP do not lead to further increases in light transmission (i.e., increases in platelet aggregation). The corollary of these observations is that use of lower concentrations of ADP would lead to the selection of lower doses of the GPIIb-IIIa antagonist.

As a result of these pilot studies, the doses of tirofiban selected for clinical trials were 10 $\mu g/kg$ given over 3 min followed by a maintenance infusion of 0.15 $\mu g/kg/min$ in patients undergoing PCI (51) and 0.6 $\mu g/kg/min$ for 30 min followed by an infusion of 0.15 $\mu g/kg/min$ infusion in patients with acute coronary syndromes (52). From a clinical perspective, the dose of tirofiban selected for patients with acute coronary syndromes proved effective at reducing a combination of death, myocardial infarction, and refractory ischemia (52) whereas the dose selected for use in PCI proved ineffective compared with a placebo infusion in patients undergoing percutaneous transluminal coronary angioplasty (without stent or thienopyridines) *(51)*. This dose (frequently referred to as the TARGET dose, after the TARGET study [Tirofiban and Reopro Give Similar Efficacy Outcomes Trial]) was significantly inferior to abciximab in patients undergoing stent placement *(53)*.

Several small trials using various modifications of the turbidimetric aggregation technique have provided mechanistic explanations for these clinical observations. In three small randomized trials, the dosing regimen of tirofiban used in the TARGET trial was compared with an 0.25-µg/kg bolus and a 0.125-µg/kg/min infusion of abciximab *(54–56)*. Two concordant findings have emerged from these studies. First, during the initial hour after administering the drugs, tirofiban led to less inhibition of ADP-induced platelet aggregation than did abciximab *(54–56;* or eptifibatide in two of the trials; *54,56*). These findings may reflect the lower (5 µM) dose of the ADP agonist that was used in the dose-finding studies of tirofiban (compared with 20 µM used for dose finding with abciximab), leading to lower levels of platelet activation and less vigorous aggregation *(23,57)*, as well as overestimation of tirofiban potency by blood collection in citrated tubes. Second, in two of the trials, considerable variability of the aggregation response was present several hours after dosing of abciximab *(54,56)*.

A fourth pilot study by Schneider et al. *(58)* has indicated that increasing the bolus dose of tirofiban from 10 to 25 µg/kg while maintaining the previously studied 0.15-µg/kg/min infusion increased the inhibition of platelet aggregation in response to a 20 µM concentration of ADP as well as an agonist of protease-activated receptor-1 (iso-TRAP) using a bedside assay of platelet agglutination (the rapid platelet function assay). After treatment with clopidogrel 300 mg, patients in this study were sequentially assigned to receive either a 20- or a 25-µg/kg bolus, each coupled with an infusion of 0.15 µg/kg/min. The 20-µg/kg bolus inhibited ADP-induced platelet aggregation by 84–89% during the first hour, whereas aggregation following administration of the higher dose was reduced by 92–95% *(58)*. After administration of the higher bolus dose, plasma concentrations of tirofiban ranged from 80 to 90 ng/mL, approximately two and a half times higher than those previously observed in patients treated with the 10-µg/kg bolus dose. Addition of exogenous tirofiban to blood samples confirmed that increasing the concentration of tirofiban from 50 to 100 ng/mL led to reduction in the ability of activated platelets to bind fibrinogen, whereas increasing the concentration to 150 ng/mL had no further effect on the fibrinogen-binding capacity (59). Although this dosing regimen of tirofiban is not yet in clinical use, a trial in which it is compared with abciximab in patients undergoing PCI is currently undergoing final design.

REFERENCES

1. Antiplatelet Trialists' Collaboration. Collaborative overview of randomised trials of antiplatelet therapy-I: prevention of death, myocardial infarction, and stroke by prolonged antiplatelet therapy in various categories in patients. BMJ 1994;308:81–106.
2. Antiplatelet Trialist' Collaboration. Collaborative meta-analysis of randomised trials of antiplatelet therapy for prevention of death, myocardial infarction, and stroke in high risk patients. BMJ 2002;324:71–86.
3. Colombo A, Hall P, Nakamura S, et al. Intracoronary stenting without anticoagulation accomplished with intravascular ultrasound guidance. Circulation 1995;91:1676–1688.
4. Yusuf S, The Clopidogrel in Unstable Angina to Prevent Recurrent Events Trial Investigators. Effects of clopidogrel in addition to aspirin in patients with acute coronary syndromes without ST-segment elevation. N Engl J Med 2001;345:494–502.
5. Furman M, Kereiakes D, Krueger L, et al. Leukocyte-platelet aggregation, platelet surface P-selectin, and platelet surface glycoprotein IIIa after percutaneous coronary intervention: effects of dalteparin or unfractionated heparin in combination with abciximab. Am Heart J 2001;142:790–798.
6. Merten M, Thiagarajan P. P-selectin expression on platelets determines size and stability of platelet aggregates. Circulation 2000;102:1931–1936.
7. Gawaz M, Neumann FJ, Ott I, May A, Rudiger S, Schomig A. Changes in membrane glycoproteins of circulating platelets after coronary stent implantation. Heart 1996;76:166–172.
8. Ott I, Neumann FJ, Gawaz M, Schmitt M, Schomig A. Increased neutrophil-platelet adhesion in patients with unstable angina. Circulation 1996;94:1239–1246.
9. Merlini PA, Bauer KA, Oltrona L et al. Persistent activation of coagulation mechanism in unstable angina and myocardial infarction. Circulation 1994;90:61–68.
10. Libby P. Current concepts of the pathogenesis of the acute coronary syndromes. Circulation 2001;104:365–372.
11. Scharf RE, Tomer A, Marzec UM, Teirstein PS, Ruggeri ZM, Harker LA. Activation of platelets in blood perfusing angioplasty-damaged coronary arteries: flow cytometric detection. Arterioscler Thromb 1992;12:1475–1487.
12. Mascelli MA, Kleiman NS, Marciniak SJ Jr, Damaraju L, Weisman HF, Jordan RE. Therapeutic heparin concentrations augment platelet reactivity: implications for the pharmacologic assessment of the glycoprotein IIb/IIIa antagonist abciximab [in process citation]. Am Heart J 2000;139:696–703.
13. Sobel M, Fish WR, Toma N, et al. Heparin modulates integrin function in human platelets. J Vasc Surg 2001;33:587–594.
14. Xiao Z, Theroux P. Platelet activation with unfractionated heparin at therapeutic concentrations and comparisons with a low-molecular-weight heparin and with a direct thrombin inhibitor. Circulation 1998;97:251–256.
15. Kleiman N, Klem J, Fernandes L, et al. Pharmacodynamic profile of the direct thrombin antagonist bivalirudin given in combination with the glycoprotein IIb/IIIa antagonist eptifibatide. Am Heart J 2002;143:585–593.
16. Hollopeter G, Jantzen H-M, Vincent D et al. Identification of the platelet ADP receptor targeted by antithrombotic drugs. Nature 2001;409:202–206.
17. Cattaneo M, Gachet C. ADP receptors and clinical bleeding disorders. Arterioscler Thromb Vasc Biol 1999;19:2281–2285.

18. Gurbel PA, Bliden KP, Hiatt BL, O'Connor CM. Clopidogrel for coronary stenting: response variability, drug resistance, and the effect of pretreatment platelet reactivity. Circulation 2003;107:2908–2913.

19. Marguerie GA, Thomas-Maison N, Larrieu MJ, Plow EF. The interaction of fibrinogen with human platelets in a plasma milieu. Blood 1982;59:91–95.

20. Marguerie GA, Plow EF, Edgington TS. Human platelets possess an inducible and saturable receptor specific for fibrinogen. J Biol Chem 1979;254:5357–5363.

21 Coller BS, Peerschke EI, Scudder LE, Sullivan CA. A murine monoclonal antibody that completely blocks the binding of fibrinogen to platelets produces a thrombasthenic-like state in normal platelets and binds to glycoproteins IIb and/or IIIa. J Clin Invest 1983;72:325–338.

22. Gold HK, Coller BS, Yasuda T, et al. Rapid and sustained coronary artery recanalization with combined bolus injection of recombinant tissue-type plasminogen activator and monoclonal antiplatelet GPIIb/IIIa antibody in a canine preparation. Circulation 1988;77:670–677.

23. Tcheng JE, Ellis SG, George BS, et al. Pharmacodynamics of chimeric glycoprotein IIb/IIIa integrin antiplatelet antibody Fab 7E3 in high-risk coronary angioplasty. Circulation 1994;90:1757–1764.

24. Simoons ML, de Boer MJ, van den Brand MJ, et al. Randomized trial of a GPIIb/IIIa platelet receptor blocker in refractory unstable angina. European Cooperative Study Group. Circulation 1994;89:596–603.

25. Kleiman NS, Ohman EM, Califf RM, et al. Profound inhibition of platelet aggregation with monoclonal antibody 7E3 Fab after thrombolytic therapy. Results of the Thrombolysis and Angioplasty in Myocardial Infarction (TAMI) 8 Pilot Study. J Am Coll Cardiol 1993;22:381–389.

26. Coller BS. A new murine monoclonal antibody reports an activation-dependent change in the conformation and/or microenvironment of the platelet glycoprotein IIb/IIIa complex. J Clin Invest 1985;76:101–108.

27. The EPIC Investigators. Use of a monoclonal antibody directed against the platelet glycoprotein IIb/IIIa receptor in high-risk coronary angioplasty. N Engl J Med 1994;330:956–961.

28. The EPILOG Investigators. Platelet glycoprotein IIb/IIIa receptor blockade and low-dose heparin during percutaneous coronary revascularization. N Engl J Med 1997;336:1689–1696.

29. The EPISTENT Study Group. randomised placebo-controlled and balloon-angioplasty-controlled trial to assess safety of coronary stenting with use of platelet glycoprotein IIb/IIIa blockade. Lancet 1998;352:87–92.

30. Smith JW, Steinhubl SR, Lincoff AM, et al. Rapid platelet-function assay: an automated and quantitative cartridge-based method. Circulation 1999;99:620–625.

31. Steinhubl SR, Talley JD, Braden GA, et al. Point-of-care measured platelet inhibition correlates with a reduced risk of an adverse cardiac event after percutaneous coronary intervention: results of the GOLD (AU-Assessing Ultegra) multicenter study. Circulation 2001;103:2572–2578.

32. Mascelli MA, Lance ET, Damaraju L, Wagner CL, Weisman HF, Jordan RE. Pharmacodynamic profile of short-term abciximab treatment demonstrates prolonged platelet inhibition with gradual recovery from GP IIb/IIIa receptor blockade. Circulation 1998;97:1680–1688.

33. Quinn MJ, Murphy RT, Dooley M, Foley JB, Fitzgerald DJ. Occupancy of the internal and external pools of glycoprotein IIb/IIIa following abciximab bolus and infusion. J Pharmacol Exp Ther 2001;297:496–500.

34. Simoons ML. Effect of glycoprotein IIb/IIIa receptor blocker abciximab on outcome in patients with acute coronary syndromes without early coronary revascularisation: the GUSTO IV-ACS randomised trial. Lancet 2001;357:1915–1924.

35. Scarborough RM, Naughton MA, Teng W, et al. Design of potent and specific integrin antagonists. Peptide antagonists with high specificity for glycoprotein IIb-IIIa. J Biol Chem 1993;268:1066–1073.

36. Scarborough RM, Rose JW, Naughton MA, et al. Characterization of the integrin specificities of disintegrins isolated from American pit viper venoms. J Biol Chem 1993;268:1058–1065.

37. Scarborough RM, Kleiman NS, Phillips DR. Platelet glycoprotein IIb/IIIa antagonists. What are the relevant issues concerning their pharmacology and clinical use? Circulation 1999;100:437–444.

38. Mondoro TH, Wall CD, White MM, Jennings LK. Selective induction of a glycoprotein IIIa ligand-induced binding site by fibrinogen and von Willebrand factor. Blood 1996;88:3824–3830.

39. Gilchrist IC, O'Shea JC, Kosoglou T, et al. Pharmacodynamics and pharmacokinetics of higher-dose, double-bolus eptifibatide in percutaneous coronary intervention. Circulation 2001;104:406–411.

40. Schulman SP, Goldschmidt-Clermont PJ, Topol EJ, et al. Effects of integrelin, a platelet glycoprotein IIb/IIIa receptor antagonist, in unstable angina: a randomized multicenter Trial. Circulation 1996;94:2083–2089.

41. Tcheng JE, Harrington RA, Kottke-Marchant K, et al. Multicenter, randomized, double-blind, placebo-controlled trial of the platelet integrin glycoprotein IIb/IIIa blocker integrelin in elective coronary intervention. IMPACT Investigators. Circulation 1995;91:2151–2157.

42. Harrington RA, Kleiman NS, Kottke-Marchant K, et al. Immediate and reversible platelet inhibition after intravenous administration of a peptide glycoprotein IIb/IIIa inhibitor during percutaneous coronary intervention. Am J Cardiol 1995; 76:1222–1227.

43. The IMPACT-2 Investigators. Randomised placebo-controlled trial of effect of eptifibatide on complications of percutaneous coronary intervention—IMPACT-II. Lancet 1997;349:1422–1428.

44. Phillips DR, Teng W, Arfsten A, et al. Effect of Ca^{2+} on GP IIb-IIIa interactions with integrilin: enhanced GP IIb-IIIa binding and inhibition of platelet aggregation by reductions in the concentration of ionized calcium in plasma anticoagulated with citrate. Circulation 1997;96:1488–1494.

45. Tardiff BE, Jennings LK, Harrington RA, et al. Pharmacodynamics and pharmacokinetics of eptifibatide in patients with acute coronary syndromes: prospective analysis from pursuit. Circulation 2001;104:399–405.

46. The PURSUIT Trial Investigators. Inhibition of platelet glycoprotein IIb/IIIa with eptifibatide in patients with cute coronary syndromes. N Engl J Med 1998; 339:436–443.

47. Ferguson JJ, Califf RM, Antman EM, et al. Enoxaparin vs unfractionated heparin in high-risk patients with non-ST-segment elevation acute coronary syndromes managed with an intended early invasive strategy: primary results of the SYNERGY randomized trial. JAMA 2004;292:45–54.

48. Rebello SS, Driscoll EM, Lucchesi BR. TP-9201, a glycoprotein IIb/IIIa platelet receptor antagonist, prevents rethrombosis after successful arterial thrombolysis in the dog. Stroke 1997;28:1789–1796.

49. Theroux P, White H, David D, et al. A heparin-controlled study of MK-383 in unstable angina. Circulation 1994;90:I-231.

50. Kereiakes DJ, Kleiman N, Ferguson JJ, et al. Sustained platelet glycoprotein IIb/IIIa blockade with oral xemilofiban in 170 patients after coronary stent deployment. Circulation 1997;96:1117–1121.
51. The RESTORE Investigators. Effects of platelet glycoprotein IIb/IIIa blockade with tirofiban on adverse cardiac events in patients with unstable angina or acute myocardial infarction undergoing coronary angioplasty. The RESTORE Investigators. Randomized Efficacy Study of Tirofiban for Outcomes and REstenosis. Circulation 1997;96:1445–1453.
52. The PRISM PLUS Study Group. Inhibition of the platelet glycoprotein IIb/IIIa receptor with tirofiban in unstable angina and non-Q-wave myocardial infarction. Platelet Receptor Inhibition in Ischemic Syndrome Management in Patients Limited by Unstable Signs and Symptoms (PRISM-PLUS) Study Investigators. N Engl J Med 1998;338:1488–1497.
53. Topol EJ, Moliterno DJ, Herrmann HC, et al. Comparison of two platelet glycoprotein IIb/IIIa inhibitors, tirofiban and abciximab, for the prevention of ischemic events with percutaneous coronary revascularization. N Engl J Med 2001;344:1888–1894.
54. Kereiakes DJ, Broderick TM, Roth EM, et al. Time course, magnitude, and consistency of platelet inhibition by abciximab, tirofiban, or eptifibatide in patients with unstable angina pectoris undergoing percutaneous coronary intervention. Am J Cardiol 1999;84:391–395.
55. Herrmann HC, Swierkosz TA, Kapoor S, et al. Comparison of degree of platelet inhibition by abciximab versus tirofiban in patients with unstable angina pectoris and non-Q-wave myocardial infarction undergoing percutaneous coronary intervention. Am J Cardiol 2002;89:1293–1297.
56. Batchelor WB, Tolleson TR, Huang Y, et al. Randomized COMparison of Platelet Inhibition With Abciximab, TiRofiban and Eptifibatide During Percutaneous Coronary Intervention in Acute Coronary Syndromes: The COMPARE Trial. Circulation 2002;106:1470–1476.
57. Kereiakes DJ, Kleiman NS, Ambrose J, et al. Randomized, double-blind, placebo-controlled dose-ranging study of tirofiban (MK-383) platelet IIb/IIIa blockade in high risk patients undergoing coronary angioplasty. J Am Coll Cardiol 1996;27:536–542.
.58. Schneider DJ, Herrmann HC, Lakkis N, et al. Enhanced early inhibition of platelet aggregation with an increased bolus of tirofiban. Am J Cardiol 2002;90:1421–1423.
59. Schneider DJ, Herrmann HC, Lakkis N, et al. Increased concentrations of tirofiban in blood and their correlation with inhibition of platelet aggregation after greater bolus doses of tirofiban. Am J Cardiol 2003;91:334–336.

Index